THIRD EDITION

WORKSITE HEALTH PROMOTION

David H. Chenoweth, PhD, FAWHP

Professor Emeritus, East Carolina University
Greenville, North Carolina

President, Chenoweth & Associates, Inc.
New Bern, North Carolina

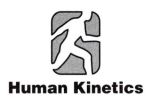

Human Kinetics

Library of Congress Cataloging-in-Publication Data

Chenoweth, David H., 1952-
    Worksite health promotion / David H. Chenoweth. -- 3rd ed.
        p. ; cm.
    Includes bibliographical references and index.
    ISBN-13: 978-0-7360-9291-3 (hard cover : alk. paper)
    ISBN-10: 0-7360-9291-9 (hard cover : alk. paper)
    1. Health promotion. 2. Industrial hygiene. I. Title.
    [DNLM: 1. Health Promotion. 2. Occupational Health Services. 3. Workplace. WA 400]
    RC969.H43C484 2011
    616.9'803--dc22

                                    2011005926

ISBN-10: 0-7360-9291-9 (print)
ISBN-13: 978-0-7360-9291-3 (print)

The web addresses cited in this text were current as of February 2011, unless otherwise noted.

Acquisitions Editor: Myles Schrag; **Developmental Editor:** Judy Park; **Assistant Editors:** Brendan Shea and Steven Calderwood; **Copyeditor:** Joy Wotherspoon; **Indexer:** Michael Ferreira; **Permissions Manager:** Dalene Reeder; **Graphic Designer:** Joe Buck; **Graphic Artists:** Yvonne Griffith and Dawn Sills; **Cover Designer:** Keith Blomberg; **Photographer (cover):** Neil Bernstein; **Photographs (interior):** © Human Kinetics unless otherwise noted; **Photo Asset Manager:** Laura Fitch; **Visual Production Assistant:** Joyce Brumfield; **Photo Production Manager:** Jason Allen; **Art Manager:** Kelly Hendren; **Associate Art Manager:** Alan L. Wilborn; **Illustrations:** © Human Kinetics; **Printer:** Sheridan Books

Printed in the United States of America   10   9   8   7   6   5

The paper in this book is certified under a sustainable forestry program.

Human Kinetics
Website: www.HumanKinetics.com

United States: Human Kinetics
P.O. Box 5076
Champaign, IL 61825-5076
800-747-4457
e-mail: humank@hkusa.com

Canada: Human Kinetics
475 Devonshire Road Unit 100
Windsor, ON N8Y 2L5
800-465-7301 (in Canada only)
e-mail: info@hkcanada.com

Europe: Human Kinetics
107 Bradford Road
Stanningley
Leeds LS28 6AT, United Kingdom
+44 (0) 113 255 5665
e-mail: hk@hkeurope.com

Australia: Human Kinetics
57A Price Avenue
Lower Mitcham, South Australia 5062
08 8372 0999
e-mail: info@hkaustralia.com

New Zealand: Human Kinetics
P.O. Box 80
Torrens Park, South Australia 5062
0800 222 062
e-mail: info@hknewzealand.com

E5134

CONTENTS

CREDITS

Part 1 opening photo: iStockphoto/Chris Schmidt

Chapter 1 opening photos: Monkey Business/fotolia.com (left); Photodisc (center).

Chapter 2 opening photos: © Jon Feingersh/Blend Images/Corbis (left); iStockphoto/Justin Horrocks (center); Stephen Coburn – Fotolia (right).

Chapter 3 opening photos: © Andersen Ross/Brand X/Corbis (left); Eyewire (center); Monkey Business/fotolia.com (right).

Chapter 4 opening photos: iStockphoto/Catherine Yeulet (left); Photodisc (center).

Chapter 5 opening photos: iStockphoto/kristian sekulic (left); Monkey Business/fotolia.com (center).

Part 3 opening photo: Getty Images/Blend Images

Chapter 6 opening photos: Monkey Business/fotolia.com (left); Photoshot (center).

Chapter 7 opening photos: Rob/fotolia.com (left); Bill Crump/Brand X Pictures (right).

Chapter 8 opening photos: Jane Doe/fotolia.com (right).

Part 4 opening photo: bilderbox/fotolia.com.

Chapter 9 opening photos: Art Explosion (left); iStockphoto/Chris Schmidt (center); Ken Pilon/fotolia.com (right).

Chapter 10 opening photos: Liv Friislarsen - Fotolia.com (left); © PhotoCreate - Fotolia.com (center).

PREFACE

The third edition of this book reflects today's diverse marketplace and the ever-evolving field of worksite health promotion (WHP). It is written for students planning careers in the field of WHP as well as for practitioners who currently plan, implement, and direct WHP programs for their organizations.

HOW THIS BOOK IS ORGANIZED

No single formula exists for planning successful health promotion programs. A program for a large company with multisite operations may look very different from a program at a small company. However, common denominators exist among successful programs. They can be affiliated with the following cornerstones: needs assessment and evaluation, healthy culture development, effective interventions, and relapse prevention.

Experts in the field have developed a framework to help program planners recognize employee needs and interests before planning and implementing appropriate WHP programs. The framework consists of five distinct yet interrelated phases (see figure 1):

1. Identification: Identifying health-related problems
2. Assessment: Assessing your employees' interests
3. Planning: Locating and applying necessary resources to establish a program
4. Implementation: Positioning, promoting, and implementing a program
5. Evaluation: Measuring the effect of a program

Based on the framework presented in figure 1, this book is divided into four parts. Each deals with an important area of WHP.

Part I, Initiating Worksite Health Promotion, presents an overview of the economic forces affecting worksites and explains how employers are responding to changing demographics, health risks for employees, rising health care costs, and health-related productivity challenges. Chapter 1 defines WHP and explains its long and rich history. Arguments for and against the concept are scrutinized. Chapter 2 covers the identification and assessment phases of the planning process.

Part II, Planning Worksite Health Promotion Programs, contains three chapters focused on front-end programming decisions. Chapter 3 explains how to establish appropriate goals, build evaluation into your program, and propose WHP plans to management. Chapter 4 describes factors to consider in establishing healthy lifestyle programs. Chapter 5 outlines various options for allocating resources and provides budgetary considerations.

Part III, Providing and Evaluating Worksite Health Promotion, contains three chapters that focus on building a healthy worksite environment, promoting and evaluating programs, and overcoming challenges of company size.

Chapter 6 describes key strategies for building a healthy worksite. It focuses on transforming an unhealthy workplace into a culture that can promote employee health and productivity. Chapter 7 discusses marketing issues and suggests ways to help programs catch on and become popular with the general workforce. Chapter 8 outlines the essentials of program evaluation and describes how to build evaluation protocols into a WHP program.

Part IV, Managing Essential WHP Considerations, consists of the final chapters of the book. They focus on building personal skills for success in different worksite settings. Chapter 9 presents an overview of various

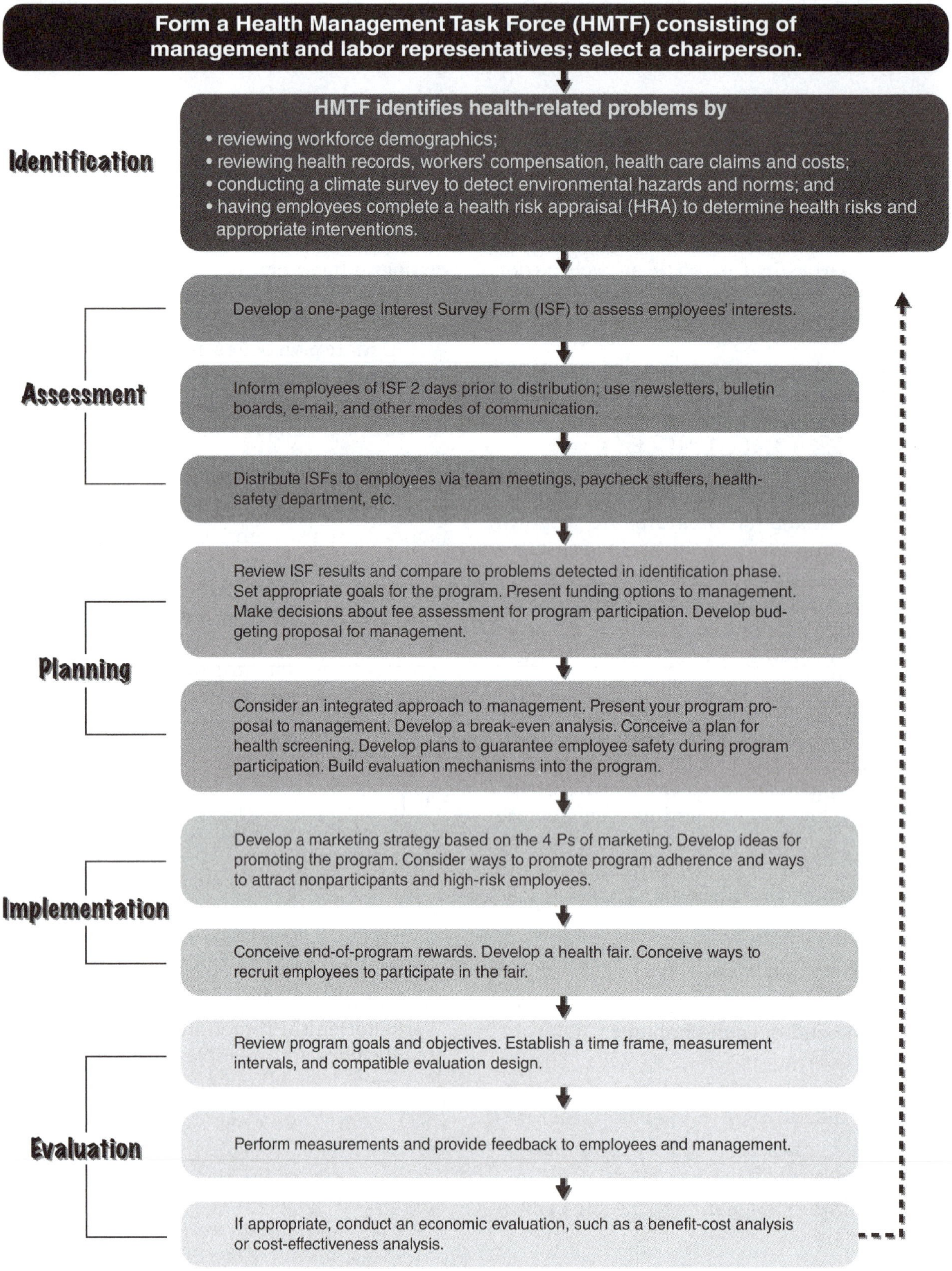

Form a Health Management Task Force (HMTF) consisting of management and labor representatives; select a chairperson.

Identification

HMTF identifies health-related problems by
- reviewing workforce demographics;
- reviewing health records, workers' compensation, health care claims and costs;
- conducting a climate survey to detect environmental hazards and norms; and
- having employees complete a health risk appraisal (HRA) to determine health risks and appropriate interventions.

Assessment

Develop a one-page Interest Survey Form (ISF) to assess employees' interests.

Inform employees of ISF 2 days prior to distribution; use newsletters, bulletin boards, e-mail, and other modes of communication.

Distribute ISFs to employees via team meetings, paycheck stuffers, health-safety department, etc.

Planning

Review ISF results and compare to problems detected in identification phase. Set appropriate goals for the program. Present funding options to management. Make decisions about fee assessment for program participation. Develop budgeting proposal for management.

Consider an integrated approach to management. Present your program proposal to management. Develop a break-even analysis. Conceive a plan for health screening. Develop plans to guarantee employee safety during program participation. Build evaluation mechanisms into the program.

Implementation

Develop a marketing strategy based on the 4 Ps of marketing. Develop ideas for promoting the program. Consider ways to promote program adherence and ways to attract nonparticipants and high-risk employees.

Conceive end-of-program rewards. Develop a health fair. Conceive ways to recruit employees to participate in the fair.

Evaluation

Review program goals and objectives. Establish a time frame, measurement intervals, and compatible evaluation design.

Perform measurements and provide feedback to employees and management.

If appropriate, conduct an economic evaluation, such as a benefit-cost analysis or cost-effectiveness analysis.

Figure 1 The WHP program planning framework.

factors confronting small and multisite businesses when incorporating WHP. Chapter 10, written mainly for students, presents practical information on academically and professionally preparing for a career in the broad field of WHP. It offers tips on selecting a strong academic curriculum as well as preparing for an internship and honing skills for a job interview.

SPECIAL CHAPTER ELEMENTS

A number of special features are contained within the text. Each chapter begins with a list of learning objectives that the reader will be able to answer after finishing the chapter. These will help students focus on specific concepts and issues to enhance their learning and application skills. Highlight boxes provide snapshots of typical WHP situations to consider as readers formulate and plan a course of action.

At the end of each chapter is a wrap-up section, which includes an element on looking ahead, key points, a glossary, and a bibliography. The key terms from the glossary are listed in bold in the text, where they are applied in realistic situations of worksite health promotion.

WHAT'S NEW IN THIS EDITION

Key features added to this edition of *Worksite Health Promotion* include the following:

- Key terms with highlighted definitions at the end of each chapter
- Updated implications of ADA, HIPAA, and GINA standards relevant to WHP
- Considerations for health coaching
- Expanded section on integrated systems for health-data management
- Options for budget development

- Competencies for intermediate-level WHP practitioners
- Expanded illustrations of evaluation designs
- Culture audit tool
- Disease management
- Present-value adjustment
- Expanded illustrations of various econometric-based evaluations
- Updated and expanded certification options
- Updated websites for interns and job searches
- Key points at the end of each chapter

These features have been added for use in readers' WHP programming efforts. The following text will enhance their personal and professional efforts in this dynamic, ever-changing field.

NOTES FOR INSTRUCTORS

Incorporate the end-of-chapter review and key points from the end of each chapter into your classroom instruction and activities. Challenge your students to describe their significance and implications for specific WHP programming issues. The "What Would You Do?" scenario can be used as a culminating in-class discussion for students or teams to develop and present their responses to the group.

The instructor guide contains a sample syllabus, a weekly in-class instructional guide, and a sample listing of guidelines for team presentations (www.humankinetics.com/ WorksiteHealthPromotion). An image bank that includes art and tables will help you fine-tune your presentations, allowing you to use graphics in PowerPoint and link information in your presentations to the text that the students have read.

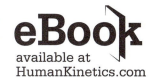

eBook available at HumanKinetics.com

ACKNOWLEDGMENTS

While I was writing and updating the three editions of this textbook during the past 12 years, many of America's finest WHP program directors and managers generously shared information with me in the hope that others could benefit from their expertise. Their ideas and strategies on screening, programming, marketing, and evaluation have given me a good perspective of the daily challenges confronting these hard-working visionaries. In particular, I owe many thanks to all the WHP professionals who provide internship and other learning opportunities to today's majors in worksite health and fitness. I have had the privilege and joy of working with many of you. In doing so, I learned a lot about the technical, political, and operational applications of your successful programs. Your inspiration and commitment to WHP is, indisputably, the impetus for even greater things to come!

Part I

Initiating Worksite Health Promotion

Chapter 1 presents an overview of the importance of worksite health promotion (WHP) programs in today's ever-changing economy, a brief history of WHP, and the ways that well-established programs enhance employees' health status and productivity. Chapter 2 provides information and tools for identifying employees' health needs and assessing their interests and motivation for participation. Collectively, these chapters present a foundation for planning appropriate WHP programs.

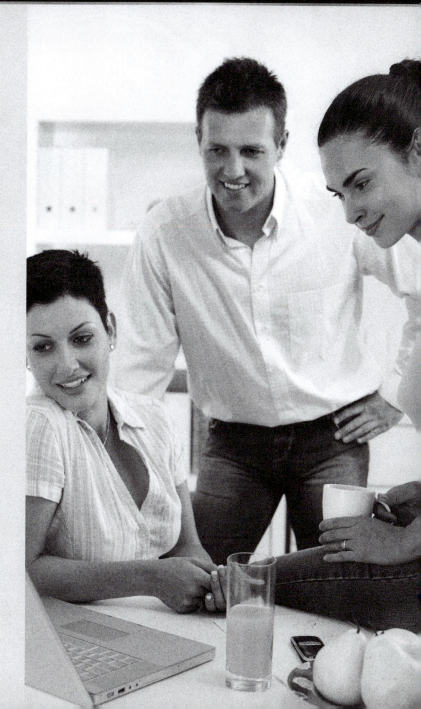

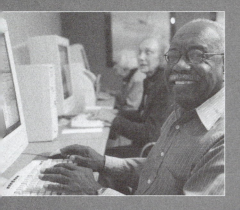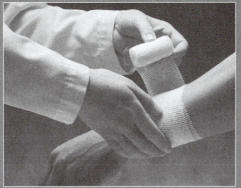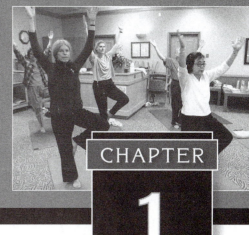

The Case for Worksite Health Promotion

LEARNING OBJECTIVES

After reading this chapter, you will be able to do the following:

✔ Describe the major factors responsible for the inflation of medical care and how rising health care costs directly affect employers and employees.

✔ Describe how major demographic, technological, and economic trends influence work performance today.

✔ Describe several significant events that characterize the history of worksite health promotion.

✔ List various factors that motivate organizations to establish worksite health promotion programs.

✔ Describe the relationship between health-risk status and health care costs.

✔ Describe the components of an integrated health-management system.

What role should worksite health promotion play in today's global economy? To answer that question, perhaps we should consider some major trends in demographics, technology, and economy over the past 50 years:

- A substantial portion of the manufacturing (industrial) sector of the economy has been replaced by the service sector.

- A substantial number of women have entered the workforce, especially in health care and education.

- The median age of many workforces has increased by as much as 10 years.

- Most worksites rely on computerized technologies rather than on physical labor.

- Commuting time to and from work has increased as much as 20%.

- The percentage of obese adults has more than doubled in some worksites.

- The percentage of working adults with chronic health conditions is at an all-time high.

- The average cost of an employer-sponsored health insurance premium for a family of four is around $16,000 per year. In the 1960s, the average cost was less than $1,500.

Collectively, the preceding trends reflect the ubiquitous influence that at-work technologies continue to have on the way in which work is done. Although new technologies certainly generate higher worker productivity in many types of jobs, technology-driven workplaces are often blamed for much of today's physically inactive, obese adult population. After all, millions of workers make their living laboring in front of computerized keyboards in predominantly sedentary jobs. And, considering today's sluggish economic landscape, even a casual observer can see that a day rarely passes without news of an employee layoff, labor strike, corporate takeover, bankruptcy, or plant closing. Although these actions can be traced to a myriad of marketplace factors, one of the most pervasive underlying forces is the relentless and rising cost of health care. Moreover, these troubling costs permeate all sectors of an economy, ranging from individual households to a nation's productivity (**gross domestic product, or GDP**). For example, health care costs consume approximately 5% of the GDP in China, Russia, and India; about 9% in Japan, Italy, and the United Kingdom; between 10% and 11% in Germany and France; and more than 16% in the United States.

Yet, in some of these nations, employers often pay much higher percentages of their revenues on health care. In the United States, for example, the business portion of the nation's total health care bill has increased from 18% in 1965 to nearly 35% today. Moreover, many companies report that the annual cost of providing employee health benefits is nearly 50% of their business profits (Pronk 2009; Loeppke et al. 1999). One of the most glaring examples of the current problem with health care costs is reflected in a study conducted jointly by the Lewin Group and Families USA. It showed these results over a four-year period:

1. Average individual wages increased 12.4%, while employees' health care insurance premiums increased nearly 36%.

2. In 26 states, health care insurance premiums for employees rose more than 40%.

3. Employer-paid premiums increased an average of 32%.

4. The number of Americans with personal health care costs exceeding 25% of their earnings rose from 11.6 million to 14.3 million (approximately 1 of every 10 working adults).

When viewed retrospectively, the preceding trends actually began in the mid-1990s (see figure 1.1). Worldwide, inflation of health care costs continues to rise at least twice as fast as general inflation (consumer price index) because many forces—demographic, economic, philosophical, cultural, political, social, and administrative—exert tremendous influence in the global economy. Collectively, these forces have driven annual increases in health care costs above the annual growth of the gross domestic product (GDP). To better understand the economic realities of this phenomenon, consider both the significant percentage growth of America's health care tab as a percentage of its GDP over the past three decades and the projected increase in the next decade (see figure 1.2). Note that the percentage of the GDP tied to health care costs has risen from less than 10% in the 1970s to nearly 17% in 2010. Furthermore, it is expected to exceed 18% by 2015. Many countries throughout the world also spend a sizable portion of their financial assets on health care (see figure 1.3). Yet, nations that spend the highest percentage of their GDP on health care do not necessarily have the longest *disability-free life spans* (see table 1.1). Specifically, this is defined as the average level of population health in terms of **disability-adjusted life expectancy (DALE).** DALE is most easily understood as the expectation of life lived in equivalent full health.

In the past, health care economists blamed about 85% of spiraling costs on medical inflation, new technological advances, more regulatory compliance, and **cost shifting** (when health care providers shift a portion

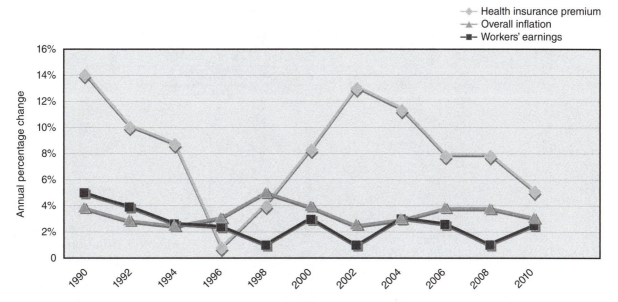

Figure 1.1 Annual percentage changes in health insurance premium, overall inflation (consumer price index), and workers' earnings.

Data from Kaiser Foundation 2009 and Families USA/Lewin Group 2004.

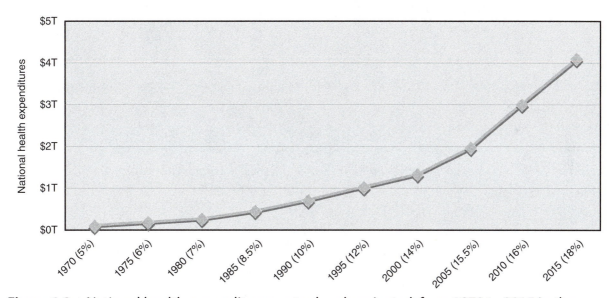

Figure 1.2 National health expenditures, actual and projected, from 1970 to 2015 in the United States. Figures listed in parentheses reflect annual national health expenditures as a percentage of the gross domestic product.

Centers for Medicare and Medicaid Services, Health and Human Services 2009.

of unpaid bills to insured employers and employees). The remaining 15% of the cost spiral was attributed to rising demand, or utilization. However, because life expectancy has increased in the past decade, utilization factors have approached the direct effect of economic factors on today's rising health care tab. This is particularly true in developing nations because greater life-expectancy rates correspond with rising health care costs.

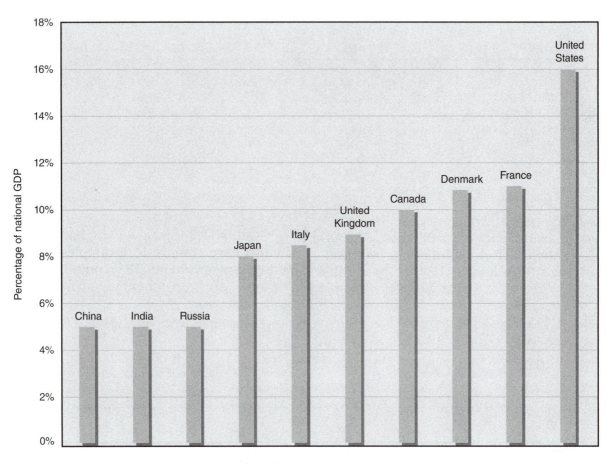

Figure 1.3 National health expenditures (NHE) as a percentage of the gross domestic product (GDP) in selected countries.

Data from World Health Organization 2009.

Table 1.1 DALE in Selected Countries by Ranking in the World Health Organization (WHO)

WHO rank	Nation	DALE at birth
1	Japan	74.5
2	Australia	73.2
3	France	73.1
4	Sweden	73.0
6	Italy	72.7
7	Greece	72.5
8	Switzerland	72.5
12	Canada	72.0
14	United Kingdom	71.7
22	Germany	70.4
24	United States	70.0
82	China	62.3

Data from World Health Organization 2000.

Since American employers collectively pay about one-third of the nation's health care tab, business owners are naturally concerned about rising medical costs. They would like to know what, if anything, they can do to contain this growing liability. Because increased demand and other utilization factors are driving a substantial portion of their costs, many employers have implemented an array of cost-containment strategies, including programs for worksite health promotion (WHP). The overriding premise for establishing WHP programs lies in the assumption that such interventions will (1) reduce modifiable risk factors, which will thereby (2) improve employees' overall health status. This change will, in turn, (3) reduce their demand for health care. This premise is explored later in the chapter.

FACTORS BEHIND RISING HEALTH CARE COSTS

Some would argue that WHP is not effective in containing, much less reducing, the health care costs of a business because many factors have contributed to the rapid rise in health care costs in addition to employee health (or lack of it).

Economic Factors

As is true with any product or service in the market, health care costs fluctuate depending on such factors as inflation, overhead, and operating expenses. When the service is providing medical or health care, some of the expenses necessary for continued operation (e.g., insurance or materials) are much greater than they are for other services. That expense is passed on, at least in part, to the consumer. If a company offers its employees the benefit of health insurance, it takes on all or part of the financial burden when the providing health care agency's costs escalate. Many companies that absorb this ever-increasing expense must look for ways to cut the costs if they are going to remain in operation. Consequently, companies are becoming more interested in the causes of health care inflation as they seek possible ways to contain costs. Let's look at some of the major forces driving today's rising costs.

- Inflation is a driving force, since the component of medical care services in the consumer price index (a measure of inflation based on the price of a group of commonly purchased goods and services, such as groceries and electricity) often rises two to three times as fast as other items. Yet, some health economists argue that high costs are necessary if we are to improve our medical care systems.

- Cost shifting adds 25% to 33% more to the average health care bill. This practice involves the hidden tax that doctors and hospitals shift to employers and paying customers to compensate for patients who cannot or do not pay their bills. A secondary type of cost shifting covers the high cost of malpractice insurance for doctors and hospitals.

- New technology leads to innovative but costly treatments. Today, although many illnesses can be diagnosed, they cannot necessarily be cured. Although maintenance programs and life-support systems may keep patients alive for long periods of time, these heroic interventions carry a huge price tag. Despite the cost, many people still believe that technology is essential for improved health and longevity.

- Catastrophic cases consume a lot of health care resources. Examples include transplant operations, HIV and AIDS cases, kidney dialysis, and complications among premature infants.

- In our lawsuit-happy society, more doctors and hospitals practice what is known as *defensive medicine*. For example, they do more procedures than necessary in an effort to protect themselves from potential lawsuits.

Demographic Shifts

The global workforce continues to rapidly change in terms of demographics. Here are four of the most dramatic changes altering the demographic landscape:

1. The workforce is aging.
2. More women are entering the workplace.
3. The proportion of people of color working in many countries is rising.
4. The number of people who have to work two jobs in different locations to make a living is growing.

These changes are particularly notable in North America, Europe, and Asia. For example, as people live longer and require more health care, the overall volume of health care services will continue to grow. One of the most important factors shaping the United States is the aging of its citizens. In fact, the concern about the baby boom after World War II that produced today's 46- to 64-year-olds is not about babies. It's about the growing percentage of older workers and their future effect on America's worksites and corporate health care costs. For example, middle-aged workers (between the ages of 35 and 54) currently make up more than 50% of America's workforce. In contrast, younger, entry-level workers—especially in the age group of 16 to 34 years—make up just one-third of today's workforce.

Eldercare is one of the fastest growing needs of many workers. Currently, out of some 40 million Americans over 65, about 9.1 million need some form of long-term care. Of those, about 2 million are living in nursing homes. The remaining 7.1 million are getting some kind of home care within or outside the health care system. Yet, less than one-third of all companies surveyed provide their employees with eldercare assistance benefits.

The realization that the mental health of its employees can significantly influence a company's bottom line has caused an increasing number of employers to take a serious look at issues raised by the demographic shifts just listed. Although some older workers can outperform their younger coworkers in terms of efficiency, as a group they still encounter greater scrutiny and discrimination from managers and younger workers, who often do not understand the aging process and do not believe that older workers can be productive in their later years.

Since 1980, the Hispanic-American population has grown more than 50% and the African-American population has grown more than 20%, greatly outpacing the 10% growth of Caucasians. This trend has resulted in more people of color in the workforce, a disproportionate number of whom work in the fast-growing, but lower-paying, service sector of the economy. Women are also entering the American workforce at an unprecedented rate, making up about 50% of laborers. These demographic shifts are occurring in many parts of the world. Japan is becoming one of the oldest societies in the industrialized world. A number of European countries (Germany, in particular) also have more rapidly aging populations than does the United States. On the other hand, Latin America, the Middle East, and some Asian countries are currently experiencing major population growth. Undoubtedly, these shifts are creating greater pressure on working men and women to successfully balance their family and work lives. Consequently, employers have a greater responsibility to provide work-life balance programs.

Major Employee Health Risks

To what extent do risky behaviors contribute to excess health care costs for workers of all ages? The following factors are according to data analysis from a large disability database (UnumProvident Corporation 2005):

- Medical costs rise an estimated 25% between ages 40 and 50.
- Medical costs rise an estimated 35% between ages 50 and 60.
- Age is a lesser factor in health care costs than the presence of such risk factors as smoking, obesity, physical inactivity, and diabetes.
- The medical-cost differential between low-risk 40- and 50-year-old workers and high-risk workers of the same ages is 3.0 and 2.8 times, respectively.
- The differential in medical costs for a low-risk 60-year-old is estimated to be 2.4 times lower than that for a high-risk 60-year-old.

Despite having a slightly longer life span than a decade ago, average Americans have not improved their health status. Despite the plethora of healthy foods and exercise options in today's marketplace, more than 60% of American adults are overweight or obese. Some studies show that physical inactivity is one of the strongest predictors of excess health care costs for American manufacturing and service workers.

According to the findings from a survey of 400 business leaders, various risk factors negatively affect employees' health status (Society for Human Resource Management

2008). For example, these are the most common risk factors in order of frequency, as ranked by the business leaders:

1. Excess stress
2. High blood pressure
3. Cigarette smoking
4. Back injuries
5. Overweight
6. Alcohol abuse
7. High blood cholesterol
8. Drug abuse
9. Depression
10. Other mental health problems

Independent studies conducted at Bank One, Ceridian Corporation, Dow Chemical, DuPont, DaimlerChrysler, General Electric, General Motors, Goldman Sachs, Osaka Gas, Procter and Gamble, Prudential Insurance, Scania, and Steelcase indicate that most of the identified risk factors are due, in varying degrees, to individual lifestyles.

HEALTH COSTS AND HEALTH PROMOTION

Considering the high percentage of unhealthy workers, what kind of effect should employers expect from their efforts to promote

COST SHARING

As many corporate benefit managers can attest, lower utilization rates for health care don't necessarily result in lower corporate medical expenses. Why? Because many of the forces that drive today's health care costs—cost shifting, medical inflation, new technology, and other economic forces—are influenced primarily by market forces, not by an employer's actions.

The time is coming—some say it is here—when the availability and cost of specific health care benefits will depend on an employee's lifestyle and risk level. Consequently, some observers speculate that WHP programs may no longer be offered primarily as a fringe benefit, but as an economic necessity. Their primary purpose may be to help high-risk and unhealthy employees reduce their risk factors in order to qualify for health insurance.

In a 2009 nationwide poll of chief executive officers (CEOs) in the United States, health care was the most pressing cost issue (43%), followed by litigation (20%) and energy prices (19%) (Kaiser Foundation 2009). In 2008, the Society for Human Resource Management conducted a survey of more than 1,200 randomly selected human-resource professionals, which showed that the top two issues were an aging workforce and rising health care costs.

In another nationwide poll of 1,500 U.S. CEOs, 90% of the respondents ranked rising costs of health-insurance premiums as their greatest economic concern (Loeppke et al. 2009). When asked how they would contain future health care costs, respondents overwhelmingly (80%) said their preferred method was cost sharing. In fact, more than half of the respondents found cost sharing to be effective in controlling health care expenses. Many employers feel that a moderate cost-sharing arrangement ($350 deductible and 10% copayment, for example) can produce substantial savings without discouraging necessary medical care. Yet, some health care economists contend that cost sharing does very little, if anything, to reduce health care inflation because it merely shifts the cost from employers to employees. In reality, they argue, cost sharing causes some people to delay seeking treatment when they really need it. Such delays can lead to needless suffering or worsening of an existing health problem. They could even result in higher health care costs. Although these arguments sound plausible, no conclusive evidence shows that the average cost-sharing arrangement ($500 family deductible and a 15% copayment) causes insured workers who really need health care to postpone treatment.

health? Independent studies conducted on employees at numerous worksites indicate the following:

- More than 50% of employer health care costs are due to potentially modifiable (lifestyle) risk factors, such as poor diet, tobacco use, physical inactivity, and obesity.
- Potentially modifiable risk factors, such as smoking, physical inactivity, and obesity, contribute to short-term health care expenses that are significantly higher.
- Workers with high-risk profiles generally have higher health care costs than those with low-risk profiles (see figure 1.4).

In particular, a study by Anderson and colleagues of 6,000 employees of the DaimlerChrysler Corporation spanning over three years showed a strong relationship between risk level and health care usage (Anderson, Brink, and Courtney 1995). Ten factors were studied: smoking, body weight, exercise, alcohol use, driving habits, eating habits, stress, mental health, cholesterol, and blood pressure. For example, smokers

had annual claim costs that were 31% higher than those of nonsmokers, persons with an elevated risk for obesity used hospitals 143% more than their low-risk peers, and persons with a poor diet had medical costs 41% higher than those with a good diet did.

Additional studies show that WHP programs, when properly administered, can contain employer health care costs. They can also favorably affect employees' quality of life, health status, and overall productivity. For example, a sampling of results shows the following:

- *Aetna.* Five state-of-the-art fitness centers keep exercisers' health care costs nearly $300 lower than those of nonexercisers.
- *British Columbia Hydro.* The company's WHP program generates a benefit-cost ratio of 3 to 1.
- *Canada Life Assurance.* The company's fitness program generated a benefit-cost ratio of 3.43 to 1 in one year.
- *Caterpillar.* WHP-program participants who completed a health-risk appraisal

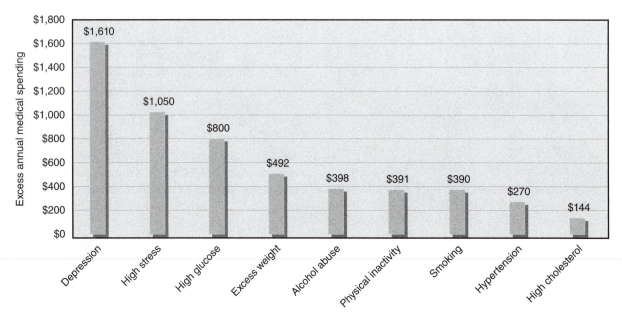

Figure 1.4 Approximate excess annual medical expenditures for high-risk and low-risk adults, excluding prescription drug costs, in 2010 dollar values.

Goetzel et al. 1998; Anderson et al. 2005; Musich et al. 2003; Goetzel et al. 2009; Long et al. 1999; Pronk et al. 1999; and Wright et al. 2002.

reduced their doctor visits by 17% and hospital days by 28%.

* *Citibank.* A comprehensive health-management program generated a benefit-cost ratio of 4.56 to 1.

* *City of Birmingham, Alabama.* Health-risk appraisal screenings and customized interventions saved the city approximately $1 million in annual medical-care expenses.

* *L.L. Bean.* Annual health-insurance premiums are half that of the national average because of a healthy workforce.

* *Coors Brewing Company.* The company saves more than $600,000 a year from its on-site fitness, cardiac rehabilitation, and recreation programs.

* *DuPont.* Absences from non-job-related illness dropped 41% at locations where a WHP program was offered. It only dropped 5.8% at 19 sites that didn't have a program.

* *Florida Power & Light.* After a WHP program was implemented, total health care costs dropped 35%, workers' compensation costs dropped 38%, and 82% of participants reported personal health improvements.

* *Johnson & Johnson.* Customized health screening saves $13 million a year in reduced absenteeism and health care usage.

* *Motorola.* WHP program participants experienced an increase of only 2.4% in health care costs compared with an increase of 18% among nonparticipants.

* *Northeast Utilities.* The Well Aware program generated a $1.4 million drop in lifestyle-related medical claims, a 31% drop in smoking rate, a 29% drop in physical inactivity, a 16% drop in mental health risk, and an 11% drop in cholesterol risk.

* *Osaka Gas.* The company's WHP program has increased productivity and morale and has decreased smoking rates and premature mortality among employees.

* *Quaker Oats.* Health-insurance premiums are approximately one-third less than the national average because of its integrated approach to health management.

* *Steelcase.* Personal health counselors motivate high-risk employees to reduce major risk factors, generating an estimated $20 million over 10 years.

* *Tenneco corporation.* Acute health care costs dropped 43% after implementing a WHP program that features a state-of-the-art fitness center and customized health-education offerings.

* *Union Pacific Railroad.* This company saves more than $3 million annually in costs related to hypertension and smoking. In 1990, nearly 33% of UPR's total medical-care costs were lifestyle related. By 2001, that number had dropped to 18.8%.

* *Washoe County school district (Reno, Nevada).* On average, WHP program participants missed three fewer workdays than nonparticipants.

* *Wisconsin Educational Insurance Group.* A medical self-care program and health-education materials produced a return on investments of 4.71 to 1.

* *Xerox corporation.* WHP program participants filed 37% fewer workers' compensation claims. Average claim costs were about $3,000 lower than those of nonparticipants.

The preceding examples are impressive in that they represent a wide range of businesses and industries (transportation, retail, manufacturing, education, services, and so on). They are also geographically diverse. This suggests that virtually any type of worksite in any location can benefit from a strategically focused program for worksite health promotion.

Despite the impressive effects cited previously, it's important to understand that worksite health promotion is only one of several prerequisites for building a comprehensive framework for health management

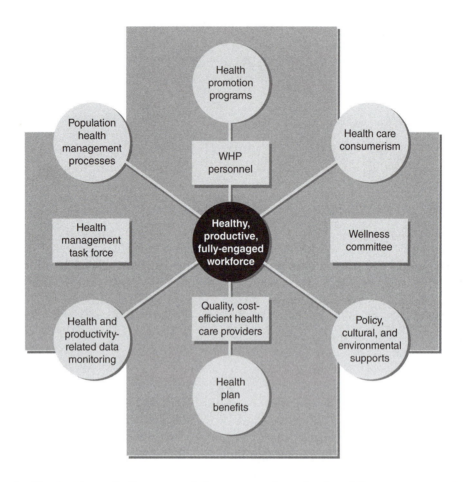

Figure 1.5 An illustration of a framework for comprehensive health management.

(see figure 1.5). Specifically, an organization's ability to cultivate a workforce that is healthy, productive, and fully engaged largely depends on whether it can develop, implement, and sustain a high-performance, integrated health-management system. Such a system consists of the following:

- Health-plan benefits that are consumer driven and cost-efficient
- High level of health care consumerism
- Data monitoring and strategic uses related to health and productivity
- Health promotion programs that are results oriented
- Policy, cultural, and environmental supports that enhance health and productivity
- Processes to manage population health

A BRIEF HISTORY OF WORKSITE HEALTH PROMOTION

What does *worksite health promotion* mean to you? The report of the 2000 Joint Committee on Health Education Terminology defined **worksite health promotion** as "a combination of educational, organizational, and environmental activities designed to improve the health and safety of employees and their families" (p. 10). Subsequently, in 2009, the International Association of Worksite Health Promotion defined WHP as "a corporate [worksite] set of strategic and tactical actions that seek to optimize worker health and business performance through the collective efforts of employees, families, employers, communities, and society at large."

One of the first worksite-based, recreation-and-fitness programs for employees evolved in 1879 when the Pullman company formed its own athletic association. Five years later, John R. Patterson, president of National Cash Register (NCR corporation), regularly assembled his employees at dawn for horseback rides before work. In 1894, he instituted morning and afternoon exercise breaks. A decade later, he built an employee gym. To top it off, in 1911, he added a 325-acre recreation park for employees. Around this time, Sears, Roebuck, and Co. also promoted healthy lifestyles to its retail workers.

In the 1930s, when the nation was recovering from the Great Depression, Milton Hershey (Hershey Foods Corporation) built an impressive recreation complex for employees that included an indoor swimming pool. The pool floor is covered in tile that Mr. Hershey purchased in Argentina while buying cocoa beans for his chocolate.

The growth of worksite programs for recreation and fitness appeared to level off for a decade until the National Employee Services and Recreation Association (NESRA, now the Employee Services Management Association, or ESM) was formed in 1941, spearheading greater interest in employee recreation programs. In 1953, Texas Instruments drafted the initial constitution and bylaws for its employee recreation program. A decade later, it established a half-million-dollar, 8-acre recreational center for employees and their families in the Dallas area. In the early 1950s, Sweden-based Scania corporation established a comprehensive support system in various departments that offered health education, skill-building courses, and support in making healthier lifestyle choices to workers in daily line operations and to more than 700 managers. In the late 1950s, PepsiCo established its physical fitness program, which eventually grew into an industry leader in the 1980s. In the early 1960s, Sentry Insurance creatively established its fitness program in the basement coal bunker at its headquarters in Stevens Point, Wisconsin. Rockwell International and the Xerox corporation also established their well-known fitness programs

in the 1960s. In 1968, American Can and NASA initiated employee fitness programs. The latter organization was one of the first worksites to publish its program evaluation findings in 1972.

The ESM Association estimates that more than 50,000 organizations exist with on-site fitness programs. Nearly 1,000 of them employ full-time program directors.

Although the bulk of WHP efforts centered on recreation and physical fitness during the first half of the 20th century, the advent of employee assistance programs (EAP) became evident in several larger worksites in the 1950s. Currently, more than 10,000 companies have EAPs. They were initially designed to help employees with alcohol problems. However, the scope of EAPs was broadly expanded throughout the 1970s to offer all employees a wide menu of services that included stress management, flexible work accommodations, eldercare assistance, family care spending accounts, personal counseling, retirement planning, and financial planning. Some companies have integrated their EAP services within a broader program for quality of work life (QWL) to administratively simplify their operations and to create a more cost-effective approach.

In 1970, the Occupational Safety and Health Act (OSHA) was created in the United States to literally clean up and regulate the worksite environment and to ensure safer practices. In addition, the act has effectively raised employers' awareness of employees' health. It probably gave some companies an impetus to expand their safety procedures into comprehensive safety and WHP programs. Two years later, Japan enacted the Industrial Safety and Health Law and related ordinances. The law is largely responsible for the significant decline in the number of serious occupational injuries over the past 40 years. Moreover, the law stipulates that health promotion is an employer's obligation.

In 1976, Osaka Gas company in Japan set up a health care system that has improved the health and physical fitness capabilities of its employees over the past 30 years. A year later, Kimberly-Clark corporation spent $2.5 million on a state-of-the-art health-management complex for employees and retirees in Neenah, Wisconsin. Two years later, Mesa Petroleum built an on-site fitness center of 30,000 square feet at the same cost that serves as the centerpiece for employee health screenings and various health promotion programs.

In the 1980s, WHP programs expanded beyond the traditional fitness-center approach, incorporating a holistic menu of wellness programs, such as stress management, lower-back care, smoking cessation, nutrition, prenatal health, weight control, annual health fairs, and weekly lunchtime learning sessions. A decade later, as personal responsibility and self-development evolved at many worksites, WHP expanded into the arenas of medical self-care, post-pregnancy accommodations (e.g., lactation rooms), ergonomic assessments, and exercise courses such as body shaping, kickboxing, spinning, self-defense, and martial arts.

Surveys conducted by the Japanese Ministry of Labor of more than 12,000 private worksites that employ at least 10 workers showed that periodic health exams were given at nearly 90% of the locations. Nearly 45% offered WHP activities. Of these worksites, 48% had sporting events, 46% had exercise programs, and 35% had health counseling.

More Canadian worksites embraced WHP in the past decade. According to a recent survey, WHP programs increased by 47% between 1997 and 2009. In particular, nearly 50% of responding Canadian worksites offered EAP programs, 48% offered training in first aid and CPR, 36% offered smoking cessation programs, and 33% provided ergonomics training.

As the 21st century approached, more worksites gradually embarked on an approach to **population health management (PHM)** to complement their WHP programs. This was based on the philosophy that an active, dynamic, and integrated approach is essential to improving health at all risk levels. In doing so, this practice eventually affects the total workforce (population). By and large, PHM recognizes that health improvement needs to occur at the individual level before it can aggregate up to the population (workforce). It must also be supported at the environmental level.

Consider the axiom of risk level to health cost as an example of how PHM can function. Within a workforce, a relatively small group of employees is responsible for the majority of corporate health care costs. For example, 20% of workers are responsible for 80% of total costs. Unless a multiyear trend of patterns comparing risk level to health costs is used, this imbalance would probably occur every year. Yet, when the entire population is examined over a period of several years, it will likely show that 50% (or more) of the high-cost cases in one year are actually low-cost cases in the subsequent year. This phenomenon is common in many worksites. Therefore, in order to address health care costs incurred by the total workforce, a total PHM strategy is needed, not just a focus on high-cost subpopulations.

As the 21st century approached, PHM strategies enabled more worksites to approach employee health management as a bona fide business strategy. Part of this strategy was based on evolving research that showed a correlation between health and certain productivity indicators, such as absenteeism, presenteeism, workers' compensation, and disability-related claims and costs. Eventually, the concept of **health and productivity management (HPM)** was born in the late 1990s. It continues to gain a strong presence today. Concurrently with the advent of HPM, several progressive companies began to integrate their PHM and HPM strategies into a health-management framework that was more dynamic and integrated (see figure 1.5).

Although most of the integrated health-management initiatives were initially developed in larger worksites, some surveys suggest that worksites of all sizes will adopt similar initiatives to foster better health and productivity for their shrinking workforces. Overall, this movement reflects the growing awareness of employers that employees are, indeed, their most valuable asset (human capital), not just workers doing a job.

Currently, nearly 6 out of 10 American worksites that have more than 750 employees offer options for lifestyle improvement or some other type of WHP program. Smaller worksites are less likely to offer such programs. For example, WHP programs are found in only 38% of worksites that employ 250 to 749 workers and in just 33% of those employing fewer than 49 people. Yet, **Healthy People 2020** recommends that worksites should provide such programs and those future programs should be comprehensive in nature, rather than offering a single intervention.

WHP historians cite fundamental differences in motivation for WHP initiatives among the United States, Japan, and Europe. For example, legislation was a driving force in Japan but not in the United States or Europe. WHP essentially emerged in Japan against the backdrop of governmental fears concerning low productivity due to the rising number of older workers. In contrast, much of the WHP initiative in the United States is driven by rising health care costs for employees. European programs stem from fears surrounding workability. Specifically, the major factors affecting workers' health were personal lifestyles in the United States and Japan and organizational factors in Europe. Consequently, WHP in the United States and Japan emphasizes intervention in personal lifestyles, while the European focus is on organization and the workplace environment.

WHY BUSINESSES OFFER WORKSITE HEALTH PROMOTION

Treating employees and fellow workers with respect and care is not just the right thing to do, it is also good business. Based on several surveys, the most common reasons given for establishing WHP interventions are reportedly to (1) attract and retain good employees, (2) keep workers healthy, (3) improve employee morale, (4) improve employee productivity, and (5) contain employee health care costs. The underlying justification for these reasons is as follows:

- *Absenteeism.* Because one-half of all unscheduled absences in the United States are attributed to minor ailments that are tied to potentially modifiable behaviors, more companies are offering specific types of WHP programs and wellness incentives to their employees. It is interesting that absenteeism and *presenteeism* (being at work but not performing up to par) are reportedly more compelling reasons for many European companies to initiate WHP initiatives than health care costs are.

- *Accessibility.* The workplace is usually a good setting in which to offer educational and motivational programs to many people at one time.

- *Aging workforce.* Every 8 seconds, another American turns 50 years of age. As workers age and experience more health problems, more employers are using age-appropriate interventions to slow the effects of the aging process and to detect problems earlier.

- *Business contacts.* Health promotion events, such as community health fairs and corporate challenge events, create new business contacts.

- *Competition.* Concern about retaining valuable employees is prompting companies to provide financial incentives and other perks that enhance morale and increase retention.

- *Growing interest.* Interest in enhancing personal health and containing health care costs is reflected in today's coverage by print and electronic media.

- *Health insurance premiums.* Employer-paid health insurance premiums for employees and dependents have doubled in the past decade, therefore jeopardizing organizations' net profits.

- *Image.* Many corporate leaders realize that successful WHP programs can boost a company's image among workers, the local community, potential investors, and industry peers.

- *Productivity.* Because healthy employees generally outperform unhealthy employees, more companies are offering health promotion programs to achieve greater outcomes.

• *Workers' compensation costs.* Up to one-half of all workers' compensation claims involve musculoskeletal strains and sprains. Because the vast majority of strain- and sprain-related injuries are tied to poor fitness levels, numerous worksites are integrating case management related to workers' compensation, work hardening (job-specific stretching and strengthening), and return-to-work protocols into a WHP framework.

Considering all of the preceding benefits that worksites can potentially gain, there is a strong business case to be made for WHP programs. Thus, employers who adopt and sustain an effectively run WHP program are positioned to reap these benefits, cultivating employees that are healthier, more productive, and more consumer oriented.

What Would You Do?

Although the growth in WHP programs has been impressive over the past 30 years, some of today's programs lack one or more of the prerequisites needed to achieve their goals in our ever-changing workplaces and economy. Common pitfalls include the following:

• Poor participation levels
• Poor leadership and associated personnel issues
• Lack of appealing programs, resources, and facilities
• Lack of appropriate incentives
• Lack of appropriately trained staff
• Lack of support and involvement by executive and supervisory management
• Lack of tailoring programs to meet the needs and wants of a diverse workforce
• Lack of options for program delivery (in person, Internet, telephone, DVDs, and so on)
• Lack of coordination with other health-related units in the organization (EAP, health and safety, human resources, and benefits)
• No flex time for employee participation
• Distrust of how personal health data may be used

Some industry leaders contend that the future growth and success of WHP programs will largely be determined by how decision makers and program personnel deal with the following issues:

• Taking steps to ensure that workers do not view WHP programs as intrusive or as an invasion to personal privacy
• Ensuring that all health screenings, policies, and incentives comply with state and federal laws
• Demonstrating the positive effect that successful WHP interventions have on employees' health, quality of life, work life, and on-the-job productivity
• Working closely with personnel in the areas of human resources, benefits, risk management, medicine, and safety to develop and administer a high-performance, integrated health-management program
• Expanding the scope of WHP programs to reach employees' dependents
• Dealing with the fact that WHP intervention requires immediate and ongoing costs, compared with economic benefits that may not occur for months or years
• Motivating all employees, especially heavy health care users, to assume more responsibility in the appropriate use of health care services
• Incorporating more rigorous evaluation of WHP efforts

In your view, which of the preceding factors is the most challenging for WHP professionals? Why? What additional factors do you think will challenge the future growth and success of WHP?

CHAPTER 1 WRAP-UP

Key Points

- Health care costs as a percentage of the nation's GDP are growing.
- Containment of health care costs is only one of several goals that many WHP programs are trying to achieve.
- Evidence is growing that health and productivity are related.
- WHP efforts have a long history, spanning from the early days of recreation to today's integration of PHM and HPM.
- When properly administered, WHP and affiliated initiatives can work in virtually any worksite.
- A high-performance integrated system is essential for achieving employee and corporate health-management goals.

Glossary

cost sharing—The arrangement in which employees and employers share a predesignated percentage of employee-incurred health care costs (deductible, copayment).

cost shifting—The additional (hidden tax) cost that health care providers shift to paying individuals and employers to compensate for treatment provided to those who cannot or will not pay.

disability-adjusted life expectancy (DALE)—The average number of years a person can expect to live free of any disability.

gross domestic product (GDP)—The total monetary value of all goods and services produced annually by businesses and industries in a nation.

health and productivity management (HPM)—The integrated management of health risks, chronic disease, and disability to reduce employees' total health-related costs, including direct medical expenditures, unnecessary absence from work, and lost productivity at work.

Healthy People 2020—A national broad-based initiative based on 10-year objectives for promoting health among all populations within a society.

integrated health management system—A comprehensive framework of various data-driven programs, policies, and incentives for health promotion, risk reduction, productivity enhancement, and health care consumerism that are implemented simultaneously to enhance the overall health, workplace quality, and on-the-job performance of employees.

population health management (PHM)—The strategic and operational processes used to generate the health outcomes of a defined group of people collectively associated with a company's efforts to improve health.

worksite health promotion (WHP)—A corporate (worksite) set of strategic and tactical actions that seek to optimize worker health and business performance through the collective efforts of employees, families, employers, communities, and society at large.

Bibliography

Aldana, S. 2001. "Financial impact of health promotion programs: A comprehensive review of the literature." *American Journal of Health Promotion* 15: 296-320.

Anderson, D., S. Brink, and T. Courtney. 1995. *Health risks and behavior: Their impact on medical costs.* Unpublished research report. Milwaukee: Milliman and Robertson.

Anderson, L., B. Martinson, L. Crain, N. Pronk, R. Whitebird, P. O'Connor, and L. Fine. 2005. "Health care charges associated with physical inactivity, overweight, and obesity." *Preventing Chronic Disease* 2: A09.

Chapman, L. 2005. "Meta-evaluation of worksite health promotion economic return studies: 2005 update." *Art of Health Promotion:* 1-16.

———. 2007. *Proof positive: An analysis of the cost-effectiveness of worksite wellness.* Seattle: Northwest Health Management Publishing.

Chapman, L., and K. Pelletier. 2004. "Population health management as a strategy for creation of optimal healing environments in worksite and corporate settings." *The Journal of Alternative and Complementary Medicine* 10: S127-S140.

Centers for Medicare and Medicaid Services, Health and Human Services. 2009. *National health expenditures accounts, 1965-2017.* Washington, D.C.

CNW. 2009. "National Wellness Survey shows Canadian organizations investing in worksite wellness." Accessed May 3, 2010. http://newswire.ca/en/releases/archive/September2009/30/c2024.html.

Families USA/Lewin Group. 2004. "Americans spending more for less health care services; workers' health costs rise faster than incomes." Accessed September 25, 2009. www.businessword.com/index.php?/weblog/comments/americans_spending_more_for_less_health_care_services.

Goetzel, R., D. Anderson, W. Whitmer, R. Ozminkowski, R. Dunn, and J. Wasserman. 1998. "The relationship between modifiable health risks and health care expenditures: An analysis of the multi-employer HERO health risk and cost database." *Journal of Occupational and Environmental Medicine* 40: 843-854.

Goetzel, R., G. Smith, S. Wang, E. Kelly, E. Mauceri, D. Columbus, and A. Cavuoti. 2009. "The relationship between modifiable health risk factors and medical expenditures, absenteeism, short-term disability, and presenteeism among employees at Novartis." *Journal of Occupational and Environmental Medicine* 51: 487-499.

Kaiser Foundation. 2009. *Kaiser/HRET survey of employer-sponsored health benefits, 1999-2009.*

Loeppke, R., M. Taitel, V. Haufle, T. Parry, R. Kessler, and K. Jinnett. 2009. "Health and productivity as a business strategy: A multiemployer study." *Journal of Occupational and Environmental Medicine* 51: 989-990.

Long, A., R. Reed, and G. Lehmann. 2006. "The cost of lifestyle health risks: Obesity." *Journal of Occupational and Environmental Medicine* 48: 244-251.

Milliman, Inc. 2009. *Milliman medical index.* Seattle: Author.

Musich, S., D. Hook, T. Barnett, and D. Edington. 2003. "The association between health risk status and health care costs among the membership of an Australian health plan." *Health Promotion International* 18: 57-65.

Pelletier, K. 2005. "A review and analysis of the clinical and cost-effectiveness studies of comprehensive health and disease management programs at the job site: Update VI 2000-2004." *Journal of Occupational and Environmental Medicine* 47: 1051-1058.

Pronk, N. 2009. "Population health management at the worksite." In *ACSM's Worksite health handbook: A guide to building healthy and productive companies*. Champaign, IL: Human Kinetics.

Pronk, N., M. Goodman, P. O'Connor, and B. Martinson. 1999. "Relationship between modifiable health risks and short-term health care charges." *Journal of the American Medical Association* 282: 2235-2239.

Rand corporation. 2009. "Current and projected health care spending." Accessed September 25. www.randcompare.org/current/dimension/spending.

Society for Human Resource Management. 2008. *Aging workforce, health care top issues in SHRM workplace forecast 2008*. Alexandria, VA.

UnumProvident Company. 2005. *Health and productivity in the aging American workforce: Realities and opportunities*. Chattanooga, TN.

Urban Transport Fact Book. 2009. *National personal transportation survey*. Accessed September 25. www.publicpurpose.com/ut-6995commute.htm.

U.S. Census Bureau. 2008. *People quickfacts, 2008*. Accessed September 25, 2009. http://quickfacts.census.gov/qfd/states/00000.html.

Watson Wyatt Worldwide. 2009. "Companies continue to add wellness programs, Watson Wyatt/National Business Group on Health Survey Finds." Accessed September 25. www.watsonwyatt.com/news/press.asp?ID=20961.

Wellness Council of America. 2009. "The 7 Cs of building a well workplace." Accessed September 22. http://infopoint.welcoa.org/blueprints/blueprint1/intro.html.

Wilkerson, G., N. Boer, C. Smith, and G. Heath. 2008. "Health-related factors associated with the health care costs of office workers." *Journal of Occupational and Environmental Medicine* 50: 593-601.

World Health Organization. 2009. *World health statistics, 2009*. Geneva, Switzerland.

Wright, D., M. Beard, and D. Edington. 2002. "Association of health risks with the cost of time away from work." *Journal of Occupational and Environmental Medicine* 44: 1126-1134.

Looking Ahead

A legendary adage reflects the essence of planning. Simply put, "failing to plan is a plan to fail." In essence, there is no substitute for high-quality planning in any venture, including a WHP program. Various program planning models exist in today's WHP marketplace, ranging in terms of complexity, cost, resources, and, of course, personnel requirements.

One of the first steps that many WHP practitioners take prior to seeking senior-level support for WHP programs is to identify the level and type of needs for employee and corporate health. Chapter 2 focuses on how an organization's health-management personnel can accurately identify employees' needs and interests in planning employee-focused programs, incentives, and policies.

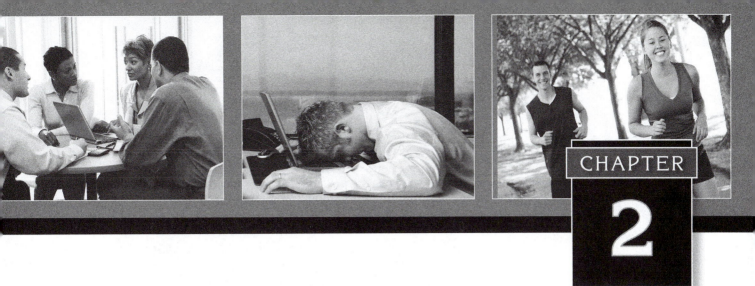

Determining Employees' Needs and Interests

LEARNING OBJECTIVES

After reading this chapter, you will be able to do the following:

- ✔ Describe the value and role of a wellness committee.
- ✔ Identify potential challenges that may occur when determining needs and interests.
- ✔ Develop an awareness of several strategies for identifying employee and organizational health needs.
- ✔ Distinguish between tools for needs identification and those for interest assessment.
- ✔ Identify several precautions when using tools for health-risk assessment.
- ✔ Describe how to compare identified needs with employee interests in order to develop an appropriate plan of action.

Under the pressures of downsizing, global competition, and rising production costs, every facet of today's business operations is being scrutinized by management. Since worksite health promotion (WHP) may be a relatively new endeavor for many businesses, it must be planned and positioned even more carefully than other business strategies. Thus, it is important to accurately determine employees' needs and interests to ensure that selected WHP programs will, in fact, achieve designated employee and employer goals. In order to do so accurately, worksite health personnel should undertake a well-crafted, step-by-step approach composed of proven techniques. Two major, interrelated phases will help achieve this goal. The first phase, *identification*, focuses on identifying, understanding, and prioritizing employees' needs. The second phase, *assessment*, focuses on evaluating, understanding, and prioritizing the level of employees' interest in specific types of incentives and WHP programs.

IDENTIFYING EMPLOYEES' NEEDS

Identification begins with forming a task force to highlight a company's demographics (for example, age and ethnicity distribution, ratio of women to men, and education levels), the existing and potential health-related problems of its workforce, and employee interest in programs to improve health and well-being.

Wellness Committees

The fate of a WHP program depends largely on the promoters' philosophy toward employee health issues. When management personnel lead healthy lifestyles themselves, they are more inclined to support health-enhancement activities at the worksite. This inclination also depends on whether they see strong employee interest in the activities. An effective way to spark enthusiasm is to involve employees in planning and implementing the program. After all, successful WHP programs are usually driven from the bottom up (by employees), not from the top down. Involving employees in all aspects of program planning and implementation gives them a personal stake in the program, greatly increasing the chances that they will commit to it.

Although the site manager or supervisor at small worksites might solicit input from individual employees about their needs and interests, this personalized approach may not always be practical for midsized, large, or multisite work settings. In these environments, it usually pays to form a committee of management and employee representatives. Although these groups have traditionally been called **wellness committees**, many WHP professionals find that the term *wellness* is often associated with a soft, fuzzy entity by employees and senior managers alike.

Thus, as WHP programs increasingly try to assume a more credible role in their company's overall health and bottom-line performance, wellness committees are realizing the importance of collaborating with other personnel, such as human resources or benefits managers, occupational health nurses or medical directors, safety managers, managers of employee assistance programs (EAPs), risk managers, designated employee representatives, and union representatives. Although the percentage of union workers has dropped substantially since the 1980s, unions remain a dynamic force in many worksites. They can enhance WHP efforts by encouraging employee participation and working closely with management.

Other key issues to consider when organizing a health-oriented employee committee include the following:

- Eligibility criteria used to select, appoint, or elect members
- Length of term served by committee members
- Ratio of management to nonmanagement members
- Desired frequency of meetings
- Group or person to whom the committee reports
- Major roles defined for the committee (planning, implementing, and so on)
- Level of influence of the committee (advisory only, policy making)
- Recognition or compensation for serving on the committee (release time from job, overtime pay if duties performed beyond normal work hours, and so on)

Once a committee has been formed, the next step is to establish protocol for the preceding issues to ensure that the group performs its duties up to par. It can then develop a sound strategy for identifying major health-related needs at the employee, worksite-environment, and organizational level.

Health-Related Data

Because employees' health needs can vary between worksites, WHP personnel should carefully assess their particular workforce for specific problems:

- What are the primary factors responsible for employee absences?
- What are the five most common medical claims filed by employees?

- What risk factors appear to negatively affect productivity on the job?
- Are smoking breaks compromising productivity?
- What has the ratio of corporate costs between medical care and prescription drugs been over the past five years?
- Is the number of lower-back injuries sufficient to justify a prevention program?
- Does the worksite culture promote personal health?
- What are the best days and times to offer particular programs?

These are just a few questions that the task force should consider exploring in this important phase.

An early task for WHP personnel is gathering appropriate data to accurately identify the scope and specificity of employee- and employer-based needs. *Scope* refers to the range and variability of needs identified at the employee, environmental, or organizational level. In contrast, *specificity* refers to the type and prevalence of identified needs. Table 2.1 illustrates a condensed version of a sample framework for needs identification. Appendix A highlights a personal health

Table 2.1 Abbreviated Framework for Needs Identification

Data	Sources	Scope	Specificity	Implications
Demographics	Human resources manager	Age range: 18-70 yrs. Female: 55% Male: 45% Management: 10% Nonmanagement: 90%	Average age: 47 Median age: 42	• Most workers are approaching middle age. • Various WHP programs needed to reach wide age range of workers.
Employee health records	Occupational health nurse	Asthma: 24% Diabetes: 8% Hypertension: 30% Migraine: 10% Obesity: 34%	• 75% of type 2 diabetics work in labor-intensive jobs. • 1/3 of hypertensive cases are unmanaged.	• What is the real impact of diabetes on productivity? • A hypertension case-management program is needed.
Health-risk assessment	WHP staff	8 of 10 lifestyle indicators rated poorly in >70% of respondents	5 highest risk indicators: 1. Mental stress 2. Physical inactivity 3. Overweight or obesity 4. Financial stress 5. Existing musculoskeletal condition	Workforce needs programs regarding • total mind-body wellness and • personal financial management.
Medical claims	Benefits manager	• Outpatient costs rising 8% each year. • Inpatient costs rising 3% each year.	• Diagnostic testing comprises 60% of all outpatient costs vs. 50% last year. • Average length of stay has dropped in 9 of 10 leading inpatient conditions.	• What factors are driving more testing? • Employee-consumerism education is needed.
Culture audit	WHP staff	Perceptions on 3 of 5 cultural indicators revealed low ratings.	3 lowest indicators: 1. Physical environment 2. On-site recreational outlets 3. Unhealthy vending machine choices	Action needed to improve the health of the worksite environment.
Productivity	All previously mentioned sources	Absenteeism: 3% Presenteeism: 15% Disability: 2%	Self-reported presenteeism is twice as high in sedentary workers as in manual laborers.	Need to explore options to motivate sedentary workers to become more physically active.

questionnaire that can be distributed to employees to gather more information during the identification phase. When feasible, analyze as many of the following types of data as possible:

- Workforce demographic profiles
- Employee health records
- Status according to health-risk assessments
- Medical care claims and costs
- Workers' compensation claims and costs
- Worksite culture or environmental health
- On-the-job productivity

When accessing any of the preceding types of data, it's important to clearly distinguish which can be acquired and analyzed at the aggregate (group) level and which should be done at the individual level. With careful up-front communication and planning, health-management personnel can work together to identify data that may reveal an employee's identity and to take the appropriate measures to protect personal privacy. Various federal laws, such as **ADA**, **GINA**, and **HIPAA**, require employers and their business partners to follow specific guidelines when accessing, acquiring, storing, and transmitting employees' personal health data. For example, it would be appropriate for a worksite's occupational health nurse and company physician to share an employee's personal health information when providing health care services. However, it is unlawful for them to share that information with a third party (e.g., WHP staff, benefits manager, human resources director, or health insurer) without specific written authorization from the employee.

Throughout the needs identification phase, data can be acquired and formatted into an aggregate (group) profile to preserve the privacy and confidentiality of employees' personal health data. In particular, using appropriate methods of data acquisition and conversion enables authorized personnel to consolidate potentially sensitive and private information, such as employee health records, workers' compensation claims, and health-risk assessment data, to protect each employee's right to privacy.

Take data on medical care claims, for instance. Since most employers at midsized and large organizations are self-insured, they use a *third-party administrator (TPA)* to administer claims payments to health care providers. At designated intervals, TPAs generally provide

> Which of the three formats do you feel reveals the most information?

an employer with aggregate (group formatted) data reports of medical-care claims. Table 2.2 shows claims and costs by **major diagnostic category (MDC)** and subcategories, which are identified by either a **diagnostic-related group (DRG)**, as shown in table 2.3, or by the code of the **International Classification of Diseases (ICD)**, as shown in table 2.4.

As implied in its abbreviation, an MDC is just that—a major or broadly defined category. Interestingly, many MDCs also represent body systems that you learned about in your 8th grade biology class (such as the circulatory, digestive, respiratory, and endocrine systems). Approximately 25 MDCs are used in the claims coding system. However, the author has seen that the number of MDC listings used by some TPAs can range from a low of 17 (when 2 or 3 MDCs are grouped into a single MDC) to as many as 27 MDCs (when a single MDC may be divided in two).

Since MDCs are broadly defined, they lack the specificity that many health managers desire in their efforts to identify needs and plan programs. As shown in table 2.5, numerous DRGs constitute each MDC. Approximately 500 DRGs are designed to reveal various groups of conditions that make up a specific group. However, ICD-coded claims are actually the most revealing type of classification, since they reflect specific types of conditions within a particular DRG. For that reason, WHP personnel prefer to receive medical claims in data formats composed of ICDs, but they often have to

Table 2.2 Sample Listing of Claims by Major Diagnostic Categories (MDC)

MDC #	# of claims	Total charges	Average charge
01 Nervous	2	$948	$474
02 Eye	5	$58,924	$11,784
03 Ear, nose, throat, and mouth	4	$1,880	$470
04 Respiratory system	15	$6,050	$403
05 Circulatory system	10	$8,900	$890
06 Digestive system	7	$5,180	$740
07 Hepatobiliary and pancreas	2	$1,960	$980
08 Musculoskeletal system	3	$13,500	$4,500
09 Skin, subcutaneous, and breasts	3	$1,050	$350
10 Endocrine, nutritional, metabolic	4	$1,806	$452
11 Kidney and urinary tract	17	$6,613	$389
12 Male reproductive system	2	$6,440	$3,230
13 Female reproductive system	2	$2,220	$1,110
14 Pregnancy, childbirth, puerperium	1	$4,500	$4,500
15 Newborns and other neonates	7	$1,575	$225
16 Blood and blood-forming cells	1	$ 870	$870
17 Myeloproliferative (neoplasm)	4	$7,000	$1,750
18 Infectious and parasitic organisms	1	$415	$415
19 Mental diseases and disorders	2	$11,900	$5,950
20 Use of drugs and alcohol	8	$3,192	$399
21 Injuries, poison, toxic effects	2	$780	$390
22 Burns	1	$9,250	$9,250
23 Factors influencing health status	4	$2,490	$622
24 Multiple significant traumas	2	$8,900	$4,450
25 Human Immune Virus infection	1	$3,400	$3,400

MDC category information from Centers for Medicare and Medicaid Services, 2009, Washington, D.C.

settle for DRGs due to the data-formatting specifications established by a particular TPA.

Data about workers' compensation claims are typically handled by the medical, safety, risk management, benefits, or human resources departments. They show the incidence and type of injuries that result in work-related absence or disability. They also indicate any employer-paid compensation to injured employees. Like data about medical-care claims, this information helps WHP personnel develop claims-driven programs that reduce accidents and injuries on the job. In addition, when workers' compensation data are integrated into appropriate analytical frameworks, evaluators can calculate savings from a successful intervention that are related to medical care and productivity.

Another popular tool for needs identification is a health culture audit (see appendix B). Some worksite personnel create their own audit tool that is tailored around the unique demographic, occupational, and cultural makeup of their worksite. Yet, numerous assessments for culture audits exist in the marketplace, ranging from one-page manual instruments to more advanced computer-

Table 2.3 Sample Listing of Diagnostic-Related Group (DRG) Claims Within Selected MDCs

DRG#	# of claims	Total charges	Average charge
MDC: Circulatory			
232 Coronary bypass with cardiac catheterization	3	$170,506	$56,835
309 Cardiac arrhythmia with complications	1	$15,240	$15,240
313 Chest pain	7	$40,474	$5,782
MDC: Mental			
881 Depressive neuroses	12	$9,016	$751
885 Psychoses	27	$42,061	$1,557
MDC: Musculoskeletal			
551 Medical back problems	23	$112,779	$4,903
557 Tendonitis/bursitis	6	$24,832	$4,138
MDC: Pregnancy			
765 Cesarean section with complications	4	$24,141	$6,035
766 Cesarean section without complications	70	$497,000	$7,100
775 Vaginal delivery without complications	81	$380,628	$4,699
793 Full-term neonate with major problems	2	$103,345	$51,672

MDC and DRG category information from Centers for Medicare and Medicaid Services, 2009, Washington, D.C.

Table 2.4 Sample Listing of International Classification of Disease (ICD) Claims Within Selected MDCs

ICD code #	# of claims	Total charges	Average charge
Neoplasm			
172.0 Skin	2	$7,192	$3,596
174.4 Breast	1	$19,484	$19,484
183.0 Ovary	1	$15,400	$15,400
188.3 Bladder	1	$16,848	$16,848
Mental			
300.0 Anxiety	4	$1,927	$481
300.4 Depression	5	$5,975	$1,195
301.3 Explosive personality	1	$998	$998
Circulatory			
402.1 Hypertension	1	$3,256	$3,256
414.0 Atherosclerosis	1	$7,777	$7,777
455.0 Hemorrhoids	1	$2,467	$2,467

ICD category information from National Center for Health Statistics and the Centers for Medicare and Medicaid Services, Washington, D.C.

Table 2.5 A Paradigm With Sample Musculoskeletal DRGs and ICDs

MDC (#)	Musculoskeletal system and connective tissue (8)		
DRG (#)	Arthopathies (553)	Medical back problems (551)	Tendonitis, myositis, and bursitis (557)
ICD	Rheumatoid arthritis	Lumbago	Synovitis or tenosynovitis
	Osteoarthritis	Sciatica	Infective myositis
	Loose body in knee	Intervertebral disc disorder	Rotator cuff syndrome

analyzed versions. Due to the variability in content, format, cost, and administration, it's important to thoroughly review various products before selecting a commercial tool.

Finally, an environmental check sheet can be used to identify existing and potential problems at a worksite, especially those resulting from working patterns or environmental factors, such as the percentage of time workers do physical labor, computer use, or perform repetitive tasks. Because each worksite and workforce is unique, the sample check sheet (see appendix C) can be customized for a specific environmental setting.

Health-Risk Assessment

Perhaps the most publicized tool for needs identification is a **health-risk assessment (HRA).** Interestingly, the genesis of today's HRA was based on a three-step concept of (1) risk identification, (2) risk assessment, and (3) risk reduction that was developed by Dr. Lewis Robbins in 1959. He and his colleagues created a patient-oriented HRA questionnaire called the health hazard appraisal (HHA) that involved a biometric screening and obtained information on a person's reported lifestyle, demographic profile, and family medical history. Using epidemiologically derived algorithms, this particular risk-assessment tool estimated the odds that a person with certain health risks would die from specific conditions in 10-year intervals.

In 1962, Cecelia Conrath, a health educator for the U.S. Cancer Control Program, and Dr. William DeMaria of Duke University suggested the term *prospective medicine* for this approach to preventive medicine. Dr. DeMaria defined **prospective medicine** as "a discipline concerned with the identification of the individual's changing risks of disease and the recognition of his earliest deviations from health" (Society of Prospective Medicine 1976). It essentially aims to promote health, prevent disease, and thus extend useful life expectancy by complementing the art of medical care with a scientific method, which reduces long-term health risks.

In the mid-1960s, the initial concept of prospective medicine was expanded to include a comprehensive concern for a total—and changing—spectrum of risk factors. Throughout the 1960s and 1970s, more risk factor research was conducted and used in a handful of HRA tools that existed in the marketplace. As the scope of HRA design added various quality-of-life measures, more tools for health-risk assessment were designed and introduced in public health, university, and worksite settings.

Initially, HRAs were administered using manually scored paper and pencil questionnaires based on very simple risk-assessment calculations. As the HRA's popularity and the number of participants grew, vendors computerized the health-risk analyses, using scoring algorithms that were more complex and sophisticated. Currently, approximately 50 commercialized HRA tools exist in a variety of types and price ranges. HRAs can be found in self-scoring formats, computerized questionnaire forms with extensive outcome reports, phone-based tools, and interactive online versions. Some

HRAs have added productivity-based questions in an attempt to simultaneously measure the effect of health risks on well-being and on-the-job productivity.

In the past, numerous employers offered financial incentives to employees who voluntarily completed HRAs. Although some employers currently require their employees to complete HRAs in order to receive company-sponsored health benefits, this may be in direct violation of ADA statutes. According to an informal opinion paper published in 2009, the Equal Employment Opportunity Commission (EEOC) ruled that a county employer's policy requiring employees to complete a HRA in order to participate in a company-funded health plan did, on record, violate ADA policy. In particular, the opinion letter states the following:

• Requiring all employees undergo a health-risk assessment that includes disability-related inquiries and medical examinations as a prerequisite for obtaining health insurance coverage does not appear to be job related or consistent with business necessity. Therefore, it violates the ADA.

• Disability-related inquiries and medical examinations are permitted as part of a voluntary wellness program. A wellness program is voluntary if employees are neither required to participate nor penalized for nonparticipation. In the county employer's case, even if the health-risk assessment had been part of a wellness program, the program was not voluntary because nonparticipants were penalized (denied health-plan coverage).

Although it is important for employers to be familiar with the positions taken by the EEOC in their informal discussion letters, they should also note that these letters are nonbinding. As such, they do not constitute official opinions of the EEOC. Nonetheless, rules established by the Internal Revenue Service (IRS) prohibit employers from collecting genetic information (family medical history) in health-risk assessments if it will be used for underwriting purposes. This includes offering employees discounts on their monthly premium contributions or lower deductibles for completing an HRA.

Certainly, making HRAs mandatory for health-plan coverage appeals to many employers who are battling rising health care costs and a volatile economy. Considering that many employers subsidize 70% to 80% of their employees' health insurance premiums, they feel they have a fiduciary right to push employees toward better health through HRA-based risk-identification and risk-awareness tools. Simultaneously, worksite health managers and policy makers generally believe the following about the EEOC:

• Its current path is illogical and misdirected.

• It has misinterpreted the intent of employers seeking to implement mandatory HRA participation.

• It misunderstands the HRA process and the level of information available to employers.

• It seems to be misinterpreting the overall value received both by employees and employers.

Meanwhile, employers need to stay up to date on this particular issue.

In order to comply with various federal laws, especially HIPAA, ADA, and GINA, the results of health-risk assessments should never be shared with employers. In order to eliminate any concerns about violation of privacy, employers should receive only the aggregate, deidentified results for their entire workforce. Moreover, if HRA results are to be used in personal (one-on-one) targeted intervention or incentive programs, consent must first be obtained from participants. In some worksite settings, this requirement may require that a third-party vendor conducts the HRA to ensure employee confidentiality. In addition, employees need to know that only authorized personnel (those providing medical services or benefits) will have access to their personal health information.

Despite their widespread appeal, HRAs are designed to complement, not replace, appropriate physical exams and other biometric-related screenings performed by qualified health professionals. A growing trend is to combine HRAs with biometric screenings. This is a good incentive to boost participation that adds a direct-measure component to the program's planning and evaluation efforts. In addition, a biometric screen can verify whether self-reported information provided by an employee is accurate. Although you may assume that employees give accurate information on HRA instruments, most employees do not know their actual body weight, blood pressure, and so on.

Common biometric screenings include blood pressure, body mass index (based on height and weight), cardiorespiratory fitness, cholesterol (total, LDL, and HDL), glucose level, flexibility, and physical strength. Because HRA instruments vary considerably, it is good to review several formats before selecting one for use in a particular setting.

Important aspects to consider when deciding which HRA is appropriate for use in your particular workplace include the following:

1. *Number and type of questionnaire items.* Some HRAs are very comprehensive, collecting information on a wide array of health risks and behaviors (e.g., biometrics, exercise, nutrition, tobacco use, stress, depression, safety, preventive exams, and medical history). These broad-scope HRAs, which may include 70, 80, or even more than 100 items, can provide a wealth of health-risk data on the employee population. However, they require more time and effort from the participants than HRAs that are more focused on primary risk factors, like body mass index (BMI), exercise, and nutrition. Stage-of-change items may be important in determining stage-based interventions at both the individual and company level.

2. *Mode of delivery.* Although most HRAs are now provided online only, some vendors may still have paper versions of the questionnaire. Since the majority of employees now have Internet access either at work or at home, web-based HRAs offer several benefits over the paper versions. These include (a) fewer response errors due to restricted response ranges, (b) faster completion time because questions are tailored to the participant (e.g., women's health questions only appear for females, smoking questions only appear for smokers), (c) ease of revising responses, (d) immediate generation of personal report when HRA is completed (as compared with paper versions that require scanning or manual data input by staff), and (e) much lower cost than paper HRAs.

3. *Time required to complete the questionnaire.* Completion time for HRAs can range anywhere from 3 to 30 minutes, depending on the delivery mode (electronic or paper) and the number of items. The less time it takes for participants to complete the HRA, the greater the chance that they will finish it and respond to all items on the questionnaire. Again, you must decide how much risk-related information you feel you need to collect. Optimally, it is probably best to use an HRA that takes no longer than 10 minutes to complete.

4. *Availability of risk reduction follow-up.* Many HRA vendors offer follow-up services that help participants reduce the risks identified in their assessment. In most cases, the HRA website provides risk-reduction resources and referral information for participants to pursue on their own. Some vendors also offer more aggressive outreach with health coaching services online or over the phone. These services are usually added on, or available at additional cost.

5. *Pricing structures and options.* Examine the HRA pricing carefully. Although online HRAs are much less costly per participant than paper versions (which can be 20 or 30 times more expensive per participant than web-based versions), the pricing structure used by the vendor can make a dramatic difference in the total cost of the HRAs for your company. Three pricing structures are generally used: (a) fees based on all eligible employees in the company, regardless of whether or not they complete an HRA, (b) fees based on employees who enroll in an online

CASE STUDY: INCENTIVES FOR PARTICIPATION

Wellness screening is one of the best ways to assess an organization's health status and to target at-risk employees. Perhaps nothing draws participation better than that certain shade of green. Saint Thomas Health Services, a comprehensive health system in Nashville, Tennessee with a staff of more than 3,400 people, designed a screening program based on financial incentives that's saving them some serious cash. As it turns out, spending money really is one of the best ways to save it.

When the incentive program was first implemented, 31% of Saint Thomas' workforce responded to the $50 incentive applied to their health benefits. Although this was quite a modest response rate, management saw promise in the initiative. They were convinced that raising the amount of the incentive would increase participation.

A Risky Investment?

In the program's second year, a point system was implemented to encourage employees to participate in the health screenings and to work toward improving their lifestyles. This wasn't just any run-of-the-mill incentive program. The benefits department at Saint Thomas assembled an award system that gave employees the opportunity to earn up to $300 toward their health benefits if they participated in the wellness screening.

Here's how it works. Employees earn points based on both behaviors and screening results. Behaviors include participation in the screening, smoking status, and whether or not they receive a flu shot. Screening results refer to the actual physical measurements from the screening, such as cholesterol and blood pressure. They can also earn points for showing improvements from their previous screening. First-year participants and those participating in nonconsecutive years receive only $50. However, those who participate in consecutive years earn anywhere from $100 to $300, depending on their physical measurements.

Improvement points are a key component of the system—they help motivate employees to change behaviors. For example, someone with a healthy cholesterol level would receive more points than someone with high cholesterol. But, if employees with high cholesterol reduced their level significantly from the previous year's screening, they would receive points for the improvement.

Show Me the Money

Even with this enticing system in place, participation rates in 1995 and 1996 were stable at best. Then something happened in favor of the participants. Congress passed HIPAA. Essentially, this federal law prohibited employers from using health status to penalize employees participating in their health plan. This meant that participants could no longer apply incentives to their health benefits. So, with unsatisfactory participation rates in mind, Saint Thomas made the decision to keep the same incentive point system, but to give the money directly to participants.

In addition to this unbeatable incentive, Dr. Porr decided that "Wellness: A Choice" would start doing its own advertising. He wanted to make it impossible to miss. He used department meetings, elevator posters, payroll stuffers, and direct mail to get the message out to everyone. Plus, the news about the cash obviously traveled fast.

Cashing In

It worked. Participation shot up to 44%. Since then, participation has climbed steadily. As the popularity of screenings increases, so does the health of many Saint Thomas employees. "Our situation is unique here. Usually, an individual's health risks increase over time. However, within our employee population, these risk factors have decreased over a seven-year period," Porr says.

Within four years, Saint Thomas' health screening program showed a solid increase in popularity, effectiveness, and bottom-line impact. With a participation rate of 52%, improved employee health, and an organizational savings of $1.6 million in health care costs, it's apparent that this company has turned a big incentive into even bigger rewards.

HRA system, regardless of whether or not they complete an HRA, and (c) fees based on only those employees who complete an HRA. These fees can be calculated based on monthly usage levels (e.g., the number of eligible employees in the HRA system database each month) or on a per-completion basis. Additional fees may also be charged for health coaching, incentive systems, data management, group reports, and other services, so make sure you ask about all the costs involved. Most vendors require a minimum one-year contract for online HRA systems. Make sure you ask the following questions:

* What population database is used as a reference for risk comparisons?
* What security safeguards are used by the HRA vendor to protect the confidentiality of participant data?
* What steps does the vendor take to maintain compliance with ADA, HIPAA, GINA, and any other applicable regulations?

We've seen much progress in the technology of health-assessment tools and applications over the past 30 years. Certainly, these developments have generated greater time, cost, and administrative efficiencies for many WHP practitioners in their assessment efforts. Yet, avoid relying exclusively on high-tech tools and protocols at the expense of personal contact with employees. Carefully consider your tools and applications in order to foster the all-important relationship between provider and client.

ASSESSING EMPLOYEES' INTERESTS

As the identification process winds down, program planners should move into *assessment*, the second phase of the planning framework. This phase focuses on the interests and intentions of employees and on ways to deal with problems recognized during the identification phase.

Interest Survey Form

A popular assessment tool is an *interest survey form (ISF)*. You can create your own ISF, use a commercially produced survey, or integrate specific questions into a HRA survey used previously in the needs-identification phase. A substantial number of employers have chosen the latter approach, integrating questions that solicit interest into an HRA tool, for reasons ranging from time efficiency and cost containment to minimizing responder fatigue and avoiding losses in productivity. In fact, several HRA tools that are commercially available include questions that assess employee interests.

In preparing an ISF, the common axiom in today's quick-paced worksite is the shorter, the better. Thus, current ISF tools are usually no more than one page in length. They often resemble a generic format, which is a good way to assess employee interests in various programs and activities. In contrast, a topic-focused ISF is appropriate when you want to identify a single risk factor (i.e., diabetes) or program element (i.e., nutrition). This one-dimensional ISF is particularly suited for worksites with an established broad-based WHP program that wish to see if employees have a level of interest in a particular topic, risk factor, or incentive that is sufficient to justify the expansion of current programming. For example, more worksites are exploring the use of financial incentives to generate more participation, especially among high-risk employees. Thus, they might consider using single-issue ISFs to assess interest in such incentives.

Since most ISFs are more generic in nature, they often include the following:

* Program options to reduce risks (blood pressure, cholesterol, exercise, nutrition, and work-life balance)
* Readiness to change levels (precontemplation, contemplation, preparation, action, and maintenance)
* Preferences in program format (seminar, class, self-help, personal coach, Internet-based)

INTEREST SURVEY FORM

Tell us where you stand!

Please check the programs that **you** would **participate in** at the worksite:

❑ Low impact exercise	❑ Medical self-care	❑ Stress management
❑ Healthy back	❑ Healthy eating	❑ Walking
❑ Blood pressure control	❑ Pregnancy planning	❑ Weight control
❑ Quit smoking	❑ Financial wellness	❑ Diabetes control
❑ Spiritual wellness	❑ Flexibility training	❑ Body sculpting
❑ Body building	❑ Circuit training	❑ Strength training

Other (please list): _____

Would you participate in any program on your **own** time? ❑ Yes ❑ No

What days would you prefer to participate? M❑ T❑ W❑ Th❑ F❑

What times would you prefer to participate?
❑ Before work   ❑ At break time   ❑ At lunch   ❑ After work

What is the biggest barrier for you to overcome in order to participate?

Comments/suggestions: _____

Please return or e-mail this survey to: _____

Thank you!

- Preferences in participation time (before work, at break time, lunch, or after work)
- Preferences in communication channels (e-mail, at-work posters, at-home mailing, staff meetings)
- Invitation to assist WHP personnel (serving on the wellness committee, on a peer-support group, or as a wellness champion)

To enhance response, inform employees of the interest survey form at least twice before distributing it. Use various delivery channels to publicize and distribute the ISF, such as the following:

- Company newsletter
- Electronic message boards
- E-mail or website
- Flyers

- Paycheck stuffers
- Worksite lunchroom or break areas
- Bulletin-board displays in key locations

Within a couple of days of publicizing the ISF, the forms should be distributed either personally to each employee or to their respective mailboxes. When using an e-mail or Internet-based ISF, it's good to publicize the survey one or two days before its actual distribution to alert respondents and to discourage them from deleting the message.

If you have received less than 50% of the forms by the due date for the survey's return, you might distribute a reminder and then extend the due date by a few days.

As was the case with the assessment of worksite environment, the results of employee ISFs can be used as a baseline measure for later evaluation. The initial

LIKERT SCALES

In a growing number of worksites, ISF feedback is being inputted into a spreadsheet (eg., Microsoft Excel) for subsequent data analysis. Of course, data used in this fashion requires that the ISF have some type of quantitative scale so numerical values can be inserted into a spreadsheet. For example, the type of continuum used in the Likert scale is particularly suitable for spreadsheet data entry and subsequent analysis:

Interest Level	Very strong	Strong	Fair	None
Points	4	3	2	1

survey results can be compared with those of a follow-up survey several months later to measure progress.

You should also consider engaging workers in focus groups or informal interviews to gather information on their interests. This can be done either before or after the survey. If you don't have the resources to survey workers, you could use this method to gather information in place of the survey.

Whatever method is used to gather information, make it as easy as possible for workers to complete and submit the information to ensure a high return rate.

Once the ISFs are returned and tabulated, program planners need to compare the feedback on the forms with the employee needs seen earlier in the identification phase. Often, the needs identified for employees and the interests expressed by the employees conflict. Suppose that after the ISF has been returned, program planners have the information in table 2.6 to work with.

As you can see, data collected during the identification phase indicates that back injuries could be a serious concern for your worksite. However, back health ranks third on collected ISFs. Since it's important that decisions be data driven, not based solely on personal opinion, program planners should consider subjecting the needs and interests to the *X test*. In this simple procedure, a line is drawn between a topic that appears in both the list of needs and the list of interests. Once you have identified similar topics in both listings, look to see if the Xs formed by crossing lines are elongated (tall) or compressed (short). Shortened or compressed Xs indicate that a topic of high need is also of high interest. Thus, it should be given priority.

> When the information and feedback gathered during the two phases differ, how should program planners decide which needs and interests should receive priority?

Table 2.6 A Comparison Ranking of Most Frequently Reported Needs and Interests

Rank	Needs to address*	Interests**
1.	Sedentary job	Fitness walking
2.	Elevated body mass index	Weight control
3.	Unhealthy snacking	Back health
4.	Circulatory claims cost	Financial wellness
5.	Musculoskeletal claims	Healthy eating
6.	High stress	Spinning (fast stationary cycling)
7.	Poor indoor air quality	Spiritual wellness

* Risks based on employee health record, environmental check sheet, health-risk assessment, medical and workers' compensation claims data, and culture audit.

** Based on interest survey form.

A second option would be to contact other local worksites with WHP programs. If they offer the specific program you're considering, they can tell you how well it has been received. Third, you could review the professional literature to determine which programs have the greatest potential for achieving a particular goal. Weigh this information, along with employee preferences and identified needs, in a feasibility grid. For example, in considering a prevention program for lower-back injuries, a review of the literature by program planners may reveal that these problems occur most frequently in employees with weak abdominal muscles, poor hip flexor flexibility, poor lower-back flexibility, or improper lifting techniques. Thus, a back-health program would have a greater effect if it were designed to do the following:

- Strengthen abdominal muscles
- Enhance flexibility in the hip flexor muscles, lower back, and hamstrings
- Motivate proper lifting

These objectives can be plugged into a feasibility grid (see table 2.7) representing the steps that must be completed in order to achieve program-specific goals. According to the sample comparison shown in table 2.7, a prevention program for lower-back injuries may have the greatest potential for improving most of the criteria.

A final option to consider when no clear-cut evidence for a particular type of WHP program exists is to offer a pilot program on a specific topic for several weeks. Based on the level of participation, you can decide whether to extend the program or to replace it with a pilot program on a different topic that garnered employee interest in the original ISF process.

Let's look again at the conflicting data we have received from the identification phase and the ISF. Data collected at the identification phase clearly show that poor nutrition is a problem that should be addressed at your worksite. However, good nutrition received lower interest on the ISF than walking. You might ask experienced WHP professionals for their input or research some case studies to see whether nutrition programs or walking programs had better success rates. If walking programs appear most promising, you might choose to launch a walking program because of its reported success elsewhere. As employees begin to experience the health benefits of exercise, you might then integrate some nutrition tips into the walking sessions as a way of improving participants' energy and stamina. On the other hand, if you had started your WHP efforts solely with a nutrition program, you might have experienced

Table 2.7 A Sample Feasibility Grid of Top Three Interests on Interest Survey Form (ISF)

Criteria	Fitness walking (1st)	Weight control (2nd)	Back health (3rd)
Process			
Appeal to employees	H	H	H
Measurability	M	H	H
Impact			
Strengthen abdomen	M	L	M
Improve back flexibility	L	L	H
Motivate proper lifting	L	L	H
Outcome			
Reduce back injuries	L	M	H
Reduce back-related medical and workers' compensation costs	L	L	H

H = High; M = Moderate; L = Low.

low participation. Consequently, you would have had a greater challenge in building interest in future WHP offerings.

From the preceding examples, you can see that properly assessing feedback from the ISF involves more than a simple quantitative evaluation. To make the best use of the ISF, you'll need to compare the results with other data and to do the follow-up research necessary for viewing the information in the most useful light.

What should you do?

Employee Motivation

Closely related to what employees are interested in is the issue of what will motivate them to follow up on their expressed interests. A simple way to determine appropriate incentives is to ask people what would motivate them to participate in a health promotion program. For example, publicize and distribute an incentive survey along with an ISF. This integrated approach is time- and cost-efficient. It also yields a higher response rate, giving you a more representative view of employees' wishes. Adapt the all-in-one survey to your own company based on preliminary projections of the budget, program offerings, and number of employees expected to participate. The survey will provide you with a basic idea of what will attract employees. You can combine this later with more precise information on resources gathered during the planning phase (see chapter 3 for discussion). Additional information on planning and using employee-driven incentives is presented in chapter 7.

Assessment is a crucial phase in the framework for planning your WHP programs. Misjudgments during this phase can have a negative effect on the program. Accurate assessments, however, can get WHP started on the right track, greatly increasing the chances for long-term success.

INCENTIVE SURVEY

Tell us what motivates you!

As you may know by now, we are planning to offer several new programs for personal health enhancement. In order to make these programs successful, we need **you** to participate. We know everyone needs an incentive to participate in new programs and activities. So, we'd like to know what incentives would motivate **you** to participate. Please take a moment to check the level of your interest for each of the following incentives. Thank you!

		Value	
Incentive	**High**	**Moderate**	**Low**
T-shirt or hat	❏	❏	❏
Exercise clothing, shoes, or other gear	❏	❏	❏
Gift certificate to local restaurant or retail store	❏	❏	❏
Free airline tickets	❏	❏	❏
Free theme park tickets	❏	❏	❏
Day off work for earning wellness credits	❏	❏	❏
"Well bucks" to exchange for gifts	❏	❏	❏
Health insurance premium waived	❏	❏	❏
$10 cash for completing health-risk appraisal	❏	❏	❏
Employer funds your health expense account	❏	❏	❏
Employer funds your health reimbursement account	❏	❏	❏
Other (list) _____	❏	❏	❏

What Would You Do?

Suppose 60% of a workforce expressed very strong preferences for walking and stress management on the ISF. Nearly 50% of all workers expressed a strong interest in eating a healthier diet. In contrast, the two most prevalent health care claims are musculoskeletal and lower-back pain (joint stiffness, in particular) and digestive ailments, ranging from gastroesophageal reflux disease (GERD) to diverticulosis. Additional reviews of medical claims showed a 25% increase in questionable emergency room visits. So, on the side of employee motivation, you have strong interest in walking, stress management, and better diet. On the side of employees' needs, you have musculoskeletal and digestive problems and many minor ailments that are apparently being treated as emergencies. Quite a hodgepodge, huh?

> **Would you offer targeted programs on a graduated basis over a 1- to 2-year time frame, combine responses related to multiple risk factors into a single intervention, or offer several targeted programs at the same time?**

Human resources, your arm of the WHP programming budget, has recently informed you that this year's budget is 20% lower than last year's. Since you would like to address all of the preceding interests and needs, what approach would you take to achieve your lofty goal?

Considering the budgetary squeeze, you are leaning toward the first option in planning your WHP programming strategy. As you sift through the mishmash of employees' interests and needs, how would you determine which of the most pressing needs is in sync with employees' interests? Are you more inclined to offer interest-based programs first, hoping to build enough early employee participation to carry over to needs-based programs afterwards? You certainly have many options to consider. What would you do?

CHAPTER 2 WRAP-UP

Key Points

- A team-oriented wellness committee composed of employee and management representatives can play an important role in determining employees' needs and interests.
- Several federal laws govern the processes that should be followed during health assessment.
- Various tools should be considered when identifying employees' needs.
- Results from different identification tools can be compared to reveal primary and secondary needs.
- Today's tools for health-risk assessment continue to evolve in terms of scope, specificity, cost, and administration.
- Employees' interests and incentive preferences can be simultaneously assessed with a single integrated format.

Glossary

Americans with Disabilities Act (ADA)—A federal law that prohibits private employers, state and local governments, employment agencies, and labor unions from discriminating against qualified people with disabilities in job application procedures, hiring, firing, advancement, compensation, job training, and other terms, conditions, and privileges of employment.

diagnostic-related group (DRG)—A group of medical conditions with similar diagnoses.

Genetic Information Nondiscrimination Act (GINA)—A federal law that prohibits discrimination in health coverage and employment based on genetic information.

Health Insurance Portability and Accountability Act (HIPAA)—Federal statutes regulating how personal health information can legally be obtained, stored, and shared between various parties.

health-risk assessment (HRA)—A procedure that uses a questionnaire, biometric screening, or other methods to assess the effect of health risks, lifestyle, and environment on overall health status.

International Classification of Diseases (ICD)—A system of codes use to classify diseases, as well as signs, symptoms, complaints, and social circumstances and injuries related to those diseases.

major diagnostic category (MDC)—A category corresponding to a single organ or body system composed of various conditions.

prospective medicine—A process in which health professionals use HRA data to identify risk level and appraise health status in order to determine appropriate interventions to improve the patient's quality of health and life.

wellness committee—A group assembled to plan, implement, or evaluate a WHP program.

Bibliography

Alexander, G. 2006. "Health risk appraisal." *Health and Productivity Management* 5: 26-29.

Hall, J., and L. Robbins. 1979. *Prospective medicine.* Indianapolis: Methodist Hospital.

Pronk, N., ed. 2009. *ACSM's Worksite health handbook: A guide to building healthy and productive companies.* 2nd ed. Champaign, IL: Human Kinetics.

U.S. Department of Health & Human Services. 2009. "The Health Insurance Portability and Accountability Act of 1996 (HIPAA) Privacy and Security Rules." Accessed October 28. www.hhs.gov/ocr/privacy.

U.S. Department of Justice. 2009. "Americans with Disabilities Act: ADA Home Page." Accessed October 28. www.ada.gov.

U.S. Equal Employment Opportunity Commission. 2009. "ADA: Disability-related inquiries and medical examinations: Health risk assessment." Accessed October 29. www.eeoc.gov/eeoc/foia/letters/2009/ada_disability_medexam_healthrisk.html.

———. 2009. "Disability discrimination." Accessed October 29. www.eeoc.gov/laws/types/disability.cfm.

Looking Ahead

Now that we've considered ways to assess employees' needs and interests, it's time to develop appropriate goals to guide programming decisions. Chapter 3 describes how to construct practical goals and customized vision and mission statements that can be used to create a strategic plan of action.

Part II

Planning Worksite Health Promotion Programs

Each chapter in this section provides information and strategies for planning employee-oriented WHP programs. Chapter 3 outlines how to create vision and mission statements, set appropriate goals and realistic expectations, and build an evaluation plan. Chapter 4 provides information on customizing healthy lifestyle programs based on sound programming philosophy. Chapter 5 highlights tips for preparing a realistic program budget, writing a sample proposal for garnering adequate resources, and positioning WHP efforts to reach as many employees as possible. Collectively, these planning-oriented chapters provide an important transition into program implementation and evaluation.

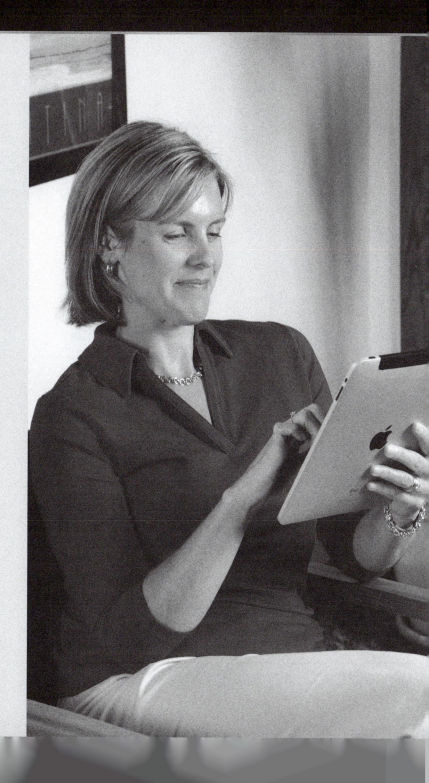

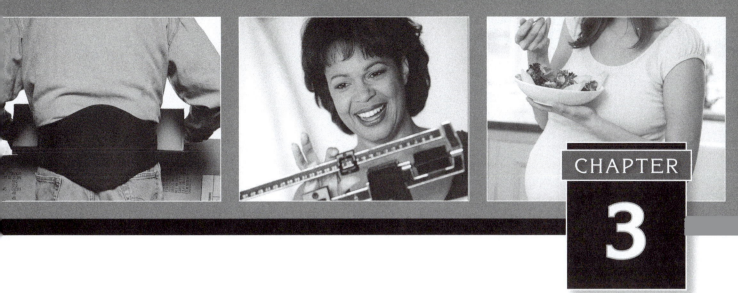

Preparing Program Goals

LEARNING OBJECTIVES

After reading this chapter, you will be able to do the following:

✔ Construct an appropriate mission statement and vision statement.
✔ List essential parts of goals and objectives.
✔ Explain the importance of evaluation within the planning phase.
✔ Distinguish between short-term and long-term objectives.
✔ List several examples of indicators of employee and organizational health.

With growing demand to generate more value with limited resources, health promotion planners must work harder than ever. This chapter presents key issues to consider during the planning phase of the comprehensive framework.

What percentage of the workday do WHP program directors spend on planning? Numerous surveys indicate that program planning may be their most time-consuming and challenging task. Therefore, their planning methods must be fundamentally sound and tailored to address the unique needs and interests of their respective worksites. Chapters 3 through 7 provide an overview of various issues, opportunities, and strategies to consider throughout the lengthy and ever-evolving planning process.

Since employees' needs and interests should drive the bulk of WHP efforts, it is essential to carefully review the results of the identification and assessment phases. For example, as you prepare strategies to deal with the needs and interests identified in phases 1 and 2, closely review the data collected in order to accurately determine the following:

1. The prevalence of the issues identified in the workforce and worksite.
2. The immediate and long-term effects of these issues on employees' health and on-the-job productivity.
3. Probable contributing factors (i.e., demographic, occupational, cultural, environmental, economic).
4. The group of workers at the greatest risk.

Let's see how this investigative process works. Imagine a company that is considering a prevention program for lower-back injuries. Program planners in this company begin by asking how prevalent the issue is. Data gathered during the first phase tell them that nearly one of every four employees reported lower-back pain over the past year. These numbers indicate a pervasive problem, so the planners proceed to the next question: What is the direct, immediate effect of the issue identified? Reviewing the data, worksite health personnel discover that one-third of employees reporting lower-back pain missed more than two weeks of work during the previous year. Moreover, when reviewing historical claims of back pain, the occupational health nurse sees that a disproportionately high number of workers who were previously affected reported workers' compensation claims within three years of their initial injury. In addition, they learn by conducting work-analysis observations that nearly one-half of the employees with back pain do not practice proper lifting methods. These results suggested that a program should be developed to specifically address back health, especially the prevention of lower-back pain. Once this decision has been made, the fourth question is asked: Which group of workers in the company needs this type of program? After reviewing data from the phase of needs identification, worksite personnel find that most workers who reported lower-back pain were men under 45 years of age who work in the departments of shipping, foundry, and quality control.

So, after asking these questions, program planners understand the following:

- A need exists for a lower-back injury program.
- The immediate effect of the problem is high absenteeism.
- The long-term effect of the problem is increased workers' compensation claims and costs.
- A major contributing factor is that many injured workers do not practice proper lifting techniques.
- The program should be targeted mainly at men under 45 working in labor-intensive jobs.

Armed with this information, you can now proceed through several important steps,

including the following (not necessarily in order):

1. Establishing vision and mission statements.
2. Setting appropriate goals for the program.
3. Making programming and resource decisions (see chapters 4, 5, and 6).
4. Funding and budgeting the program (see chapter 5).
5. Deciding whether to establish an integrated program (i.e., operate WHP within an existing department such as human resources) or an independent arrangement in which the program exists on its own (see chapter 7).
6. Incorporating reliable methods to evaluate the WHP program (see chapter 8).

The following sections discuss each of these steps in detail.

ESTABLISHING VISION AND MISSION STATEMENTS

The operating structure of an organization is a significant factor to consider when planning and implementing WHP programs. Each organization has its own unique way of sustaining business functions for success. In order to understand the operating structure used by a particular organization, a Socratic approach is helpful for defining and clarifying key factors to consider in this important endeavor. Questions that can be used to achieve this goal include the following:

- What are we doing?
- Why are we offering this particular product or service?
- How are we serving the needs of our customers?
- With whom are we partnering to provide this service?
- Who is responsible for each phase of product development, marketing, and delivery?
- When are specific services provided to customers?
- Where are we providing these services?

By answering the preceding questions, WHP program planners will have a better understanding of how their organization functions as they proceed with their work.

Of course, a WHP program should reflect its organization's vision and mission (see figure 3.1). An organization's **vision statement** is a short, succinct, and inspiring statement of what the organization intends to become and to achieve at some point in the future. It is often stated in competitive terms. For example, a sample vision statement for an organization would read something like this:

To be the leading worldwide clothing brand in the women's sportswear manufacturing business.

At the WHP level, a vision statement reflects the goals of worksite health personnel and the organization's identity. Since health and productivity issues are gaining popularity in many worksites, many WHP planners are developing vision statements similar to this one:

To have the healthiest and most productive workforce in our industry.

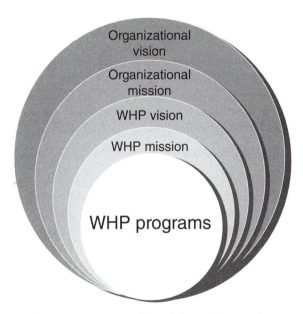

Figure 3.1 Illustration of the relationship between the vision and mission of an organization and its worksite health promotion program.

In order to achieve its corporate and WHP-specific vision, an organization needs to develop and implement a sound mission. A **mission statement** describes the step that moves your strategic planning process from the present to the future. The mission statement is usually a multidimensional statement because it reflects the organization's philosophy, purpose, goals, and commitment for achieving the vision. For example, the following mission statement was developed by WHP planners in one large industry:

The employee wellness program provides opportunities, services, and resources for employees, spouses, and retirees to make healthy lifestyle choices. Its purpose is to help improve health-risk status and control health-related costs, with special emphasis on less-fit and at-risk participants.

The preceding statement consists of the following dimensions:

- Who we are (employee wellness program)
- What we do (provide opportunities, services, and resources)
- General population (employees, spouses, and retirees)
- Objective or prerequisite (healthy lifestyle choices)
- Employee health goal (improve health-risk status)
- Organizational or corporate health goal (control health-related costs)
- Target population (less-fit and at-risk participants)

Although the preceding dimensions are common to many organizations, some program planners may decide to limit the scope of their goals. Thus, they may include only a portion of these elements. In such cases, the preceding mission statement could be condensed as follows:

The wellness program provides opportunities, services, and resources for employees, spouses, and retirees to make healthy lifestyle choices.

SETTING APPROPRIATE GOALS

It's important to set and develop **goals** relevant to the scope and specificity of your target population. For purposes of convenience, let's continue to use the example of a company in which lower-back injury has been recognized as a pervasive problem among employees. During this first step of the planning phase, the company's WHP program planners need to establish goals that are realistic enough to attain and yet demanding enough to bring about a clear improvement in the problem area.

Both the research literature and common sense tell us that improper lifting technique is connected to back injury or pain. In our case study, almost half of the employees with back injury or pain do not consistently use proper lifting technique. Thus, it is reasonable to assume that reports of back injury and pain could decrease as much as 50% if all employees lifted properly. If this were the case, would a program outcome of reducing lower-back injuries by 50% be an appropriate goal? Probably not. Although 50% sounds like a high percentage under most circumstances, in this case, the desired effect should be higher. Considering how relatively simple it should be to reduce the number of lower-back injuries by nearly half with a single intervention of proper lifting technique, a good program for lower-back health should strive for a success rate of 75%. This would mean that 25% of all back injuries would need to be addressed through interventions other than teaching proper lifting technique. Thus, each case must be evaluated individually to establish a suitable goal for each program.

Goal Criteria

Goals that clearly reflect the scope of key Socratic elements should be SMART (Kotelnikov 2009):

- *Specific.* Specificity is reflected to the extent that various Socratic questions are asked: Who is involved, what do I want to achieve, where is the action occurring, when is the action occurring, and why am I doing this action?
- *Measurable.* Tangible criteria are used to quantify progress.
- *Attainable.* The goal can be attained with a reasonable amount of knowledge, skills, and resources.
- *Realistic.* The goal can be achieved within a person's preparation time and commitment.
- *Timely.* The goal can be achieved within a reasonable time frame.

Because you are developing your evaluation goals in connection with specific programs, you must think not only about goals that are exclusively concerned with evaluation but also about the general goals of the WHP programs. Proper attention will make your evaluation goals that much easier to develop. In particular, the overall quality of your evaluation efforts will be greatly enhanced when you develop evaluation goals tailored around programs that (1) are compatible with stakeholders' health-related needs, interests, and values and that (2) include a time frame that sufficiently allows an intervention to achieve the desired effect.

Let's take a couple of goals that are not very useful for either planning or evaluation. By applying the preceding criteria, let's revise them so they will be more useful for a quality evaluation. Suppose that your two goals are as follows:

- Improve the cardiorespiratory health of female employees.
- Improve employee productivity.

Now, one by one, add the elements defined in each of the criteria to transform these vaguely stated goals into valuable directives for planning both programs and evaluation.

1. Compatibility With Stakeholders' Health-Related Needs, Interests, and Values

When creating your goals, you must be certain that the stakeholders will support them. Say, for example, that after you decided on your goals, you ran a survey of the 400 women in your workforce. You learned that the primary health concern of 350 women was preventing breast cancer. In that case, you would have a hard time selling a program for cardiorespiratory health. If you had limited funds and could afford only one major program for women, you would want to change the focus of your first goal to reducing personal risk of breast cancer among female employees. Of course, you would have saved yourself some trouble if you had surveyed the stakeholders in your women's health program before you decided on your goal. We will assume that you had surveyed major stakeholders already about employee productivity. Thus, the second goal will remain the same.

2. Quantifiability

Although both of your goals are now compatible with the interests of your stakeholders, neither is particularly useful yet because neither contains anything that can be quantified. In order for a goal statement to be measurable, it must contain an *outcome variable*. An outcome variable, also known as a *dependent variable,* represents an observable property that varies. That is, it takes on different values, depending on the effect of the intervention (independent variable). You can improve your incomplete goals by assigning each of them a quantifiable (dependent) variable that could help measure progress toward the general goal. Consider the following as examples:

• Reduce personal risk of breast cancer among female employees, as shown by at least a 50% reduction in risk-factor prevalence for breast cancer in the female workforce.

• Improve employee productivity by reducing tardiness and absenteeism by at least 30%.

You can see that the second version of each goal includes a measurable factor. You can also see from the two examples that it is not possible to write measurable program goals in the absence of baseline data. You cannot, after all, tell whether an improvement has occurred if you do not know the original value. Thus, if no baseline exists for the area being measured, the first goal should be to establish one. For your goals, for example, you would first need to know the current risk-factor status for breast cancer of the female workforce. Second, data about absenteeism are needed, such as the average tardiness rate every 6 months and average absenteeism rate every 6 months for the last 3 years. In the case of certain program-evaluation goals, the baseline could be established in the first evaluation time frame.

3. Measurability

Now that you have qualified your goals, the next step is to be sure that you have the means to measure them. Continuing with our example, you must ask yourself what resources are available for measuring the risk of breast cancer, tardiness, and absenteeism. For example, will breast-cancer risk be assessed using personalized health-risk appraisals, self-reported feedback, clinical screening, or medical-claims data? Do departmental supervisors have the proper tools to easily monitor tardiness and absenteeism?

4. Sufficient Time Frame for Intervention

To know how to plan and evaluate, you must also include some kind of time frame in your goals. Consider these examples:

• Improve the health of female employees, as shown by at least a 50% reduction in the number of women classified as high risk for breast cancer within six months.

• Improve employee productivity by reducing tardiness and absenteeism by at least 30% in four months.

Now you have a defined target at which you can aim. Without a definite deadline, your measurement of progress is not very meaningful. Knowing how you're doing within a time frame can help you decide whether to change your tactics for greater effect or to set your sights higher than your original goal.

5. Realistic Achievability

Be wary of creating false expectations for yourself or others. Although the goals developed so far are compatible with stakeholders' personal goals and feature both measurability and a chronological definition, you must also be sure that they can be realistically achieved. You can form a good idea of what is realistic in your situation by studying similar programs and learning what their results have been. You can also study the factors that have affected their success rates. In doing so, look for significant differences between your situation and those of similar programs. For example, consider differences in educational level, age of participants, number and types of risk factors within the target population, and culture. Consulting an expert is also a useful strategy. After doing your homework for your two hypothetical goals, you discover that they are not actually realistic. Based on what you have learned, then, make the following revisions to your goals:

- Improve the health of female employees, as shown by a reduction of at least 25% in the number of women classified as high risk for breast cancer within one year.

- Improve employee productivity by reducing tardiness and absenteeism by at least 10% in six months.

Some evaluation experts recommend that once you establish objective goals, you lower your sights a few percentage points to compensate for differences you may have overlooked. If

How do you do this?

you have a general idea of what you'd like to accomplish in your WHP program, applying the five criteria to those general ideas will yield goals that are quantifiable, measurable, realistic, chronologically defined, and compatible with your stakeholders' interests. Such goals are indispensable for valid evaluation as well as for program development.

Measurable Objectives

Once program goals have been developed, it is time to establish measurable **objectives**. Objectives are stepping stones, or rungs in a ladder, that enable program planners to

achieve a particular goal. Evaluators should be particularly interested in this because properly written objectives facilitate and enhance the evaluation process and results.

When constructing objectives, strive to do the following:

- Establish short-term objectives for monitoring progress in the initial phase of the intervention. For example, "At the end of one month, at least 75% of all original participants will be actively involved in personalized risk-reduction programs."

- Establish long-range objectives to determine whether initial levels of progress have been sustained. For example, "At the end of six months, at least 50% of all participants achieving initial risk-reduction goals will have maintained or exceeded that level of success."

- Avoid the temptation to establish a long list of objectives, especially if the intervention to be evaluated is a short-term endeavor, if evaluations have not been conducted in the past, or if an evaluation will be used as a basis for a more formalized and thorough assessment. Too many objectives can add unnecessary procedures that increase the costs of conducting an evaluation.

- Include objectives that identify specific resources needed to achieve the goal. For example, "Develop a network of personal health coaches for employees identified with a chronic health condition."

- Specify time frames when appropriate. For example, "All participants will be screened on a quarterly basis at minimum and more frequently if they are classified as high risk."

An effective tool commonly used in worksite settings to organize and align objective-driven tasks into an operational framework is a **Gantt chart**. The Gantt chart focuses on the sequence of tasks necessary for completing specific objectives within a particular project or program. Each task on a Gantt chart is represented as a single horizontal bar on an X-Y chart. The horizontal axis (X-axis) is the time scale over which the program will occur. Therefore, the length of each task bar corresponds to the duration of the associated objective, or the time necessary for completion. Arrows are often used to signify a transitional time frame for completing each of the relevant objectives. The relationship usually shows dependency—one objective cannot begin until another is completed. The resources necessary for completion are also identified next to the chart. This is an excellent tool for quickly assessing the status of a project or program. The Gantt chart illustrated in figure 3.2 was created in a simple calendar-based platform. However,

a more elaborate version of the chart can be developed using Microsoft Project or similar software applications.

Any seasoned WHP professional will testify that properly written objectives are invaluable in planning the evaluation process. Suppose, for example, that the primary goal of a program to enhance prenatal health is to increase the percentage of healthy babies at least 20% within 12 months (sample objectives for a prenatal health program appear on this page). You can see that if all of the objectives are achieved, the goal with which

PROGRAM OBJECTIVES FOR PRENATAL-HEALTH ENHANCEMENT

- *Objective 1.* Identify the population at risk. In this case, the population is female employees and dependents who experienced a pregnancy complication in the past two years.

Evaluation planning decision. During weeks 1 through 4, contact the organization's health insurer or third-party claims administrator to obtain medical claims data on the number of all pregnancy-related complications.

- *Objective 2.* Conduct an analysis of pregnancy-related claims data from the past two years to identify specific types of pregnancy-related complications. Review specific complications with the International Classification of Diseases and diagnostic-related groups.

Evaluation planning decision. During weeks 5 and 6, develop a framework in which to record the number of each type of complication that has occurred in the past two years.

- *Objective 3.* Develop an expanded prenatal screening and health-education program with financial incentives.

Evaluation planning decision. During weeks 7 and 8, develop a framework to track participation in the screening and education program.

- *Objective 4.* Inform all women of the new program and incentives using bulletin boards, paycheck stuffers, e-mails, and newsletters.

Evaluation planning decision. During weeks 9 and 10, prepare a format to list distribution activities.

- *Objective 5.* Provide orientation sessions, including a comprehensive health screening to identify women at risk of pregnancy complications. Construct a format for collecting baseline data.

Evaluation planning decision. During weeks 11 and 12, establish a two-group, quasi-experimental evaluation design.

- *Objective 6.* Initiate on-site programs and additional referrals to personal physicians for selected women, if necessary.

Evaluation planning decision. During weeks 13 through 18, record the names and numbers of on-site participants and off-site referrals.

- *Objective 7.* Monitor health status of at-risk women at appropriate (risk-based) intervals. Provide customized interventions for each woman.

Evaluation planning decision. During weeks 24 through 30, compare baseline health-status levels to 6-month and 12-month levels. Analyze changes between intervals to determine the intervention's effect.

Objective/task	Resources/venues	Personnel	Duration	September	October
Conduct focus group interviews with employees	Environmentally suitable area for interviews	Mary Ann Roberto	21 days	⟶	
Review interview results and prioritize	Tool for tabulating input from employees	Mary Ann Roberto	7 days	⟶	
Determine programs to meet employees' top 3 needs and interests	WHP staff meeting in suitable venue	WHP staff	14 days		⟶

Figure 3.2   An abbreviated Gantt chart.

they are associated will have been reached. Note that some of these objectives are not directly related to evaluation (e.g., "Initiate on-site programs and additional referrals"), yet the programs required by the objectives (i.e., the effectiveness of the on-site and additional referral program) will need to be evaluated. You should plan for those evaluations at this stage. The program objectives tell you what data you will need to collect, how often you will need to analyze it, and what instruments you will need to use. Each objective is followed by appropriate evaluation planning decisions you may make based on that objective.

Unfortunately, some WHP program planners make the mistake of designing an evaluation after the health promotion program is underway, rather than during the planning phase. This often leads to rushed evaluation procedures that yield unreliable results. Because crafting the evaluation is so important, chapter 8 is devoted to that subject. Carefully consider the information you find there. Proper evaluation planning at this stage is essential for the program to achieve its potential.

ANTICIPATING REALISTIC RESULTS

Assuming appropriate goals have been set in the first place, the best way to evaluate a program's success is to compare the results with its goals. Of course, results cannot be judged until after the program has been completed. Because evaluation procedures need to be set up early, we need ways to predict the possible results of a program. Two good ways to gauge the potential effect of health promotion programs are to do the following:

1. Talk to other WHP professionals who have implemented similar programs.
2. Review the literature to see what types of programs have had a positive influence.

For instance, reviewing the data in table 3.1 on specific outcome variables should give you a reasonable idea of which programs may generate short-term, intermediate, or long-term impacts. Therefore, you can establish realistic standards to evaluate your respective programs.

Variables directly related to employee health status and behavior are called *employee health indicators*. Variables closely related to an organization's health and productivity are called *organizational health indicators*. A sampling of each category can be seen in the sidebar on page 50.

Some indicators may be defined and measured according to a specific company's operations, philosophy, and record-keeping practices. Take absenteeism, for example. Some companies classify absences as either unscheduled or scheduled. Unscheduled absences are those that employees may be able to influence through their own actions. In contrast, scheduled absences are those which employees have previously arranged

Table 3.1 Variables Directly Related to Employee Health Status and Behavior

Program	Variables		
	Short term (<1 yr.)	Intermediate (1-2 yrs.)	Long term (>2 yrs.)
Back health	Absenteeism Back injury trend Presenteeism	Health care usage Short-term disability	Health care costs
Employee assistance program (EAP) and quality of work life (QWL)	Absenteeism Health status Mental health Work satisfaction	Accidents Health care usage Productivity	Health care costs
Injury prevention	Accident and injuries Productivity Short-term disability Work satisfaction	Health care costs Workers' compensation costs	
Medical self-care	Self-care behavior Health care usage	Health care costs	
Nutrition	Dietary improvement	Health status Productivity	
Physical fitness	Absenteeism Health status Health insurance* Productivity	Health care usage Health care costs	
Prenatal health	Absenteeism Health care usage Health care costs Health status Productivity		
Smoking control	Health status Health insurance* Productivity Property insurance*	Absenteeism Health care usage	Health care costs
Stress management	Coping skills Health care usage Health status Productivity	Health care costs	

*Cost borne by employers

HEALTH INDICATORS

Employee health indicators	Organizational health indicators
Blood pressure	Absenteeism
Body fat percentage	Accidents and injuries
Body mass index	Health care utilization
Body weight	Health care costs
Cholesterol level	Long-term disability
Coping skills	Presenteeism
Eating habits	Productivity
Emotional health	Short-term disability
Flexibility	Turnover
Safety belt usage	Workers' compensation costs
Substance use	
Tobacco use	

or can apply to their company-approved sick days. Here are some typical examples:

Controllable Absences (Unscheduled)

- Falsely calling in sick
- Faking an injury
- Poor health or illness
- Work injury due to negligence

Uncontrollable Absences (Usually Scheduled)

- Caring for a sick child or dependent
- Inclement weather
- Jury duty or military duty
- Maternity or paternity leave
- Mechanical or machinery breakdowns

Because WHP programs have very little, if any, effect on factors that prompt scheduled absences, program goals and evaluation procedures should focus on factors that prompt unscheduled absences. For example, a tangible goal relevant to occupational injury would be to reduce the number of on-the-job injuries by 10% within one year. Evaluating the degree to which this goal is achieved would require that the number of past, present, and one-year injuries be tracked. See chapter 8 for a complete discussion of evaluation procedures.

What Would You Do?

Senior management recently gave all midlevel managers, including your boss, a mandate to demonstrate that every employee service program is closely aligned with the organization's vision and mission statements. Its current vision is to become the world's leading supplier of computers to business and industry. Its mission is to provide a culture for workers to be the most productive and cost-efficient in the industry. Although the company's mission is void of any direct reference to employee health, your boss asks you to prepare a WHP vision and mission focused on productivity. Yet, you feel a person's health and productivity are strongly related. Thus, you would like to incorporate something about health and productivity in either your vision or mission statement. You realize the need to diplomatically convince your boss to see your side. How would you consider sharing any published research as evidence to justify your position? Would you research what other companies in the industry have done in this area? Describe your plan of action.

CHAPTER 3 WRAP-UP

Key Points

- An organization's vision and mission statements should be considered when developing a WHP program.
- Clearly defined goals and objectives are essential for effective WHP programming and evaluation.
- WHP goals should be specific, measurable, attainable, realistic, and time specific.
- Objectives should always be measurable and directly related to major tasks.
- Evaluation methods should be considered when planning program goals.

Glossary

Gantt chart—A visual platform used to assign, track, and monitor various objective-based tasks required to complete a project.

goal—An observable and measurable end result with one or more objectives to be achieved within a specified time frame.

mission statement—A statement indicating an organization's philosophy, purpose, and goals for achieving its vision.

objective—Actions that must be successfully completed in order to achieve a particular goal.

vision statement—A short, succinct, and inspiring statement of what an organization aspires to become.

Bibliography

Corporate Health Promotion. 2009. "Worksite health promotion: Formulate a detailed action plan." Accessed October 28, 2010. http://corporate-health-promotion.com.

CPI-HR. "Population health management: Enhancing people and profit." Accessed October 28, 2010. http://cpihr.com/documents/PopulationHealth Management.pdf.

HR Management. 2010. "Corporate wellness." Accessed October 28. www.hrmreport.com/article/Corporate-Wellness.

Justice, G. 2010. "What makes a corporate wellness program effective?" *Corporate Wellness Magazine*, June 11.

Kotelnikov, V. 2009. "Corporate vision: Mission, goals, and strategies." Accessed October 30 2010. www.1000ventures.com/business_guide/crosscuttings/vision_mission_strategy.html.

Top Achievement. 2009. "Creating S.M.A.R.T. Goals." Accessed November 4. http://topachievement.com/smart.html.

Writing Help Central. 2009. "How to write a vision statement." Accessed October 30. http://writinghelp-central.com/corporate-vision-statement.html.

Looking Ahead

Now that goal-setting procedures are underway, it's time to establish healthy lifestyle programs based on employees' needs and interests. Chapter 4 presents a strategic plan for developing employee-centered programs that can be tied to tangible and measurable goals.

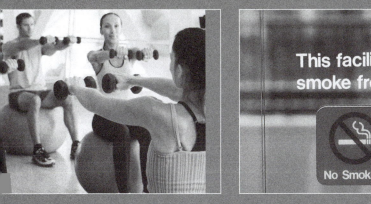
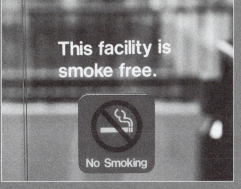
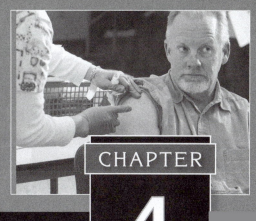

Establishing Healthy Lifestyle Programs

LEARNING OBJECTIVES

After reading this chapter, you will be able to do the following:

✔ Cite major factors to consider in selecting specific types of WHP programs.

✔ Describe why the traditional programming approach, focused primarily on risk factor reduction, is gradually being replaced with a more holistic approach that is centered on lifestyle.

✔ Describe several advantages of creating programs with integrated health themes.

✔ List several ways to create healthier eating options at a worksite.

✔ Illustrate a step-by-step process for establishing a worksite no-smoking policy.

• ✔ Describe how strong medical self-care and consumerism skills among employees are essential for achieving organizational goals of health care cost containment.

Although numerous reasons for providing WHP programs are listed in chapter 1, several federal health promotion provisions that were signed into law in 2010 are particularly noteworthy. These provisions, which may have exciting potential for this industry in the coming years, include the following:

• Development of a national health promotion plan

• Enhancement of health promotion research

• Technical assistance to enhance evaluation of WHP programs

• Grants to pay a portion of the cost of comprehensive WHP programs for small employers

• Regular periodic surveys of prevalence and components of WHP programs

• In 2014, permission for employers, with some safeguards, to offer employees health insurance premium discounts of up to 30% (up from 20%) based on positive lifestyle practices or participation in health promotion programs (the DHHS will study the benefits of increasing this amount to 50%)

PROGRAMMING PHILOSOPHY

Each worksite has unique needs that require specific WHP programs and resources. This portion of chapter 4 presents a programming philosophy as well as a basic overview of various programs, such as physical fitness, back health, weight control, prenatal health, smoking cessation, HIV and AIDS education, medical self-care, disease management, and financial wellness. By omitting other programs from this discussion, the author is not suggesting that programs highlighted on the following pages are necessarily more important than programs not included. The program overviews included in this chapter are provided solely to highlight different administrative, cultural, environmental, political, financial, and ethical issues under consideration by decision makers. The author encourages WHP personnel to offer programs that best meet the specific needs and interests of their respective employee populations. Please note that despite the absence of program overviews based on stress management and spirituality, employ-ers may wish to integrate these themes into their major programs (see table 4.1).

Many successful WHP programs exist throughout the world. Although some industry insiders contend that the United States has more of a culture for research and documentation, WHP programs in other countries are equally, if not more, successful because of their supportive worksite cultures. Yet, the means to achieve such outcomes can vary from continent to continent. For example, WHP programs in the United States have traditionally focused on behavioral change and risk-factor identification. Critics of this approach contend that this particular strategy doesn't breed sufficient opportunities for building a supportive organizational culture and environment. Unfortunately, these are often sacrificed for short-term results.

In contrast, companies in Europe, Japan, and Scandinavia are well known for building supportive environments at the worksite and community level that provide ongoing incentives and opportunities for enhancing personal health. Consider, for example, the famous North Karelia case study in which a community-wide health promotion initiative

Table 4.1 Examples of Integrated WHP Programs

Integrated themes	Physical fitness	Weight management	Smoking cessation	Holistic health
Nutrition	Eating for energy	Eating to lose excess fat	Avoiding foods that trigger smoking	Eating right to enhance physical, mental, and spiritual health
Exercise	Moderate or vigorous	Moderate or vigorous	Moderate or vigorous	Moderate or vigorous
Stress management	Proper breathing	Stress tips to avoid junk foods	Tips to avoid smoking triggers	Tips to minimize daily stress
Confidence building (mental health)	Setting realistic goals and overcoming barriers	Setting realistic goals and overcoming barriers	Setting realistic goals and overcoming barriers	Increased ability to have an active lifestyle
Consumer health	Purchasing appropriate clothes/shoes	Choosing a diet for long-term weight control	Selecting effective and safe aids to stop smoking	The power of self-directed consumerism in your life
Spirituality	Achieving a mind-body connection	How the mind influences the waistline	How a smoke-free lifestyle creates a stronger mind-body connection	How a healthy lifestyle creates a stronger mind-body connection
Financial wellness	How regular physical activity results in less demand for health care	How a lower body weight results in less demand for health care	How a smoke-free lifestyle saves more than $1,000 per year (not including health care savings)	How a healthy lifestyle results in less demand for health care

involving schools, worksites, and community groups resulted in a significant decrease in heart disease throughout the Finnish population. This endeavor is only one of many examples that demonstrate the successful effect of a strong, environmentally based health promotion intervention on status and behavior related to personal health.

Traditionally, WHP efforts have focused primarily on controlling or eliminating risk factors known to predispose people to specific diseases. In doing so, worksite professionals identify unhealthy habits and try to motivate employees to replace them with healthier ones. Employees are encouraged to join programs that reward them for changing their behaviors. They are told they will subsequently decrease their chances of contracting certain diseases and dying prematurely if they do so. The science behind this approach to health promotion reflects the biomedical model of health and disease with roots in the scientific revolution of the 17th century. This myopic view of WHP has been particularly prevalent in the United States, where a disproportionately high level of personnel and monetary resources have been devoted to managing chronic diseases, such as diabetes, cardiorespiratory disease, congestive heart failure, chronic obstructive pulmonary disease, cancer, and asthma. By and large, this **disease management** (DM) approach has typically been used to concentrate on employees at high risk for a particular disease. Health plans then monitor and control the patient's care to assure appropriate and cost-effective treatment (Rager et al. 2008).

Although this approach has been somewhat effective in reducing health care in the short term, it has done little to provide sustained cost control at the organizational level. Moreover, it does not address the very critical need for disease management for persons with comorbidities (multiple conditions). While chronic illness and disease is still the main emphasis of DM programs, more of these programs are also addressing a wider array of conditions, including common health problems that have been previously excluded from DM efforts (e.g.,

migraines, allergies, prenatal problems, autism, musculoskeletal conditions, sleep disorders, depression, and anxiety).

In companies of all sizes, an increasing number of employee DM programs are comprehensive, multicomponent systems that address an expanding array of chronic diseases, encompass other conditions (i.e., condition management), and take a proactive approach to the prevention of health problems (i.e., health promotion). This integrated model of health management promotes and supports collaboration and intercommunication among all major on-site and off-site stakeholders (refer to figure 1.5 in chapter 1). It can be successfully developed when decision makers share a global view of employee health issues and, concurrently, realize that a typical work force consists of adults representing a broad continuum of risk-level prevalence and severity. In cultivating this contemporary view of employee health, WHP practitioners can eventually develop an approach to **comprehensive (*global*) health management** that, when properly implemented, can successfully meet the needs of their respective employee populations (Rager et al. 2008). Essentially, this approach consists of an integrated system of customized programs, policies, incentives, activities, and health care services provided to all workers, not just those employees with high-risk profiles or chronic conditions.

In addition to the growing shift toward integrated WHP programming, we're also seeing a transformation from traditional programs based on risk factors to a more holistic approach that addresses body, mind, and spirit. One of the leading authorities in this movement is Jon Robison, PhD, who has written extensively on the evolving field of holistic health. Dr. Robison contends that in moving from a biomedical model to a more holistic model, the focus of health promotion should be on the relationship among the spiritual, biological, psychological, and social dimensions of the human experience that are critical to a true understanding of health and healing. In their book, *The Spirit and Science of Holistic Health*, Dr.

Robison and coauthor Karen Carrier provide a definitive and thought-provoking look at holistic health promotion and offer compelling reasons for reinventing the field in the modern age.

Shifting the focus of traditional health promotion to a more holistic approach essentially means more emphasis can be placed on the supportive factors for overall health and happiness, not just risk factors for illness and disease. These supportive factors relate to various biological, psychological, emotional, spiritual, financial, intellectual, and environmental attributes.

Take the dimension of spirituality, for instance. By recognizing the significant role that spirituality plays in a person's health, various WHP programs have incorporated this dimension of wellness into their respective programs. For example, the United States Postal Service was one of the first organizations to do so in the early 1990s by offering a lecture series, "Roadblocks on the Human Path," including creative anger management, prolonged grieving, and the art of forgiveness. WHP staff members at Mercy Hospital in Mason, Iowa, offer numerous seminars in stress and spirituality, including "spiritual appetizer" breaks (visualization, meditation, and back-to-nature programs). And Conoco Oil in Houston, Texas, continues to offer a balance of mind-body-spirit programs as well as various theme days, including random acts of kindness, attitude of gratitude, Earth Day, patience, and serenity (based on the Serenity Prayer).

In summary, in order to make sound programming decisions, take time to understand the needs and interests of your population, assess your resources, and determine what types of incentives, activities, and ongoing programs will yield the highest dividends for managing employee and organizational health. Financial resources are also a major factor to consider in programming decisions. Chapter 5 provides some insights on how to make the most of your financial resources.

INTEGRATION VERSUS SEPARATION

Sooner or later, most WHP practitioners wonder how they should provide programs to reach those in greatest need. Depending on their particular circumstances, some practitioners choose to offer single-topic programs at the same time or in a staggered fashion. Other practitioners prefer to integrate various health themes into a single program. In these days of tighter budgets, increased productivity demands, and heightened expectations to do more with less, more WHP practitioners are moving toward more **integrated programming.** They reason that a single multifaceted program is not only more cost effective than a one-dimensional (single-topic) program, but also more likely to generate greater long-term results if participants can adopt lifestyles around a true holistic approach to body, mind, and spirit. Table 4.1 illustrates several examples of how various themes can be integrated into selected programs.

EXERCISE AND PHYSICAL FITNESS

One of the most pressing challenges WHP practitioners face today is how to motivate employees to exercise on a regular basis. The Surgeon General's Report on Physical Activity and Health advises at least 30 minutes a day of moderate exercise (e.g., walking at 3 to 4 miles, or 5 to 6 km, per hour). Currently, less than 1 of every 3 American adults meets this standard. In 2005, the Department of Health and Human Services (DHHS) and the United States Department of Agriculture (USDA) jointly released the Dietary Guidelines for Americans 2005, which recommends at least 30 minutes of physical activity of moderate intensity (not counting usual activity) on most days of the week. However, it states that for most people, greater health benefits can be obtained either by engaging in activity that is more intense or by exercising longer. The recommendations encourage not only cardiorespiratory conditioning, but also doing stretches for flexibility and resistance exercises or calisthenics for muscle strength and endurance. To prevent weight gain, DHHS recommends 60 minutes of moderate to vigorous exercise on most days of the week. To drop pounds, moderate-intensity exercise, lasting 60 to 90 minutes per day, is advised.

For the first time since exercise patterns have been monitored, the percentage of inactive adults exceeds the percentage of active adults. This startling fact extends to the workplace. In hopes of encouraging employees to exercise, many employers provide *physical fitness programs (PFP)*. They are motivated, in part, by the following:

- Growing evidence showing that regular exercise can reduce the risk of heart disease, cancer, stroke (the leading causes of death), obesity, and many other conditions.
- Increasing evidence of a direct relationship between physical activity and on-the-job productivity.
- Growing financial stress due to paying billions of dollars to treat employees' illnesses and disorders that could have been prevented with a physically active lifestyle.
- Growing awareness that millions of working baby boomers expect them to provide opportunities for physical activity at the worksite.
- Greater publicity on the profound financial effect of physical inactivity on their health care and productivity costs.

If you are interested in calculating the economic cost of physical inactivity in your community or organization, check out the cost calculator at the following website: www.ecu.edu/picostcalc.

More WHP programs are shifting their focus from PFPs based on fitness centers to a holistic, wellness-oriented approach that is centered on lifestyle. By doing so, worksites are no longer perpetuating their historical emphasis on physical health, cardiorespiratory conditioning, and strength training. This approach may involve a resource or support center that encourages employees to explore a broad range of life issues (relationships, financial wellness, rest and play, aging, mind-body healing, spirituality, and so on). Moreover, a holistic approach to exercise programming creates experiences to explore the connection among mind, body, and spirit through movement, rather than exercising solely to reshape the body, lose weight, or compensate for overeating.

Although some of today's more publicized PFPs operate in modern, state-of-the-art, multimillion-dollar fitness centers, most worksites do not have the need, much less the financial resources, for constructing such facilities. Many of these sites instead provide small, on-site fitness centers, establish walking trails around the perimeter of the worksite, or subsidize employee memberships to local health clubs.

Exercise Precautions

Of course, when employers sponsor on-site or off-site PFPs for employees, they assume some level of risk. Thus, it's important for employers to have appropriate risk-management protocols and policies in place before sponsored programs or activities begin. For example, one key risk-management issue relates to exercise precautions that should be taken to ensure that participating employees are fit enough to safely engage in any exercise program.

Although heart attacks during exercise are rare, most health clubs and worksite fitness centers take certain precautionary measures to handle such possibilities. The most common safeguards involve staff members trained in and capable of administering cardiopulmonary resuscitation (CPR), as well as an in-house communication system that can immediately notify emergency medical personnel in case of a life-threatening event.

Automated external defibrillators (AED) are also generating much attention as more states consider passing laws for exercise facilities. Although the bulk of the early mandates were directed primarily at commercial health clubs, some industry insiders feel that WHP programs will follow. And with a noted study published in the *Journal of the American Medical Association* showing that CPR is often performed inadequately by even trained medical professionals, pressure to make AEDs more readily available will continue to mount in all exercise facilities (Balady et al. 2002).

Adding to the pressure being felt by some legislators—and eventually commercial and corporate fitness directors—is increasing activity on the judicial side of the equation. So far, several states have passed legislation mandating the placement of AEDs in health clubs. The American Heart Association (AHA) strongly advocates the placement of AEDs in targeted public areas, such as sports arenas, gated communities, office complexes, doctor's offices, and shopping malls. When AEDs are placed in the community or a business or facility, the AHA strongly encourages that they be part of a defibrillation program. Furthermore, the International Health, Racquet and Sports-club Association (IHRSA) supports AED legislation that contains necessary liability protections (use and nonuse) for health-club owners and their employees, reasonable staffing requirements for staffed and unstaffed clubs, and adequate compliance time.

Equipment and Facility Considerations

Designing and equipping a healthy worksite requires considerable planning and coordination between the company and outside vendors. When considering current options for exercise equipment, employers need to look closely at their budgets and the marketplace, review product literature, and consult with other worksite personnel on best practices. Some early decisions about facility planning and equipment purchasing could make or break your program, so research as much as you can before making a choice.

Purchasing equipment may take the most planning and budgeting expertise. Equipment costs vary widely, depending on brand name, durability, computerized features, and shipping expense. In general, stationary bikes cost between $300 and $3,000. Multistation weight systems go for $1,000 and up. Climbing machines range from $1,000 to $4,000, rowers from $300 to $1,500, and elliptical and treadmill units from $400 to $5,000. With such a huge range in quality and price of equipment, it is foolish not to shop around. Here are some tips for purchasing equipment:

- Purchase equipment designed for institutional use.
- To cut shipping costs, buy from a local firm or manufacturer whenever possible.
- To save up to 50% of the retail price, buy carpet directly from the manufacturing mill.
- Ask distributors if they provide free equipment instruction.
- Closely compare maintenance requirements of mechanized equipment and computerized equipment.
- Check a firm's stock inventory, credit plan, warranty, service contract, and whether or not the manufacturer has product liability insurance.
- Ask vendors for the names of other companies who have purchased their equipment, and solicit opinions before buying.
- Invite sales representatives to visit your worksite to discuss your particular needs.

Additional information on maintaining exercise equipment is provided in appendix D.

NUTRITION

It seems like every WHP program includes some type of nutrition information or activity. These interventions range from a simple visual display at the annual health fair and monthly lunch-and-learns to a year-round comprehensive program. Whatever type of nutrition intervention is adopted at a particular worksite, its odds of being successful are greatly enhanced when the worksite culture is supportive. For example, Scherer Brothers Lumber Company, a Minnesota-based company of 150 employees, made its worksite healthier by removing candy machines and adding fruit dispensers, replacing caffeinated coffee with decaf, and offering healthy snacks free of charge (Workplace Wellness Programs 2009). The changes were welcomed by most workers, as evidenced by increased sales receipts and healthy snack consumption.

By strategically using the worksite environment as a strong motivating force, WHP personnel can promote healthier eating and weight control for employees in several ways:

- Distributing and publicizing educational materials in the cafeteria and near canteens, vending machines, or break areas.

- Offering heart-healthy entrées, a salad bar, and other healthy options.

- Affixing "healthy choice" labels to foods that are low in fat, calories, sugar, salt, and cholesterol.

- Offering a weekly menu of nutritious bag lunches that employees can prepare.

- Offering discounted prices on heart-healthy entrées in the cafeteria.

- Gradually easing out the junk food from vending machines and replacing it with natural fruits, unsweetened fruit juices, low-fat dairy products, and other nutritious foods. (Do not get rid of all junk food at once.)

- Placing weight scales and body mass index (BMI) charts in company restrooms for employees to regularly monitor their weight.

- Providing free body-fat measurements at quarterly intervals. (Skin-fold calipers are relatively inexpensive and relatively accurate when administered by trained personnel.)

- Publicizing the positive effect that a nutrition program can have on employees' health status. (For example, at L.L. Bean Company, 70% of the 77 heart club members lowered their cholesterol levels by 14% and their risk of heart disease by 23% within eight months of participation in on-site nutrition education.)

As with any WHP program, nutrition programs and activities should be designed around employee interests, work schedules, and available distribution venues. Many worksites continue to offer different versions of weekly or monthly lunch-and-learn sessions, in either face-to-face lunchroom (classroom) settings or in one or more electronic venues (e.g., closed circuit television or in-house webinar). In addition, employers may wish to consider online nutrition education for their employees. Some of these programs can be purchased for a fee by commercial providers, whereas others are offered at little or no fee by nonprofit organizations. Thus, it's important to research all of your options before you decide which, if any, outside resources to use in your nutrition-education programs.

A good resource to use in nutrition education is the dietary guidelines for Americans (http://health.gov/dietaryguidelines), which provides science-based advice to promote health and to reduce risk for chronic diseases through diet and physical activity. The dietary guidelines are published jointly every five years by the DHHS and the USDA. Timing is an important consideration to promote healthy eating. For example, lunchtime is a good opportunity to offer lunch-and-learn seminars on such issues as cholesterol reduction, hypertension control, and diabetes control. March is national nutrition month, an excellent time to introduce new programs for shaping up for the summer. Several resources for consideration can be found on the website of the American Dietetic Association (www.eatright.org).

WEIGHT CONTROL

Worldwide, over one-half of all workers are overweight or obese and about two-thirds of all workers eat unhealthy diets. A high-fat diet is a major risk factor for problems associated with many health care claims (circulatory, digestive, cancer, and metabolic). Obese employees have significantly longer hospital stays and higher health care costs than their coworkers. Given these facts, it's little wonder that weight control is a prime target area for WHP.

Developing countries are adopting lifestyles that have existed in the United States and western Europe for decades, such as working at sedentary jobs, driving cars, eating poorly, and generally being physically inactive. These habits are leading to a global epidemic of obesity. An interesting case study involves the Arabian Gulf countries, which, overall, don't have major aging problems because they have fairly young populations. Yet, their newly acquired lifestyles have dramatically changed their patterns of illness and disease. For example, rates of obesity and diabetes in the United Arab Emirates (UAE), Saudi Arabia, Kuwait, and Qatar are increasing dramatically. In particular, the prevalence of diabetes in the UAE is estimated to be at least 15%, about twice the rate in North America and Europe. Although these wealthy nations are building high-tech medical clinics, no amount of money or technology in the world can reverse the debilitating effects of these lifestyle trends. Essentially, only lifestyle changes can improve this situation.

Consider your options and goals before purchasing any program resources. For example, a multifaceted program of screenings, exercise sessions, competitions, and follow-up counseling sessions may be a cost-effective approach to help high-risk employees with multiple health problems. Weight-control programs may consist of small-group sessions, large-group lectures, self-management tips, or weight-loss competitions. Yet, in reality, most weight-control programs produce little, if any, long-term success because they don't help participants regain a normal relationship with food by addressing key factors, such as chronic dieting, body dissatisfaction, and cultural weight prejudice.

Many WHP personnel choose to integrate nutrition education and weight-control information into a single program. If you prefer this approach, it's good to create a fairly comprehensive program that teaches employees such key tenets as (a) the role of good nutrition in achieving weight control, (b) how to plan nutritional meals, and (c) how to be a savvy consumer. To achieve all of these goals, Apple Computer's broad-

EFFECT OF WORKSITE PROGRAMS ON WEIGHT CONTROL

What effect does a weight-control program have on employees? Here are some examples:

- *Campbell Soup Company.* 233 employee participants in Campbell's "STRIP" (spare-tire reduction incentive program) lost a total of 3,078 pounds (1,396 kg) within three months.

- *Dow Chemical.* The company's "Walk-A-Weigh" program, which was offered in 23 countries and in nine languages, had more than 5,000 participants. It featured a nautical theme on the importance of physical activity and weight management. More than two-thirds of the participants reporting their results cumulatively lost 9,460 pounds (4,291 kg).

- *DuPont.* DuPont's weight-loss program produced an average loss of 5.5 pounds (2.5 kg) per participant. Furthermore, 85% of them maintained the loss for at least three months.

- *Lockheed Martin Missiles and Space Company.* Employees lost a total of 14,378 pounds (6,522 kg) in the company's three-month "Take It Off" program, at a cost of only $.94 per pound.

- *Businesses in Lycoming County, Pennsylvania.* Three independent weight-loss competitions between various industries and banks produced an average weight loss of 12 pounds (5.5 kg) per participant.

based approach is made up of the following components:

- *Week 1.* Participants' body-fat composition is assessed using skin-fold calipers. The goals of the course are outlined and assistance provided to employees as they set realistic, specific goals.

- *Week 2.* A nutrition overview is provided. Particular emphasis is placed on the differences between protein, fat, and carbohydrate, followed by an overview of essential vitamins and minerals for good health.

- *Week 3.* A discussion focuses on the importance of exercise for good health, illustrating the difference between aerobic exercise and anaerobic exercise.

- *Week 4.* Menu planning is this week's primary focus, with a particular emphasis on how to plan healthy, low-fat meals and how to modify favorite recipes to reduce fat, sodium, and cholesterol. A preliminary overview of how to read nutrition labels is also provided.

- *Week 5.* Tips are presented on how to eat healthy food in different settings, such as restaurants, meetings, and parties.

- *Week 6.* All participants bring in a healthy dish and enjoy it at lunch while the group watches a video by a registered dietician. The video provides a virtual tour of a supermarket, highlighting healthy food options in each aisle.

BACK HEALTH

Back injury is one of the most common injuries at the worksite and is the primary cause of absenteeism in many companies. Nearly 2% of the U.S. workforce files a claim for a lower-back injury each year. Most are classified as a minor strain of lower-back muscles. These claims cost employers about $600 per injury in medical care and lost productivity. However, more serious back injuries, such as bulging discs, intervertebral disc disorder, or fractured vertebrae, can cost around $30,000 per case. These types of back and spinal injuries constitute up to 50% of all

workers' compensation claims and, in some cases, can lead to long-term disability.

By establishing on-site programs, many companies are reducing the incidence and cost of lower-back injuries. Research indicates that the most successful lower-back programs include these three major components:

- Injury prevention and health promotion
- Intervention and treatment for injured employees
- Rehabilitation and a return-to-work protocol

Treatment and rehabilitation of injured workers is usually provided by occupational health nurses, physical therapists, massage therapists, and other allied health care personnel, but WHP professionals often play a major role in the promotion of back health.

Perhaps the most effective incentive for promoting healthy backs at the worksite is constant support from management, supervisors, and coworkers. Here are some ideas for promoting healthy back practices at your worksite:

- *Awareness and knowledge.* Make employees aware of the risk of back and spinal injuries by providing company- and industry-specific data, teaching the structure and function of the spine and lower back, and providing instructions on how to identify high-risk tasks by showing slides or videotapes of employees performing work functions. You can reinforce important learning and behavioral concepts with poster campaigns, paycheck stuffers, monthly safety meetings, and other highly visible methods. Display posters of easy stretching routines at key locations. Use the company newsletter and e-mail communications to illustrate spinal anatomy and tips on proper body mechanics for lifting, pulling, and pushing.

- *Practice.* A trained leader teaches employees proper body mechanics for lifting, bending, carrying, pushing, pulling, and reaching. Employees practice prework stretching and strengthening routines on a

IMPACT OF WORKSITE PROGRAMS ON PREVENTING BACK INJURIES

What effect can on-site back-injury prevention programs have on employees? Here are a few examples of the payoff in some organizations:

- *Biltrite Corporation (Chelsea, MA).* Within one year of operation, the company's back program produced a 90% drop ($150,000 savings) in workers' compensation claims.

- *Capital Wire and Cable (Plano, TX).* The company saved more than $83,000 within 20 months of instituting a new program for lower-back health.

- *Coca-Cola Bottling Company (Atlanta, GA).* Plant employees perform a 10-minute routine before work to prepare for the rigors of loading and unloading beverage trucks. Accidents have dropped 83%, producing an annual savings of more than $250 per employee in lost time and replacement costs.

- *Lockheed Martin Space Systems Company (Sunnyvale, CA).* The company reported a drop of 67.5% in costs due to lower-back injuries within 14 months of implementing its back-health program.

- *Pepsi Bottling Group (Riviera Beach, FL, and Pompano Beach, FL).* The company reported that lower-back injuries dropped from 146 to 13 within two years of a mandatory prework stretching program.

- *Swedish factory workers.* A weekly 30-minute session of group calisthenics combined with a 10-minute talk on lower-back health resulted in fewer lower-back injuries as well as a decline in sick-leave absences.

daily basis with their immediate supervisor and coworkers.

- *Implementation and follow-up.* All employees are trained to lead their coworkers in daily prework stretching and strengthening exercises. Offering these sessions on company time is a good way to show employees that their employer is investing in their health while building a cohesive, team-oriented workforce. Consider using extrinsic incentives to encourage employee participation in prework stretching and warm-up routines. For example, injury-free employees at regular intervals (3, 6, 9, and 12 months) can enter a sweepstakes to win one or more prizes, presented at designated company functions or at the end of the year, or to receive semiannual financial bonuses from any savings due to back-injury prevention.

PRENATAL HEALTH

The average total cost for prenatal care services and an inpatient hospital delivery without complications is approximately $8,000 in the United States. However, a pregnancy with complications can cost more than $100,000 (Machlin 2007).

Statistics show the percentage of unhealthy infants born in most countries is an international challenge, even in the largest industrialized nations. For example, China's infant death rate is more than 20 per 1,000 live births. The rate for the United States' rate is 6.2, while the rates in Canada (5.0), Australia (4.7), Scandinavian countries (less than 3), and Japan (2.8) reflect some of the lowest in the world (Central Intelligence Agency 2010). In the United States, 1 of every 8 babies is born prematurely and 1 of every 14 babies is born with a low birth weight. Medical care costs for premature infants are more than $5 billion a year. The hospital bill for one premature infant can be as high as $500,000, whereas a baby born with breathing or feeding problems may require more than $60,000 of health care services in a single month (Machlin 2007). Given these numbers and their effect on increasing insurance premiums, it only makes sense that employers develop aggressive programs on prenatal care as a part of their WHP efforts.

A typical program for prenatal-health education consists of the following components:

- *Prepregnancy counseling.* Employees interested in learning about their genetic predisposition are encouraged to meet with an occupational health nurse to discuss various influential issues, such as age, family history, pregnancy history, lifestyle, and health status.

- *Identification.* Employees who believe they are pregnant are asked to visit the company's on-site nurse or personal physician for a pregnancy (urine) test.

- *Referral.* If an employee is pregnant, she is informed of the company's health care (maternity) benefits and referred to her personal physician. To qualify for maternity health care benefits, pregnant employees and dependents are required to attend on-site prenatal-health classes.

- *Education.* In conjunction with regular visits to their personal physicians (or on-site physician), pregnant women participate in the company's program for prenatal-health education, which is taught by a certified professional. One-hour programs are offered every two weeks on company time, and they typically include two phases:

  - *Information phase.* This includes prenatal care, nutrition, substance use and abuse, discomforts of pregnancy, fetal development, signs and symptoms of labor and birthing, and recommendations of postnatal home care.

  - *Clinical phase.* This includes one-on-one screenings and discussions to assess each woman's blood pressure, weight, water-retention level, and urine-test results.

In between classes, informal sessions are held for women who are in the latter stages of pregnancy or who are considered high risk because of excess weight, hypertension, or a history of difficult childbirth.

The Colorado Department of Health Affairs estimates that at least $9 could be saved for every dollar spent on prenatal care. If long-term costs were included, the savings could be as much as $11 for every dollar spent. Numerous companies, including CIGNA, First Chicago Bank, and Oster-Sunbeam, have reported impressive cost savings from prenatal-health education. For example, CIGNA's "Healthy Babies" prenatal program generated an average savings of $5,000 per birth by providing high-risk expectant mothers with educational materials and rewarding early and regular prenatal care. In fact, 80% of program participants had normal births without complications, while only 50% of nonparticipants had standard births.

A high participation level of pregnant employees (especially those at risk) is vital to the overall success of any program for prenatal-health education. Although many companies have mandatory participation policies (to qualify for 100% of employer-paid maternity benefits), employees tend to take a more genuine interest in prenatal programs that include personal incentives. Some of the more successful incentives include the following:

- Offering programs on company time
- Waiving the first year's health insurance deductible and copayment if the

FINANCIAL EFFECT OF PREGNANCY COMPLICATIONS

To better understand the financial impact of pregnancy-related complications on some employers, consider what happened at two Oster-Sunbeam (O-S) worksites. In one year, four severely ill babies were born to employees at one O-S worksite. Medical costs for the four infants totaled $500,000 (PHC4 2003). The next year, at the other O-S worksite, three more babies were born prematurely. One infant's lengthy hospitalization exhausted the company's major medical insurance allocation and resulted in the termination of coverage. Soon after, the company established a prenatal program that has slashed the average cost per birth by 90%.

Within a year of establishing the new program for prenatal-health education, the cost per maternity case at the company's plant in Coushatta, Louisiana, dropped from $27,242 to $2,893. The average cost per case at the plant in Holly Springs, Mississippi, dropped from $3,500 to $2,872. Moreover, only one premature birth has occurred at either plant since the start of the program. Obviously, not all complications are preventable. However, the O-S case study and many similar cases reflect the influence that quality on-site interventions for promoting prenatal health can have on potentially avoidable complications.

expectant mother attends all scheduled prenatal classes

- Offering monetary rewards (e.g., $100) for attending all scheduled prenatal classes and screening sessions
- Paying a higher percentage (e.g., 100% versus 80%) of the health care bill for participating mothers

Since the actual effectiveness of specific incentives varies from worksite to worksite, incentives should be tailored to employees' needs and interests, the worksite culture, and an employer's financial situation. Management can make a significant effect on mothers and babies by taking the following actions:

- Sponsor a meeting of management and supervisors to announce company support of a program for prenatal health promotion (i.e., March of Dimes' "New Beginnings"). Explain the purpose, clarify the benefits to the company and the employees, and gain commitment for your program.
- Involve employee representatives and supervisors in your efforts. Solicit their help to recruit employees, promote the program, and offer ideas on how to get the message out.
- Send a personalized letter of invitation to every employee announcing your company's support.

- Appoint one or more employees or volunteers to be representatives for programs for healthy mothers and babies. Have special buttons, name tags, or T-shirts made for these representatives. Responsibilities may include giving presentations to employee groups and meetings, placing articles or announcements in company newsletters, changing bulletin boards and posters, and creating novel ways to promote the programs. Provide recognition and support for these representatives and rotate their appointments occasionally to prevent burnout and to give others a chance to contribute.
- Publicize your maternity-related health policies and benefits and emphasize the importance of early prenatal care.
- Link your company name and logo with the prenatal program. For example, "ABC Company and New Beginnings: Working Together for Healthy Moms and Healthy Babies." Companies are discovering that investing in programs for prenatal and maternal health pays off. Each high-risk pregnancy that is avoided saves tens, if not hundreds, of thousands of dollars for employers and society. This translates into healthier families, communities, and workforces in the future.

THE SOUTHERN REGIONAL CORPORATE COALITION TO IMPROVE MATERNAL AND CHILD HEALTH

One of the most ambitious worksite-based initiatives for promoting prenatal health is the Southern Regional Corporate Coalition to Improve Maternal and Child Health. Established in 1986 by the Southern Governors' Association's project on infant mortality, the coalition consists of 29 employers from 17 southern states. Coalition studies suggest that employers will create a healthier and more productive workforce, as well as cut their own expenses, if they do the following:

1. Include benefits for maternal and infant health in their insurance packages with incentives to encourage families to use preventive services, such as prenatal care for pregnant women.

2. Review their maternity leave policies and grant such leave for pregnant women without compromising a successful return to work.

3. Engage in public and private partnerships to develop health care public policy to encourage good maternal health.

4. Provide educational programs for employees and their families on preventive health care for mothers and children.

Items 1 through 3 here generally are the concern of human resources and benefits managers. However, WHP personnel are often responsible for writing and implementing educational programs on prenatal, infant, maternal, and child health.

SMOKING CONTROL

One of the most visible examples of corporate commitment to employees' health is reflected in the growth of smoking control policies at many worksites. Nearly three-fourths of all medium and large worksites throughout North America have smoking control policies, and most of these organizations also offer smoking cessation programs. In addition, more European worksites became smoke-free after Italy, Malta, and Ireland established indoor clean-air policies in 2005.

Many factors are responsible for the growing push for smoke-free worksites. First, federal agencies are addressing the issue in various ways. The *2004 U.S. Surgeon General's Report* attributes an estimated 420,000 deaths each year to cigarette smoking, making it one of the nation's leading causes of preventable death. In 1990, the Environmental Protection Agency (EPA) officially classified secondhand smoke as a significant indoor pollutant and a class-A carcinogen. And, the *2006 Surgeon General's Report: The Health Consequences of Involuntary Exposure to Tobacco Smoke* concluded that exposure to secondhand smoke can cause disease and premature death in nonsmoking children and adults.

Second, antidrug campaigns are spreading into worksites and targeting both illegal drugs and legal drugs, such as cigarettes (nicotine). Third, more nonsmokers are requesting that their employers establish smoke-free working environments. Fourth, more business owners are becoming aware of the economic costs of smoking employees. Smokers are absent an average of 2 to 5 days more per year than nonsmokers. They incur approximately 15% higher health care costs than nonsmokers. Fifth, there is overwhelming evidence that smoking employees incur greater costs in terms of medical care and lost productivity than nonsmoking workers. Finally, a growing body of statutory, regulatory, and judicial developments does the following:

- Grant employees in some jurisdictions the right to sue employers if smoking is permitted in a workplace.
- Stipulate that employers can be held partially accountable for employee pain, discomfort, and illness caused by tobacco smoke in the workplace.
- Rule that no legal grounds exist for claims that smoking at work is a constitutional right.

Additional factors influencing efforts at controlling worksite smoking include ensuring the purity of manufactured products, preventing property and equipment damage, and enhancing a company's corporate image to shareholders and the public.

Program and Policy Planning

Early employer initiatives to reduce smoking focused on policies and programs delivered at the worksite. Overall, policy-level changes are effective in reducing the prevalence of worksite smoking at least 10% more than worksites without such policies.

POLICY BENEFITS OF SMOKING CONTROL

Potential benefits to employers who establish smoking control policies include, but are not limited to, the following:

- Lower premium costs for health, life, and fire insurance and workers' compensation
- Fewer health care claims and costs from smoking-related conditions
- Less absenteeism from smoking-related illnesses
- Less property and equipment damage and lower maintenance costs
- Fewer accidents and reduced fire risk
- Greater productivity (avoiding down time used for smoking breaks)
- Fewer premature disabilities and deaths from cigarette smoking

Actual benefits depend largely on factors such as the extent of smoking control measures, the amount of smoking and physiological damage to the heart, lungs, and blood vessels before such measures are implemented, the percentage of employees who smoke off site, the general health of workers, and coexposure to other occupational hazards, such as asbestos and coal dust.

Worksite-based programs for smoking cessation include self-help manuals, physician advice, health education, cessation groups, and competitions. Although effective, these programs have been plagued by low participation rates. Incentives have been mildly effective in increasing participation rates, but this does not necessarily translate to improved cessation rates.

Some tools for quitting smoking and some common brands and prices are as follows:

Nicotine Replacement Therapies

- *Gum and lozenges.* Nicorette, which can be purchased over the counter, is $4.50 for 10 pieces.
- *Inhaler.* This is a plastic cylinder with a cartridge that delivers nicotine when you puff on it. A package of 42 cartridges is $45.
- *Nasal spray.* A prescription is required for Nicotrol NS. It costs $5 per day for average use (13 doses) or $15 per day for maximum usage (40 doses).
- *Patch.* NicoDerm is available both over the counter and by prescription. It costs $4 per day.

Prescription Drugs Without Nicotine

- Bupropion, which is marketed under the brand name Zyban and also sold as the antidepressant Wellbutrin, costs $2 per day (the generic version is $1.17 per day).

Counseling

- Free quitting hotlines, both state and federal (1-800-QUITNOW).
- Private telephone-based counseling (average cost of $200 to $300 for 4 to 6 intensive phone conversations).
- Group counseling in smoking cessation is offered through public health departments, nonprofit groups such as the American Cancer Society, and commercial groups such as SmokEnders and SmokeStoppers (session prices range from $50 to $350).

When planning a smoking-control policy, authorized personnel should properly structure and communicate the strategy for establishing smoke-free initiatives at the worksite. For example, more worksites are integrating their smoke-free efforts with proposals for clean-air policy proposals and the theme of protecting the health of employees. This minimizes the potential for heated debates, personal conflicts, and friction between smoking employees and management.

So-called *half-and-half policies* (banning smoking at workstations only) are essentially counterproductive because they force smokers to leave their work areas to smoke, resulting in lost productivity. In contrast, a total worksite policy for clean air can eliminate such violations and help smokers who are trying to quit. Removing all cigarette vending machines from the worksite and providing smoking cessation programs with financial rewards usually helps smokers who really want to quit to do so successfully. Some employers reportedly give employees at least six months' notice before implementing the policy.

On-site programs for smoking cessation exist most commonly in large companies (more than 1,000 employees), but they have better success rates in smaller worksites (fewer than 250 employees). In larger, dispersed worksites, facilitators can be easily identified. Social relationships within the worksite also tend to be stronger. In larger worksites, employees from the same department should be placed in the same cessation groups to maintain interpersonal relationships and group cohesiveness. Starting a support group of former smokers often encourages recent quitters to keep it up.

To help build the business case for covering smoking cessation, a group of health care economists from Kaiser Permanente's center for health research and from the industry group America's Health Insurance Plans developed a modeling tool to help companies determine how quickly they will see a payoff. The model is based on a large study that showed financial benefits from smoking cessation programs come in as little as two years. Researchers examined six years of medical data from 200,000 members of Kaiser Permanente Northwest to determine the effect of common anti-smoking interventions—basically having a doctor recommend and advise patients to quit, either alone or in conjunction with counseling, nicotine replacement therapy, or other medication. The researchers concluded that modest investments of just $.18 to $.79 per plan member each month began to save money after two years. After five years, a net monthly savings existed between $1.70 and $2.20 per member.

This research is likely to better justify making an investment in smoking cessation because most people stay in a health plan for at least three years. The smoking cessation ROI calculator can be accessed at the following website: www.businesscaseroi.org/roi/default.aspx.

By examining the demographics of your organization and reviewing health-risk appraisal data, you can compare your workforce's smoking rate and note whether the subgroups mentioned earlier match your experience. You can then decide whether to apply the percentage rate by the respective subgroups.

The three general elements of a successful intervention program are as follows:

1. Receiving consistent and repeated advice from a team of supporters to quit smoking.
2. Setting a specific end date.
3. Providing follow-up visits.

Additional modalities specifically for physicians include the following:

1. Support and mention of current programs offered at the worksite or in conjunction with the health care provider.
2. Referral to community group counseling.
3. Advice from more than one clinician (if available).
4. Using chart reminders to identify those who smoke.

Interventions provided at the worksite or by the health care organization should contain the option of three core elements. A combination of these three elements may not be the best for all smokers. However, to increase the probability of higher success and reduced relapse rate, the combination of these three strategies should be considered.

The first strategy centers on education and counseling. The education component should focus on the health effects of smoking, the importance of gaining support at work and at home, and moving the smoker to the action phase (e.g., setting a quit date). Once the participant is in the action phase, the counselor should work through the following priorities:

- Build readiness to quit.
- Build support needed to quit.
- Build skills needed to quit.
- Identify a quitting date.
- Assess success at various time intervals (depending on the client) after the quitting date.
- Prevent relapse.

The second strategy centers on nicotine replacement therapy (NRT). Once the quitting date arrives, the participant should use an NRT, such as nicotine gum, lozenges, or nicotine patches, in combination with counseling. When used correctly and in combination with education and counseling, nicotine replacement products increase long-term rates for smoking cessation by about one-third. Consequently, quitting rates up to 30% are commonly reported from NRTs, especially with combined interventions (Stead et al. 2008; Diefenbach 2003). Overall, a 4-mg dose of the nicotine-replacement product seems to be more effective than the 2-mg dose for people highly dependent on nicotine. The evidence suggests that nicotine-replacement products are most effective in combination with continuous counseling. Participants should receive proper instruction on how to use these products as part of the ongoing counseling.

At this time, limited evidence exists that a third type of intervention strategy can be used in combination with the education, counseling, and nicotine-replacement strategies. It centers on a brand of sustained-release tablets (Zyban), a non-nicotine prescription aid for smoking cessation.

Initially developed and marketed as an antidepressant (Wellbutrin), this drug affects the part of the brain that inhibits addictive behavior. In some studies, Zyban was used in conjunction with individual counseling for smoking cessation. Overall results indicate that Zyban is a successful intervention in approximately 20% to 40% of all users (Schnoll et al. 2010; Science Daily 2006).

Self-help programs delivered through the mail and the Internet offer the potential to reach greater numbers of employees and their spouses or partners with cessation treatment. Although the overall effectiveness may be lower than individual- or group-based programs, the overall effect is higher given the greater reach. Self-help interventions (written materials in particular) generally produce low initial quitting rates, but they are effective in helping quitters sustain their efforts and in assisting nonquitters to make additional attempts. For example, the American Lung Association's self-help guide, *Freedom From Smoking,* and the follow-up version, *A Lifetime of Freedom From Smoking,* are designed for employees who want to quit on their own. Self-help kits (e.g., SmokeStoppers) have produced one-year quitting rates as high as 32%. It is ironic that 81% of current quitters and more 90% of formerly successful quitters reportedly quit on their own without aid.

Growing Internet programs for smoking cessation have reported varying quitting rates. Preliminary research from specific smoking-cessation websites shows that the quitting rate achieved through Internet-based programs may be just as high as traditional, face-to-face programs. However, they have not been evaluated rigorously enough to render reliable quitting-rate estimates. However, some preliminary, uncontrolled studies of a highly used site (www.QuitNet.com) show one-year quitting rates in the range of 40% to 50% (Sarna et al. 2009; Healthways 2010).

Group-cessation methods (multicomponent, behavior-based programs) may produce one-year quitting rates of 30% to 40%, but they often attract a small percentage of employees. In contrast, incentive- and competition-based programs may attract good participation and produce more favorable quitting rates. However, these programs are typically based on self-reported behavior that should be verified with biochemical measures, such as thiocyanate or carbon monoxide testing. In a survey of more than 200 adult smokers, respondents preferred smoking cessation programs that included the following:

- Ways to quit smoking for life
- Endorsement by doctors
- Ways to deal with potential weight gain
- Relaxation techniques to use while quitting
- Healthy substitutes for smoking

When evaluating the effect of worksite smoking-cessation programs, it is important to define *quitting rate, long-term abstinence,* and any other key terms or concepts that can be subjectively quantified. *Quitting rate* is commonly defined as a percentage or ratio of the number of employees who quit successfully to the number of employees who started the intervention. A minimum period of one year is generally accepted for judging long-term abstinence. Also, be wary of vendors and proposals who promise quitting rates of more than 40%. Ask vendors for the names and phone numbers of past and current clients who can verify claims.

Sample Implementation Schedule

The following overview is a step-by-step plan for organizations who want to expand a partial restriction policy into a policy for a totally smoke-free environment.

- *Months 1 through 3.* In the first month, form a smoking-issues committee that consists of managers and labor representatives who are nonsmokers, smokers, and former smokers. Consider hiring an outside consultant to facilitate committee meetings and various phases of the project. In months 2 and 3, study the smoking issue by reviewing the company's current policies, other companies' policies, federal laws (e.g., EPA and OSHA), legal liability implications with a corporate attorney, and local, state, and provincial ordinances.

• *Months 4 and 5.* In the fourth month, assess employee attitudes and behaviors relevant to smoking. Develop a simple questionnaire to assess employees' smoking status, attitudes toward the current policy, and recommendations to expand the policy. An easy six-point number scale could be used:

1. Smoking permitted in all areas
2. Designate several smoking areas
3. Designate one smoking area
4. Ban smoking indoors
5. Completely smoke-free workplace
6. No smokers hired (policy prohibited in some states)

During the fifth month, develop a draft of the proposed policy. Review employee responses and construct a policy for a preliminary review by senior management. If the policy is not accepted, revise it accordingly and resubmit it.

• *Months 6 and 7.* Use the sixth month to obtain mainstream support. Meet with key supervisors and middle managers to inform them of the policy and to encourage their support. Announce the new policy in the seventh month by sending a memo from the human resources or personnel department to inform all employees of the purpose of the policy and the dates it will gradually go into effect.

• *Months 8 and 9.* During the eighth month, implement partial restrictions to reflect the locations cited in the survey. For example, restrict smoking to designated break areas only. This is also a good time to remove all cigarette machines from the worksite. Devote the ninth month to educating employees on the hazards and costs of smoking. Use various communication methods (e.g., newsletter, message boards, and health fairs) to inform employees of the health risks and financial costs of smoking.

• *Months 10 through 12.* Over the next three months, begin to offer smoking cessation programs to interested employees and spouses. Review the section on program and policy planning earlier in the chapter to determine appropriate interventions, participation fees, program schedules, and incentives. Now is the time to send a memo to all employees outlining the entire policy

IMPACT OF WORKSITE PROGRAMS ON SMOKING CONTROL

These examples from well-known companies illustrate potential benefits of smoking-control programs and policies.

• *Speedcall Corporation (Hayward, CA).* After the company's president offered each employee a $7 weekly bonus for not smoking at the worksite, the number of smoking employees dropped from 24 to 5 within a year.

• *Dow Chemical (Texas Division).* 24% percent of the company's smokers competed in a smoking cessation competition. Those quitting for at least one year entered a raffle for a fishing boat. At prize time, nearly 80% of the entrants had quit smoking.

• *Japan.* A radiator manufacturing company used a multifaceted approach, consisting of individualized physician counseling, periodic motivational visits by the occupational health nurse, leaflet distribution, and group discussion. Overall, smoking rates dropped between 8.4% and 12.9% at two follow-up evaluations (Kadowaki and Kanda 2006).

• *Unum life insurance company (Portland, ME).* The company reported an estimated health care savings of $200,000 in the first year of its worksite smoking ban.

• *Pacific Bell (Seattle, WA).* The percentage of smoking employees dropped from 28% to 20% within two years of its worksite smoking ban. Visits to the company's health clinic for respiratory problems dropped 13% and respiratory absences dropped 20%. Collectively, productivity and medical care savings exceeded $500,000.

and reminding them of the dates the policy will go into effect. The policy can now be implemented with clearly defined protocols on monitoring. Schedule monthly meetings over the next six months to solicit committee members' feedback on the new policy.

AIDS EDUCATION AND HIV DISEASE PREVENTION

Acquired immunodeficiency syndrome (AIDS) is a growing problem throughout the world. The World Health Organization (WHO) estimates that several million adults are infected with HIV (human immunodeficiency virus). Although men are stricken in greater numbers, women are contracting HIV at a proportionately higher rate. The Centers for Disease Control and Prevention (CDC) estimate that 1 of every 260 Americans has HIV, so it is likely that many American worksites have at least one employee who is HIV positive. Workers in health care settings dealing with body fluids are particularly at risk. Thus, such facilities have developed regulations in response to Healthy People 2020, which stipulates that regulations to protect workers from exposure to blood-borne infections, including HIV infection, should extend to all facilities where workers are at risk of occupational transmission of HIV.

In the early 1990s, the average life expectancy of a person with HIV or AIDS was projected to be about two years. Yet, since then, medical treatment for persons with HIV had steadily improved, enhancing the quality of life for those diagnosed with the disease. In fact, HIV disease is gradually changing from being considered a terminal condition to being viewed as a chronic, treatable illness, at least in some cases. Thus, the increasing number of people who currently have HIV disease will live longer and, in many cases, will continue to work. Consequently, employers are paying more for medical care, disability pay, and associated productivity losses from illnesses and premature deaths related to HIV and AIDS, which alone cost more than $125 billion a year in the United States. According to the CDC, the estimated cost of lifetime hospital care for an infected person can be more than

$60,000, and even more for total health care costs. For example, the CDC estimates that for every HIV infection that is prevented, an estimated $355,000 is saved in the cost of providing lifetime HIV treatment.

Faced with the rising health care costs of treatment for HIV and AIDS, more employers and insurers are betting on managed-care programs to help slow these cost increases. The key to managed care for HIV disease is to reduce inpatient hospitalization, which is the most expensive component of traditional AIDS care. Case management (individualized care at home or in an outpatient facility) is the most common type of managed care used in treating HIV disease. According to some insurers, it is capable of saving as much as $50,000 per case. Furthermore, home treatment is less expensive, more psychologically comforting, and less likely to expose the patient to other infectious agents that exist in a hospital setting. This type of managed care certainly merits consideration as a cost-control strategy. Yet, to effectively deal with this complex and evolving phenomenon, companies will have to establish education and prevention activities that appeal to as many employees as possible, especially to those in greatest need.

To date, numerous companies, including Syntex, Bank of America, AT&T, Eaton, Transamerica, and Pacific Telesis, have developed specific personnel policies to deal with HIV disease in the workplace. Bank of America is one of the most progressive companies in this area. It makes certain accommodations (flexible work hours, for example) for an employee with HIV disease, as long as the person's condition does not impair the department's efficiency. Another progressive step is treating HIV and AIDS as any other serious disease, allowing infected employees to work as long as their health permits.

During the mid- to late 1990s, advances in HIV treatments led to dramatic declines in AIDS-related deaths and slowed the progression of HIV to AIDS. However, in recent years, the rate of decline for both cases and deaths began to slow, and in 1999, the annual number of AIDS cases leveled off. The decline in AIDS-related deaths has also slowed considerably. Employers should address the issue of HIV infection before the first case is reported at the worksite because the employees' level of objectivity and receptivity is probably the greatest at that time. Waiting to educate employees on HIV and AIDS issues after a coworker has been infected may only intensify general anxiety throughout a workforce.

Employers who have made a corporate commitment to provide education on HIV and AIDS have received favorable response from employees, especially when information and education has been integrated into existing health benefits and internal communications. The Business Leadership Task Force, composed of 15 major employers in northern California, has taken a leadership role in providing education about HIV and AIDS at various worksites since 1983. A number of task-force members, such as AT&T, Bank of America, Chevron, Levi Strauss, Mervyn's department stores, Pacific Telesis, and Wells Fargo, have developed a videotape, *An Epidemic of Fear*, to use in corporate information and education campaigns about HIV and AIDS. In addition, several companies that are task-force members provide the following:

- Informational pieces for managers to use that are developed by HIV-AIDS experts
- Informational sessions for employees, workers with HIV, and their relatives
- Articles in company newsletters related to HIV and AIDS
- Video presentations that employees may borrow for home viewing

RESPONDING TO AIDS: TEN PRINCIPLES FOR THE WORKPLACE

The Citizens' Commission on AIDS for New York City and northern New Jersey has drafted guidelines to help employers manage AIDS in the workplace. "Responding to AIDS: Ten Principles for the Workplace" has been endorsed by more than 370 companies and organizations. The principles are as follows:

1. People with AIDS or HIV infection at any stage are entitled to the same rights and opportunities as people with other serious or life-threatening illnesses.

2. Employment policies must, at a minimum, comply with federal, state, and local laws and regulations.

3. Employment policies should be based on the scientific and epidemiological evidence that people who are HIV positive or who have AIDS cannot transmit the virus to coworkers through ordinary workplace contact.

4. The highest levels of management and union leadership should unequivocally endorse nondiscriminatory employment policies and educational programs about HIV disease.

5. Employers and unions should communicate their support of these policies to workers in simple, clear, and unambiguous terms.

6. Employers should provide employees with sensitive, accurate, and up-to-date information about risk reduction in their personal lives.

7. Employers have a duty to protect the confidentiality of employees' medical information.

8. To prevent work disruption and rejection by coworkers of an employee with AIDS or HIV infection, employers and unions should educate all employees before such an incident occurs and as needed thereafter.

9. Employers should not require HIV screening as part of preemployment or general workplace physical examinations, but they can provide the phone number and location of local anonymous testing sites.

10. In those special occupational settings where a potential risk of exposure to HIV may exist—for example, health care workers who may be exposed to blood or blood products—employers should provide specific, ongoing education and training in universal precautions about blood and body fluids as well as the necessary equipment to reinforce appropriate procedures for infection control.

Although various approaches are being used at worksites, some experts feel that peer-to-peer education among employees is most effective.

MEDICAL SELF-CARE AND HEALTH CARE CONSUMERISM

The average person in the United States sees a doctor about five times a year and takes about seven different prescriptions per year, yet at least 80% of all outpatient physician visits for new health problems are essentially unnecessary. They could have been treated just as effectively through medical self-care. According to the National Center for Health Statistics, fewer than 30 different conditions account for as much as 90% of all physician visits:

Asthma	Hay fever
Backache	Headache
Bronchitis	Heartburn
Chest pain	Influeza (flu)
Cold	Ingrown toenails
Cough	Laryngitis
Cuts or scrapes	Nausea or vomiting
Depression	Premenstrual syndrome
Diarrhea	Sinusitis
Earache	Sore throat
Eczema	Sports injuries
Fatigue	Sprains and strains
Fever	Urinary tract infections

Many of the preceding conditions are usually minor ailments and, thus, are responsive to medical self-care interventions.

As more workers continue to use a high volume of health care services, many worksites have resorted to greater cost-sharing arrangements with employees and dependents. However, this move has not slowed health care utilization rates in most workforce populations. And, in those worksites reporting lower utilization, total health care costs often increase due to more employees using higher-priced specialty services for chronic conditions. Moreover, cost-sharing has done little, if anything, to motivate employees and dependents to adopt healthy lifestyles, properly use their health care benefits, or learn to apply self-care regimens in treating minor ailments. In the mid-1980s, a handful of worksites keenly observed this evolving phenomenon and adopted medical self-care and consumerism programs. Since then, many worksites have become enlightened on the need to cultivate a culture of employees who understand and adopt these skills in their personal lives.

For maximum effect, medical self-care and consumerism efforts should be directed toward both employees and their dependents. Early in the movement of medical self-care and consumerism, one of the most common strategies used by employers involved distributing resources to employees, such as self-care books, newsletters, and videocassettes. These resources are primarily designed to help workers do the following:

- Identify when a health problem is a minor condition that can be treated through self-care and when it is a true emergency (approximately 55% of all visits to emergency departments are not urgent).
- Learn how to use self-care measures to treat minor ailments.
- Compare health care providers on important quality and cost criteria.
- Ask the right questions of their health care providers.
- Understand cost sharing and key features of health insurance, such as who pays for what (premium, deductible, and copayment) and what types of alternative health care providers are in the plan.

Reports at worksites using medical self-care and consumer-education interventions indicate they are saving $3 or more for every $1 spent on such efforts. For example, employees at Berk-Tec, a small manufacturing company in Lancaster County, Pennsylvania, learned self-care techniques and lowered their company's health care costs in one year. By using a self-care guide, the 938 employees saved nearly $22 per person. Their dependents saved nearly 18%. Combined reductions in doctor visits and emergency-room usage led to savings of $39 per employee, a 24.3% drop in costs over the previous year (National Wellness Institute 2005; Workplace Wellness Programs 2009).

Medical self-care interventions operating at many multisite organizations include core communications, such as self-care books, newsletters (from an employer or health plan), educational seminars, Internet-based resources, subject-specific videotapes, and other promotional materials. Recently, some self-care vendors have offered customized self-care guides based on a company's most common health problems. For example, based on the most common employee health risks and types of health care claims indicated on a check sheet, the vendor will design a self-care guide.

One of the fastest-growing resources used to target and support high-risk employees is a telephone-based counseling service. This particular type of service is consumer focused. Its goal is to assist workers in making better health care decisions at home and with their personal health care provider.

The telephonic service can be offered to all workers. It includes targeted messages to specific risk-specific sectors of the workforce (e.g., people with chronic conditions, high-frequency health care users, or recently injured or disabled workers). This particular type of service is often staffed by health-plan-certified case managers and advisers to provide chronic-disease management and disability-management services to individual employees.

Of course, the more preventive care and health services are integrated within the organization, the greater the effect. For example, employees in 285 Wisconsin school districts with access to a 24-hour telephonic nurse-advice line, a self-care reference book, and health-education materials generated a health care savings of 4.75 to 1 (Workplace Wellness Programs 2009).

Whether an employer is a single-site operation or has multiple site operations, it is good to reach as many employees as

THE QUAKER OATS HEALTH MANAGEMENT PLAN

One of the earliest and most successful worksite-based health-management programs that included medical self-care and consumerism was implemented by the Quaker Oats Company in the early 1980s. Its integrated plan, which serves as a model for many worksites, includes the following features:

- A company-produced booklet (*Informed Choices*) that helps employees and dependents decide on when to seek health care, how to compare providers on quality and cost criteria, how to select a health care provider, and what questions to ask a provider.
- Financial incentives within a health expense account in which Quaker Oats allocates a fixed amount of money that employees can use toward their health insurance premium, deductible, or copayment. Unused money at the end of the year is applied to the following year's allocation.
- "Live Well, Be Well" is a health promotion program that offers on-site health screenings, seminars, and personal self-enhancement activities. Participants can earn financial rewards for completing a health-risk appraisal and adopting healthy lifestyle practices.

Before adopting its integrated approach, Quaker's health care costs rose about 20% a year. Since then, Quaker's health care costs have risen an average of about 7% a year.

possible with an intervention. Thus, many worksites introduce or enhance their medical self-care and consumerism programs for several weeks during the annual health-plan reenrollment.

Popular topics highlighted in these programs include the following:

- Allergy education
- Asthma management
- Back care
- Customizing health-risk assessments
- Diabetes management
- Fatigue management
- Home remedies for flu and colds
- Managing high blood pressure
- Men's health issues
- Women's health issues

To affect as many people as possible, it is important to provide visible support and to engage family members into as many facets of the medical self-care and consumer campaign as possible. Since many employers have multisite operations, they should partner with local health plans to provide local staff support and reduce funding of the program.

Finally, when employers customize these programs around the needs, interests, and educational backgrounds of their employees, they are likely to build a strong employee-employer partnership in the war against rising health care utilization and costs.

FINANCIAL WELLNESS

If you take a look at your favorite news media, you're likely to read about some disturbing financial trends. Health care costs are on the rise, affordable health insurance is virtually impossible to obtain, employee wages are shrinking, and many employees aren't taking full advantage of benefits that can help them ease these worries. Understandably, at least 1 in 4 American workers

is seriously distressed about a personal financial situation. This often translates into problems with productivity, attendance, and retention—all factors that affect the bottom line. Studies have shown that up to 80% of financially distressed workers spend time on personal financial issues instead of working (Marquez 2009).

With today's tough economy taking a toll on workers and companies, more and more employers are seeing the value of programs for financial wellness. Responding to employee requests and growing research linking finance and health, employers are adding a wide variety of financial-education initiatives to their programs, including budgeting, college funding, and retirement planning. Although some of these initiatives appeared in a few EAP-related programs in the 1990s, many worksites have expanded the scope of these programs to include a greater emphasis on financial wellness in the past decade. Administratively, some companies have chosen to offer financial-wellness programs outside the realm of an EAP, either as a stand-alone program to attract employees who are interested in financial wellness alone or as a marketing strategy to motivate participants from financial-wellness programs to explore other WHP programs.

Although the links between financial health and overall health may not be as compelling as other WHP areas, a study of 79,070 employees cited finances as second only to work as the leading source of employee stress (The Financial Wellness Group 2009). Respondents with higher stress levels were 2.6 times more likely to experience five or more days of absenteeism than employees with low stress levels. Moreover, additional studies involving 46,026 employees in various worksites showed stress as one of the strongest predictors of high health care costs.

Integrating the concept of financial health into WHP can help employers provide a wider array of employee-friendly programs, add more perceived value to the health-benefits plan and, consequently, contain their total health care costs. Moreover, it creates a strong incentive for WHP practitioners to engage traditionally hard-to-reach employees. For example, smokers might not be interested in attending a smoking cessation program because they aren't ready to quit. However, if they attend a program on financial health that discusses the costs of cigarettes and the potential health care costs associated with smoking, they might be more willing to participate in a cessation program.

Also, by integrating financial education with wellness programs, employers can help employees make better decisions about how they spend their health care dollars. For example, more employees may realize that it makes sense to invest more of their paychecks into their retirement or flexible spending accounts. For example, the United States has a 401(k) connection. The 401(k) retirement plan may be a good place to initiate financial-wellness programs for employees. Currently, only about 50% of employees fully fund their 401(k) plans, and one-third don't participate at all. This can become a serious problem for some corporations because 401(k) regulations require minimum participation rates. Also, legal experts warn that employees who retire with inadequate retirement funds might sue their employer because they were not adequately informed of the need to make contributions to a 401(k) plan. Financial-education programs at your worksite may be more easily justified if you can show increased 401(k) participation.

A second factor worth consideration is the strong potential for high participant interest. According to a survey funded by the National Institute of Drug Abuse, 60% of 10,308 employees from nearly 40 organizations wanted counseling, workshops, or more information regarding finances. Because such a wide range of personal-finance topics exist, it is likely that most, if not all, employees would be interested in at least one financial topic if it were marketed properly.

A third factor that compels numerous organizations to offer financial-wellness initiatives is that such programs may attract high-risk populations. For example, various surveys conducted by vendors of financial-wellness programs indicate that more than 50% of the participants were classified as high risk. Furthermore, more than one-third of these people expressed a strong desire to act on their risk factors within the next 30 days after attending financial-wellness workshops. Exit surveys indicate that workshops making a connection between money and health are likely to motivate participants to take such actions.

A fourth potential benefit from offering financial wellness at the worksite relates to attracting underserved populations. Surveys conducted on participants in financial-wellness programs indicate that as many as 35% of attendees report they seldom or never attended other wellness workshops (The Financial Wellness Group 2009). This number represents a substantial portion of the traditionally underserved population. These workers typically have lower incomes and are highly interested in personal finances.

While many financial wellness initiatives are established internally, there is some momentum for collaborations between the private and public sectors in this arena. For example, the Center for Economic Progress is working to help employees of local employers to gain access to important programs and benefits they may not be aware of. In cooperation with the Chicagoland Chamber of Commerce, the city of Chicago, and RealBenefits, the Center partners with numerous local employers to bring health insurance screening and enrollment, tax assistance, financial education, and savings and credit education to hundreds of Chicago workers.

What Would You Do?

You have just completed a survey of more than 100 corporate clients for your employer, a large managed-care company. The survey was designed to assess what types of WHP programs each client would prefer to receive from your staff. Approximately 40% of the clients expressed interest in a traditional offering of health fairs, a walking program, and group lunch-and-learn sessions. The remaining 60% of clients prefer more personalized and spiritual offerings. Despite the contrasting preferences, your WHP colleagues prefer the one-size-fits-all philosophy. They are leaning toward offering the traditional entrée to all clients.

However, you would like to tailor WHP offerings to each client's preference, despite knowing that it will cost your organization more up front to do so. Aside from the issue of customer satisfaction, what other factors should you and your WHP colleagues consider in making your final decision? Does any credible research suggest that your approach is the best option? Where does your supervisor stand on this issue? Is it possible to promote both options, considering your budgetary, staffing, and facility resources? What would you do?

CHAPTER 4 WRAP-UP

Key Points

- Each worksite's unique needs require specific WHP programs and resources.
- Progressive-minded employers understand the importance of providing holistic WHP programs and activities.
- Traditional single-topic WHP programs can appeal to and positively influence more employees by adopting an integrated (multifaceted) design.
- The overall level of success achieved by a particular WHP program depends on the ability of WHP practitioners to strategically align supply-side resources to the specificity of the demand-side needs and interests of employees.

Glossary

comprehensive *(global)* health management—An integrated system of programs, policies, incentives, activities, and health care services provided to improve the health status, on-the-job productivity, and overall well-being of all employees.

disease management—A system of coordinated health information, health promotion, and health care interventions and communications for populations with chronic health conditions.

integrated programming—Combining individual health strategies into a single multidimensional program.

Bibliography

Balady G.J., B. Chaitman, C. Foster, E. Froelicher, N. Gordon, and S. Van Camp. 2002. "Automated external defibrillators in health/fitness facilities. Supplement to the AHA/ACSM recommendations for cardiovascular screening, staffing, and emergency policies at health/fitness facilities." *Circulation* 105: 1147-1150.

Centers for Disease Control and Prevention. 2009. "HIV in the United States." Accessed November 27, 2009. www.cdc.gov/hiv/resources/factsheets/us.htm.

Center for Economic Progress. 2009. "Employees' financial wellness." Accessed November 27. www.economicprogress.org/index.php/c/Newsroom/d/Employees%27_Financial_Wellness.

Central Intelligence Agency. 2010. World Fact Book. www.cia.gov/library/publications/the-world-factbook/geos/us.html. Accessed November 1.

Cherry, D., D. Woodwell, and E. Rechsteiner. 2007. *National ambulatory medical care survey: 2005 summary.* Hyattsville, MD: National Center for Health Statistics.

Diefenbach, L., and P. Smith. 2003. "What is the most effective nicotine replacement therapy?" *Journal of Family Practice* 52: 492-494.

Disease Management Association of America. 2009. "Definition of disease management." Accessed November 29. www.dmaa.org/dm_definition.asp.

EUROPA press releases. 2009. "Commission calls for smoke free Europe by 2012." Accessed: November 28. http://europa.eu./rapid/pressReleasesAction.do?reference=IP/09/1060.

Healthways. 2010. "Wyoming advances tobacco cessation: Integration simplifies quit process and program." Accessed October 29. www.healthways.com/search/searchresults.aspx?searchtext=wyoming.

Machlin, S. R., and F. Rohde 2007. "Health care expenses for uncomplicated pregnancies." *Research Findings* 27: Agency for Healthcare Research and Quality, Rockville, MD.

Marquez, J. 2009. "Employers add financial components to wellness programs." *Workforce Management Online.* Accessed December 1. http://workforce.com/section/02/feature/26/43/99.

National Wellness Institute. 2005. "On promoting medical self-care and wise health consumerism." Ask the Experts Newsletter2 (4), 1-3.

Office of the Surgeon General. 2006. "The health consequences of involuntary exposure to tobacco smoke: A report of the surgeon general." Accessed December 1, 2009. http://surgeongeneral.gov/library/secondhandsmoke/report.

Office of the Surgeon General. 2006. The health consequences of smoking: A report of the surgeon general. Accessed December 1, 2009. http://surgeongeneral.gov/library/smokingconsequences/Index.html.

PHC4. 2003. "Promoting maternal health in the workplace." *FYI* 21:1-2.

Rager, R., J. Leutzinger, J. Hochberg, W. Kirsten, and D. Chenoweth. 2008. "Employee disease management in U.S. and global workplaces." *Disease Management & Health Outcomes* 16: 87-94.

Rx List: The Internet Drug Index. 2009. "Zyban drug information: Uses, side effects, drug interactions and warnings." Accessed November 27, 2009. www.rxlist.com/zyban-drug.htm.

Sarna, L., et al. 2009. Nurses trying to quit smoking using the Internet. *Nursing Outlook* 57: 5, 246-256.

Schnoll, R., et al. 2010. "A bupropion smoking cessation clinical trial for cancer patients." *Cancer Causes Control* 21: 6, 811-820.

Science Daily. 2006. "New kind of drug could increase number who quit smoking." Accessed October 29, 2010. www.sciencedaily.com/releases/2006/05/060503100419.htm.

Stead, L., et al. 2008. "Nicotine replacement therapy for smoking cessation." *Cochrane Database of Systematic Reviews* 1: 1-3.

Surgeon General's Report on Physical Activity and Health. 1996. Washington, DC: U.S. Department of Health and Human Services.

Tharret, S., K. McInnis, and J. Peterson. 2006. *ACSM's health and fitness facilities standards and guidelines.* (3rd edition). Champaign, IL: Human Kinetics.

The Financial Wellness Group. 2009. "Financial wellness in the workplace." Accessed November 28. http://thefinancialwellnessgroup.com/employer-features.php.

U.S. Department of Labor. 2008. "Quick stats on women workers." Accessed December 1, 2009. http://dol.gov/wb/stats/main.htm.

Workplace Wellness Programs. 2009. "Workplace wellness program ROI." Accessed October 29, 2010. http://workplacewellnessprograms.org.

Looking Ahead

Now that we've considered a strategic plan for developing employee-centered programs and activities that promote health, it's time to consider funding and resource issues. Chapter 5 presents an overview of various strategies for planning a budget, staffing options, preparing realistic proposals, and crafting a prospective break-even scenario.

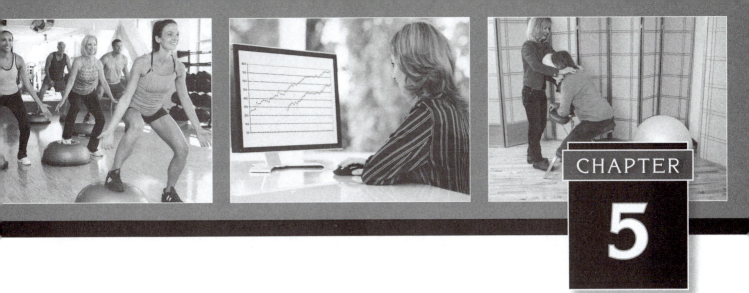

Funding and Resource Considerations

LEARNING OBJECTIVES

After reading this chapter, you will be able to do the following:

- ✔ Identify several options to consider in deciding how to fund a WHP program.
- ✔ Generate a list of pertinent questions you would use to assess the feasibility of outsourcing options.
- ✔ List the major components of a proposal.
- ✔ Describe the major steps used in preparing a break-even analysis.
- ✔ Describe potential advantages of an integrated WHP program.

Some of the most important decisions in getting WHP programs under way involve identifying and using appropriate financial resources. This chapter addresses financial considerations for making wise use of your resource allocations. In most program settings, these considerations center on selecting appropriate personnel and equipment, outsourcing, budgeting, and including relevant cost items into a proposal. In weighing each of these issues, review your program's vision, mission, and goals to ensure that you make sound and realistic financial decisions throughout all phases of program planning and implementation.

In addition, it's important to clearly establish a strong **business case** for your WHP program as you explore funding options. Most funding sources, whether it's the in-house human resources department or an external grant-sponsoring organization, require objective and compelling justification for a program before they make a financial commitment.

> **Why is it important to build a strong business case?**

In building a strong business case for your program, consider the following questions and take appropriate action:

- Prepare risk-factor prevalence, health-related lost productivity, and health-cost trend data on your workforce.
- Demonstrate why your workforce needs a WHP program (e.g., aging workers with existing health conditions that impair on-the-job productivity).

- Explain how a well-developed and effectively implemented WHP program provides a real, value-added component to the employee benefits package.

- Highlight how other organizations that are occupationally similar to your company have benefited from WHP programs in terms of lowering employee health risks, boosting morale and productivity, and containing health care costs.

- Prepare a practical WHP-program framework that incorporates key Socratic dimensions, such as the following questions:

  ➡ *What* features constitute the program?

  ➡ *Why* is this particular program necessary?

  ➡ *Who* (personnel) will provide the program?

  ➡ *How* will the program be provided in a cost- and time-efficient manner? (Funding options should be addressed at this time.)

  ➡ *Where* will the program be offered?

  ➡ *When* will the program be offered?

  ➡ *With whom* will WHP personnel work in providing the program?

In building a strong business case for WHP, it's essential to thoroughly explore on-site and off-site resources, personnel, and funding options. This preliminary work will enhance the quality of short-term and future planning decisions. Consequently, the odds are greatly increased that a viable and cost-effective program will be established and sustained over a period of time to successfully achieve employee and organizational goals.

ALLOCATING RESOURCES

The availability, utility, and cost of resources often influence the scope of WHP program offerings. Scope refers to the range or breadth of program offerings. For example, when WHP personnel have a variety of on-site resources at their disposal, they're more likely to offer activities or programs that promote health for all types of employ-

ees, regardless of their individual health status, level of interest, or readiness to act. In contrast, when WHP practitioners have limited on-site resources, the scope of their programs and activities are often restricted. Yet, even in a resource-constrained environment, savvy practitioners can usually provide employee-valued programs and activities with some creativity and ingenuity (see chapter 6).

When speaking of resources, it's common to immediately think of on-site facilities, personnel, equipment, and in-house funding sources. Yet, in these times of limited resources, it makes good business sense to explore the potential role that off-site facilities, external providers, and ancillary funding sources may play in your WHP programming.

Location

In many worksites, health promotion programs and activities do not need to be confined to a single location. However, an organization's goals and resources largely influence the types of programs that can be feasibly implemented. Issues, such as operational costs and the desired effect, are influenced to some extent by site selection. Traditionally, WHP practitioners felt that if an organization was more interested in keeping programming costs as low as possible than in achieving a high level of effectiveness, it should offer programs and activities at off-site facilities. In contrast, if effectiveness was most important to an organization, they felt it would benefit most from on-site programs, especially if the company had more than 500 employees.

Whether WHP interventions are offered on-site, off-site,

> Do you think this approach is appropriate in today's worksites?

or a combination thereof, it's important to consider the structure, function, and goals of specific programs and activities prior to selecting an appropriate location. For example, think through the following questions:

- Will health-risk assessments or fitness screenings be conducted? If so, how could they be administered in the most time-efficient manner, while preserving privacy and confidentiality?

- Will formal educational and instructional activities require a classroom setting?
- Will participants be sitting, standing, or moving during the program or activity? If so, how much space is needed?
- Will participants need certain types of equipment or access to computer terminals to participate?
- Will the lunch-and-learn sessions require special partitioning in the cafeteria?
- What amount of time for daily or weekly participation is needed for participants to achieve their goals?
- Do most employees live close to an off-site facility that might be more appropriate?

Seminar programs, with topics such as stress management, nutrition, weight management, medical self-care, and smoking cessation, are best provided in quiet, classroom-type settings with no distractions. Conference rooms, employee lounges, and cafeterias are also popular locations to offer such programs, especially at low-usage times. For example, Sentry Insurance in Stevens Point, Wisconsin, converted an unused area into a quiet room that was specially equipped with sofas, soft lights, and soothing music to ease employees' stress.

Space efficiency is particularly important for worksites with limited facilities. In order to be as effective as possible, choose appropriate on-site or off-site areas that can offer the most usable space for the least expense and inconvenience. For example, a good way to identify the most viable location for programs and activities is to use a feasibility grid, such as the one shown in table 5.1. This

Table 5.1　Sample Feasibility Grid Framework

Activity or program	Conference room	Cafeteria	Warehouse or outside	Fitness center	Health clinic	Workstation (e-mail)	EAP (on-site or off-site)
Health screening				✓	✓		
Health-risk assessment				✓	✓	✓	
Preexercise screening				✓			
Prework stretching			✓			✓	
Physical fitness			✓	✓		✓	
Walking			✓	✓			
Nutrition	✓	✓				✓	
Weight management	✓	✓				✓	
Back health			✓	✓	✓	✓	
AIDS and HIV prevention	✓				✓	✓	✓
Prenatal health	✓				✓		
Smoking cessation	✓	✓			✓	✓	✓
Disease management					✓	✓	✓
Medical self-care	✓	✓			✓	✓	
Employee assistance					✓		✓
Stress management	✓				✓	✓	✓
Spiritual health				✓		✓	✓
Financial wellness	✓					✓	✓

can help planners determine the most efficient use of existing resources. The key is not only to use existing space more efficiently, but also to take advantage of unused space at the most accommodating times. This principle applies to both on-site and off-site options. For example, some companies pool their finances to rent or lease a community fitness center, school gymnasium, church meeting rooms, or other suitable venue. Many companies without on-site exercise facilities choose to subsidize memberships for their employees at commercial fitness clubs.

Personnel

The essence of every successful WHP program lies in the quality of its personnel. You will encounter wide variation in your level of responsibility and budget size, depending on the size of your company and your position within it. Given the programs determined by the wellness committee during the identification and assessment phases, what types of personnel are needed to implement and sustain the program? In larger worksites, the wellness committee can examine the issue of whether more professional staff are needed or can be afforded. For example, depending on the budget, one of your options may be to provide current staff members with financial support to attend appropriate professional conferences, earn continuing education units, or earn some enhanced certifications (see chapter 10).

Because smaller companies must do with little or no professional staff, relying instead on volunteers or outsourced personnel, can any existing employees be identified to fill some of this gap? Does anyone in the company have any health-related expertise or skills that, for example, enable them to lead daily stretching sessions or break-time walking groups? Opportunistic small companies often engage in reciprocal relationships with local colleges and universities to fill the personnel gap. For example, university professors and graduate students conduct on-site WHP activities and research in small businesses in exchange for using the worksites as venues for formal training and research.

Whether an organization chooses to use professional staff, in-house volunteers, off-site providers, or a combination approach, it is essential for all personnel to work together as a team in order to meet employees' needs and interests.

Consultants and Independent Contractors

As many worksites continue to experience downsizing, aging workers, and greater efficiency demands, employers are calling on external vendors and health promotion consultants to assist them in one or more of the capacities shown on page 84.

Because few organizations know about a provider's capabilities until a project is actually under way, a vendor or consultant should be selected with a great deal of consideration to ensure a proper fit among all parties. For example, in selecting a consultant, organizations should do the following:

- Identify why a consultant may be needed.
- Check to see whether all internal resources have been fully tapped and whether an employee or someone on staff may be able to solve the problem.
- Solicit bids (detailed proposals) from several consultants.
- Develop a list of criteria to use in judging all candidates. (Common criteria include fees, availability, experience, type of clientele served, specialties, opinions of references, and the ability to customize services.)
- Interview the top candidates in person, by video conference, or phone conference. Solicit feedback from all staff members
- Avoid consultants who charge up front or who appear to be inflexible.

When an organization uses a consultant or any other resource on a part-time basis, all parties must clearly understand each entity's role and legal relationship. It is important to avoid any misunderstanding as to who qualifies as an employee or an independent contractor. The Internal Revenue Service (IRS) applies a standard known as the **20 Factor Test** to determine whether workers are employees or independent contractors (Miami Dade College Human Resources Department 2009). The 20 questions are as follows:

1. Do you provide the worker with instructions as to when, where, and how work is performed?
2. Did you train the worker to have the job performed correctly?
3. Are the worker's services a vital part of your company's operations?
4. Is the person prevented from delegating work to others?
5. Is the worker prohibited from hiring, supervising, or paying assistants?
6. Does the worker perform services for you on a regular and continuous basis?
7. Do you set the hours of service for the worker?
8. Does the person work full-time for your company?
9. Does the worker perform duties on your company's premises?
10. Do you control the order and sequence of the work performed?
11. Do you require workers to submit oral or written reports?
12. Do you pay the worker by the hour, week, or month?
13. Do you pay the worker's business and travel expenses?
14. Do you furnish tools or equipment for the worker?
15. Does the worker lack a significant investment in tools, equipment, and facilities?
16. Is the worker insulated from suffering a loss as a result of the activities performed for your company?
17. Does the worker perform services solely for your firm?
18. Are the worker's services unavailable to the general public?
19. Do you have the right to discharge the worker at will?
20. Can the worker end the relationship without incurring any liability?

The IRS considers any affirmative answer to be evidence of an employer-employee relationship that would prevent classification as an independent contractor. Since the early 1980s, many independent contractors have been hired for worksite health and fitness settings because, in large part, such relationships create immediate savings to an employer's bottom line. For example, by using an independent contractor, an organization is not required to pay FICA (Federal Insurance Contributions Act, for Social Security), FUTA (Federal Unemployment Tax Act), or state unemployment taxes on the worker. In addition, the independent

WORKSITE ASSIGNMENTS FOR HEALTH PROMOTION CONSULTANTS

Preprogram	Programming	Valuation
Feasibility studies	Database development	Benefit-cost analysis
Risk management	Program planning	Cost-effectiveness analysis
Staff development	Incentives design	Break-even analysis
Facility design	Marketing	Forecasting
Information technology	Integrative operations	Metric outline reporting
Health-claims analysis	Online program delivery	Health and productivity management

contractor is not eligible to receive company-paid benefits, such as health insurance, paid personal leave, disability, and vacation. Typically, independent contractors are not covered by an organization's general liability insurance policy. Thus, the organization should require all independent contractors to carry appropriate liability insurance, show evidence of current coverage, and make sure the organization is listed as an additional insurer on the policy when appropriate.

Outsourcing

One of the fastest-growing movements influencing today's WHP landscape is *outsourcing*. Outsourcing is typically referred to as a contract service or vendor contract. A survey of 927 companies conducted by The Wyatt Company indicates that nearly one-third of employers outsource some or all of their human resources and benefits programs (Meltzer 2009). Moreover, many employers continue to outsource their health promotion operations in order to efficiently downsize, focus on their core businesses, and improve their profit margins. Additional reasons for such outsourcing relate to the following areas:

• *Experience.* Outsourced vendors generally have the expertise needed to efficiently administer WHP.

• *Employee trust.* Employees are generally more candid with a health coach or other WHP practitioners about their health than with someone who's employed by the company.

• *Legal protection.* Outsourcing firms assume most, if not all, of the fiduciary responsibility to preserve and protect an employee's right to privacy and confidentiality regarding potentially sensitive matters (e.g., risk-factor status, lifestyle-related risk factors, health-related productivity, health care usage, and cost patterns).

Despite the high level of WHP outsourcing that has prevailed since the early 1990s in many sectors, health care employers tend to maintain in-house WHP operations. Health care systems typically have a good supply of trained WHP staff and well-defined systems in place to protect private health informa-

---

COMMONLY OUTSOURCED HEALTH PROMOTION AND FACILITY-MANAGEMENT SERVICES

HEALTH PROMOTION SERVICES

Disease and condition management

Employee health screening

Health promotion seminars

Health fairs

Health coaching

Toll-free self-care services

Health promotion and benefits integration

Health-awareness programs

Newsletter publishing

Health-risk appraisals

Online and web-based program delivery

FACILITY MANAGEMENT

Preopening promotions and publicity

Conducting a grand opening event

Establishing computerized entry and exit systems

Conducting fitness evaluations

Supervising all exercise activities

Conducting recreational programs and leagues

Sponsoring on-site health fairs

Implementing customized incentive programs

Designing and managing web pages

STAFF DEVELOPMENT

Hiring, training, and placing staff members

Certifying staff

Training instructors

tion, in keeping with ADA, GINA, and HIPAA regulations.

Since no nationally recognized guidelines exist for selecting vendors, it is important to screen providers, especially those who sell products or render services in the following areas: body-fat testing, employee assistance programs (EAP), preexercise stress testing, nutrition analysis, weight management, smoking cessation, and stress management. Here are some suggested questions to ask and qualifications to check:

1. What types of resources (personnel, equipment, and facilities) does the provider have to serve the company's needs?

2. Is the provider certified by a reputable association?

3. Does the provider have a program or service that appears to be philosophically sound and easily understood? Are written goals, objectives, and policies clearly presented?

4. Does the provider have a reasonable fee schedule? Is it willing to offer discounts to firms with small budgets?

5. Does the provider demonstrate substantial expertise in the area? Can it provide a list of past and current clients?

6. Is the provider willing to provide a complimentary demonstration of the product or service?

7. Can products and services be customized to meet specific needs?

8. Does the provider maintain records in compliance with ADA, GINA, HIPAA, and OSHA?

9. Does the provider have a formal process for evaluating its performance?

10. Does the provider possess professional liability insurance? If so, what is the policy coverage level?

When considering outsourcing options, employers typically consider three factors: cost, service, and value. Although cost information is the easiest to obtain, it takes more effort to accurately gauge the value and service from potential vendors, especially if you haven't previously dealt with a vendor. Thus, it's essential to develop a list of relevant quality-assurance questions to ask vendor candidates before making your final decision. In general, assessing the overall cost-service-value proposition of a product, such as purchasing a treadmill or medical self-care booklet, may require several up-front questions about cost. However, if the human element enters this proposition, such as when selecting health coaches or health-screening personnel, then service-oriented criteria should command the bulk of the investigative questions.

Commercial Health Promotion Materials

In the past decade, many employers have cut their workforces, thereby creating greater workloads for fewer people. Naturally, this downsizing has placed greater pressure on many organizations to stay competitive while using fewer human resources. In response, more organizations are providing their health promotion staff members with kits, guides, and newsletters to better meet employees' needs. You will need to examine both the situations in which you might use such materials and the materials themselves. For example, large or multisite organizations can purchase multiple copies of specific resources to use in hard-to-reach locations or as stand-alone programs where no full-time health promotion staff exists. Multisite operations may have a designated employee at each site acting as a health promotion facilitator to distribute resources and motivate coworkers to promote their personal health. Worksites with WHP practitioners may choose to purchase multimedia program kits for a designated employee (or outside vendor) to implement on a part-time basis (e.g., a take-home video on how to facilitate on-the-job stretching breaks with supplementary wall posters and employee information sheets on work-station stretching routines).

Many employers negotiate arrangements with their health plans to provide health promotion and preventive-care services to employees and dependents at designated intervals (e.g., semiannual health fairs). In a nationwide survey conducted by The Henry J. Kaiser Family Foundation, nearly 87% of the companies surveyed reported that most of the WHP benefits they offer are provided through their health plans (Kaiser 2010). One of the fastest-growing examples of how worksites are using their technology networks is the increase of Internet- and intranet-based WHP programs, which employees can access online, 24 hours a day, from work or home.

Whether an organization is starting a new WHP program or looking for ways to enhance an existing one, it is important to shop around to ensure that the resources selected can be tailored to a particular worksite. For example, assess your target population's needs and interests before purchasing a particular kit or program that may or may not meet your goals and objectives. Although some programs are limited to a single topic, such as exercise or back health, other programs may provide several topic-specific kits, including an array of complimentary resources such as the following:

- Educational videos for employees and dependents to view at home or in designated work areas (e.g., worksite wellness library or multimedia break room)
- A program announcement memo that can be scanned, faxed, or e-mailed simultaneously to all employees
- A suggested time line for conducting specific phases when implementing certain activities
- A ready-to-use article on a specific topic to reprint in the company newsletter
- Reproducible table tents (folded index cards containing brief health messages to be placed on cafeteria tables)
- Large two-color posters for program announcement
- Small display posters for program announcement
- Reproducible handouts and quizzes

- Facilitator guide explaining how designated staff members or vendors can incorporate specific kits within a suggested time frame
- Bimonthly facilitator newsletters (tips on implementing certain activities)
- Participant and program evaluation forms

In today's fast-paced, tech-oriented world, a wide variety of communication resources are available to WHP personnel. Table 5.2 lists various health-education resources to inform, educate, motivate, and support employees in their quest for good health. Your choice of tools from this chart depends on a number of variables, including the target group's needs and interests, access to services, and preferred learning styles. Learning style is particularly important to consider in selecting communication resources because people learn in different ways. In addition, tool selection must factor in your program goals and objectives, resources, and budget. Analyze which tools are likely to achieve the greatest return on your investment and use different communication tools to reach as many people as possible.

When reviewing the table, avoid the temptation to select only one or two tools indicated to achieve a certain goal. Remember, successful WHP programs combine tools to achieve definable results that, when implemented, result in a cohesive intervention strategy that supports individual health decisions.

FUNDING WHP

For most companies, the decision to implement a WHP program comes down to funding. Unfortunately, in many worksite settings, WHP programs are viewed as non-essential, added-cost commodities, and thus must operate with limited or conditional funding. Sometimes planners can dodge this situation by positioning their programs in places where they will receive more visibility and management support. For instance, in

Table 5.2 Examples of Communication Tools for Health Promotion

Products and services	Communication goals						Cost per employee
	Generate awareness	Increase knowledge	Teach skills	Motivate change	Reinforce behavior	Support behavior	
Articles	3	3	1	2	2	1	Copy costs
Audiotapes	1	3	3	3	3	2	$3-$12
Books and workbooks	2	3	3	2	2	1	$4.25-$12
Booklets	2	3	3	2	2	1	$1.50-$3.75
Brochures	3	3	2	2	3	1	$0.65-$2
Calendars	3	1	1	2	2	1	$3-$9
CD-ROMs	1	3	3	3	3	1	$10-$50
Computer programs	1	3	3	2	2	1	$20-$200
Group education programs	1	3	3	3	3	3	$0-$140
Health-risk appraisal	3	2	2	3	2	2	$2-$30
Incentives	1	2	3	3	3	2	Varies
Interactive videos	1	3	2	3	3	1	$50-$100
Internet and intranet	2	3	2	2	2	3	Time to generate or productivity costs
Magazines and journals	3	3	3	3	3	1	$1-$2/issue
Memos	2	3	1	3	2	1	Copy costs or time to generate
Newsletters	3	2	2	2	3	2	$0.20-$0.30/issue
One-on-one coaching and counseling	1	3	3	3	3	3	$50-$125/hr
Paycheck stuffers	3	1	1	2	3	1	$0.15-$0.50
Postcards	3	1	1	2	3	1	$0.15-$0.50
Posters	3	1	1	2	3	1	$1.50-$6.00
Self-help and support groups	1	3	3	3	3	3	Lost production time if done on company time
Tabletop displays	3	2	1	2	3	1	$0.50-$1.50
Telephone-based services	1	3	3	3	3	3	$0-$25
Videotapes	2	3	3	3	3	1	$5-$150

Rating: 1 = low effect on communication goals; 2 = moderate effect on communication goals; 3 = high effect on communication goals.

Elin Silveous and George Pfeiffer, printed with permission. *Worksite Health,* Winter 1995, pp. 26-27.

many companies, WHP programs are housed in human resources, benefits, personnel, medical, or safety departments. Thus, they operate within a single departmental budget, rather than on a separate budget. A program may or may not do well under such an arrangement. If, for example, the department within which the WHP program is located experiences an unexpected expense, crucial dollars for funding health promotion may be cut or completely eliminated. This risk is worth taking in the view of many program directors, especially if a separate budget can be requested within the department to ensure adequate resources. In any case, the strategy of receiving greater funding for health programs by integrating them with another department is worth considering.

When employer-sponsored funding is insufficient, some employers try to offset part of the expense by charging employees some type of out-of-pocket fee for participating. For instance, a survey of midsized and large companies with on-site fitness centers reportedly charged employees annual fees that ranged from $80 to more than $500, although most charged between $150 and $250 per year (VanWormer and Pronk 2009, 240-246). While some worksites contend that fees are a financial necessity that actually boosts participation rates, other companies choose to charge a very modest fee (e.g., $5 per month) or no fee at all, hoping that free access will be an incentive.

Several alternate funding strategies that may exist for organizations who wish to look beyond conventional funding arrangements include the following:

- *Grants.* Numerous organizations offer short-term grants for employers starting new WHP initiatives. You may obtain grant information by contacting your local health department, state health department, regional health associations (such as the American Heart Association, American Lung Association, and American Diabetes Association), and federal agencies (such as the Centers for Disease Control and Prevention, National Institutes of Health, National Institute of Environmental Health Sciences, and Occupational Safety and Health Administration).

- *Pooling.* Some worksites, especially smaller employers in a defined geographic area, merge to form a business consortium, or pool, in which each worksite pays a set fee to a single vendor for selected services (e.g., employee health screenings, health fairs, on-site mammographies, and employee assistance programs).

- *Health plan.* Many worksites, especially midsize and larger employers, possess the leverage to negotiate complimentary or discounted WHP programs from their health plan. Commonly negotiated services include health fairs, health screenings, flu vaccinations, and specific theme-oriented events (e.g., Great American Smokeout, Breast Cancer Awareness Month). Of course, with today's aging workforces, many midsize and large employers are pressing their health plans to provide additional risk-reduction services, such as health coaching, disease management, customized health-risk assessments, and so forth.

PREPARING A BUDGET

Preparing and controlling a budget is essential to the success of a WHP program. Depending on the size of the program, a WHP practitioner may have full budget responsibility or may need to work with someone within the company who has budgeting expertise and responsibility. Regardless of the situation, the health promotion practitioner should be familiar with the company's budgeting process as well as with standard budgeting principles. In preparing a program budget, it's important to consider key factors, such as the following:

- *How others within the organization view WHP.* It is important to gain as much information and insight about how your department, programs, and services fit into the overall mission and goals of the organization. Thus, it pays to regularly review the WHP vision, mission, and goals to see whether they truly reflect the organization's vision, mission, and goals.

- *How recent programs and budgets have performed.* In taking stock of recent activities, it is important to ask key questions. Which programs appear to produce the highest value for the least expense? Could an underachieving program yield greater value with some additional funding, realignment with or integration within another program, more focused, population-specific marketing, or different day and time offerings? What piece of the budget should be scrutinized further at regular intervals (e.g., staff, incentives, marketing, evaluation, equipment, and so on)? Either a benefit-cost analysis (BCA) or a cost-effectiveness analysis (CEA), highlighted in chapter 8, can be a useful tool to help you make these decisions.

- *Using program-analysis outcomes.* Head-to-head evaluations of specific programs can be used to create cost projections for each line item on your budget, such as salaries, equipment purchases, facility operations, marketing, and office supplies.

- *Soliciting input from all staff members.* Expenses for each department should be assessed at regular intervals. Consider using the principles of **zero-based budgeting (ZBB)** so all department heads are encouraged to think about and justify what they are doing. This type of budgeting requires staff members to build their case for each expense item, starting with a zero-based dollar amount.

- *Allowing for flexibility.* It is essential to be flexible when creating a budget to allow for inevitable changes in participation, operational cost variations, staff compensation increases, seasonal influences, and other fluctuations that distinguish expectations from reality. Thus, it is important to keep notes throughout the year to monitor any changes that will help decision makers identify possible reasons for any aberration and make appropriate adjustments in next year's budget.

- *Keeping everything in perspective.* Budgetary control is time consuming. Budget goals are important, but they should not come at the expense of programming goals. For example, is it really worth spending several days to research, analyze, and justify a new $300 program when your total budget exceeds $100,000? A spirit of common sense and practicality will help budget makers maintain a level of objectivity that is crucial for effective budget preparation.

When planning a budget, WHP practitioners are likely to be faced with one of two distinct situations. The first one, **top-down budgeting,** may be the least desirable, but is likely the most common planning process. The main premise behind the top-down approach is that health promotion practitio-

ners are given a finite dollar amount to run their operation. As you can imagine, this type of defined monetary allowance generates various questions, such as the following:

- Which programs are most important?
- Should we keep the long-running programs that keep going up in price?
- How do we fund new initiatives?
- Is it more cost-effective to deliver our existing (or new) program with in-house staff, to contract with an outside vendor, or to negotiate complimentary or discounted services with our health plan?

The other common process for budget planning is the bottom-up approach, sometimes referred to as zero-based budgeting (ZBB). With a ZBB approach, you essentially start with zero funds and build a case for each item in your proposal. Unlike the traditional (incremental) budgeting approach, in which previous funding amounts are assumed to continue, ZBB requires that every WHP resource be listed with a justification of its cost. Fundamentally, ZBB assumes no current commitment from decision makers. All items must be subjected to some level of benefit-cost analysis. Although WHP practitioners may prefer this approach, it also generates a bevy of important questions. Moreover, this approach invariably generates the fear of leaving out an initiative because you are concerned it will not be approved. On the other hand, if you propose a program that carries an excessive budget, it may bring more scrutiny on all itemized components.

WHP practitioners using the bottom-up budgeting process must also be prepared to explain and justify why specific initiatives are proposed. Was the proposed initiative selected because it's part of the newest fad? Is it top management's preference? Is it to head off a competitor's newly publicized employee health initiative? Or, is it because it has the strongest potential to generate a positive *return on investment (ROI)*? Thus, whether a top-down, bottom-up, or combined approach is used in preparing a WHP budget, various factors should be carefully considered.

WHP budget makers need to develop a sound proposal for decision makers. In general, a proposal is more likely to be accepted if it includes some level of cost itemization and shows how proposed programs and resources can meet company needs. For example, research conducted by staff members at one worksite showed probable costs for conducting a program for lower-back stretching and flexibility, as reflected in table 5.3. Based on the comparison shown in the table, the projected benefit

Table 5.3 Direct Cost of Items and Projected Benefits of Prework Stretching

Direct costs	Daily	Weekly	Monthly	Yearly
Personnel (program leader)				
Time required (hrs.)*	0.167	0.835	3.34	40.08
Hourly wage ($)	× 15.00	× 15.00	× 15.00	× 15.00
Total personnel cost ($) =	2.50	12.52	50.10	601.2
Productivity (employees)				
Work time for program (hrs)*	0.167	0.835	3.34	40.08
Employees' hourly wage ($)	× 13.50	× 13.50	× 13.50	× 13.50
Number of employees	× 300	× 300	× 300	× 300
Total productivity cost ($) =	676.35	3,381.75	13,527.00	162,324
Total cost of personnel and productivity				$162,925
Projected benefits (1-Year Effect)				
Health care spending				
Number of employees				300
Company's back-injury rate last year (20%)				× .20
Number of employees reporting back injury				60
Average cost per back-injury claim ($)				× 3,015
Total cost of lower-back injury claim ($) =				180,900
Productivity loss				
Number of disability days per back injury				3.5
Number of back injuries				× 60
Number of disability days for back injuries				210
Average cost of lost productivity per day** ($)				× 138.24
Total cost of lost productivity per year ($) =				29,030
Total costs of health care and productivity loss				**$209,930**
Estimated effect of program (90%)*				× .90
Estimated cost avoidance (benefit)				**$188,935**
Total costs of personnel and productivity				−$162,925
Net savings				**$26,012**

*Time required reflects an average of 10 min. per day for the program facilitator to prepare the worksite and perform the stretching and flexibility routine.

**Based on average hourly compensation (wage of $13.50 per hour and company-paid benefits of $3.78 per hour) multiplied by 8 hours (average workday).

***Based on selected findings reported in the professional literature.

($188,935) exceeds the projected program costs ($162,925), suggesting a program for lower-back health on company time would be a worthy investment.

WHP program developers should determine budgetary needs based on the types of resources required for a new or existing program. In setting up a budget, program planners need to distinguish between variable and fixed expenses to forecast appropriately. For example, variable expenses are costs that vary from month to month (e.g., utilities, advertising, certification renewals, and equipment purchases). In contrast, fixed expenses are costs that are consistent throughout the year (e.g., personnel salaries, facility and equipment leasing, and maintenance).

Because new programs may require greater start-up expenses for new personnel, staff training, facilities, equipment, and materials, you can use an expense-management grid to evaluate budgeting options (see table 5.4). When developing a customized grid for a particular worksite, first list the major expense categories for a specific program or activity across the top of the grid. Second, list specific options on the left side of the grid. Third, review the available literature, conduct a survey of the local market, or talk with other worksite health professionals to help you identify major issues. Finally, use all this information to identify possible relationships on the grid. For example, results from a market survey may indicate that it is more time- and cost-effective to hire a local physical therapist on a part-time basis to conduct lower-back health seminars at a worksite rather than to pay to train and certify a staff member for this task.

Table 5.4 Expense Management Grid

Expense categories	Personnel	Facilities	Utilities	Equipment	Materials	Maintenance	Advertising
Major issues							
Options							
Full-time							
Part-time							
Services negotiated							
Services contracted							
Services donated							
On-site operation							
Off-site operation							
Purchase new							
Purchase used							
Bartered							
Leased							
Donated							
Rented							
Other (list)							

Because the direct worth of expense items varies from site to site, program planners should consider various options to determine the most efficient way to use specific resources. Some typical questions during this phase include the following:

- Is it more economical for in-house personnel to operate in on-site facilities and programs compared to with an outside (contract) vendor? What is the cost difference?

- Is new equipment needed, or will used equipment do? If used or leased equipment is suitable, what type of warranty can be obtained? How often will the equipment need to be replaced?

- Is it more cost-effective to pool our resources with those of local worksites to sponsor a health fair or employee health expo?

- Can we barter with the local college or university to have their faculty and graduate students conduct employee-health screenings in exchange for using our worksite as a research venue?

- Will an in-house EAP be as appealing to employees as an external EAP?

- What is the best use of specific resources available from local health agencies (e.g., American Heart Association, American Cancer Society, American Lung Association, March of Dimes, or the county health department)?

- Do in-house staff have the time and skills to conduct an evaluation as quickly and objectively as an outside firm?

Prior to preparing a formal budget proposal for key decision makers to review, WHP practitioners should familiarize themselves with three strategies that may help with budget justification. The common denominator in all three strategies is program planning.

The first strategy is to ensure that your program can provide short-term and long-term results. Planning programs that produce results at different intervals will ensure that practitioners always have some data to present to management. For example, back-injury prevention, medical self-care, prenatal programs, and flu-vaccination campaigns are just some examples known to produce positive short-term results. In contrast, verifiable cost savings from risk-factor reduction and exercise programs are more likely to produce long-term outcomes. By rotating the availability of these programs or the level of effort, emphasis, and resources, you can avoid situations in which no data is readily available for key decision makers. By and large, this programming flexibility enhances your ability to provide interval-based results that can be an effective strategy for budget justification.

The second strategy consists of securing an agreement from management when cost justification data is presented. If using this strategy, it will need to be presented during the proposal phase for program planning. This decision needs to be well documented. Periodic reminders may be necessary.

The third strategy for budget justification involves the sharing of data on a frequent basis, perhaps monthly or quarterly. The expectation from this approach needs to be clear from the onset. It is common for WHP practitioners to track and report different types of participation data (e.g., utilization, penetration, adherence) on a monthly basis. Yet, employee risk factor or health data on behavior change are usually reported at quarterly intervals. In contrast, cost justification data (e.g., medical, workers' compensation, productivity) require longer time frames to accurately measure and verify. These should be announced at certain times to receive ample attention. For example, highlighting this data before the annual process for budget approval or when an economic downturn possibly threatens the WHP budget may be a smart, strategic decision. Using this strategy in conjunction with the second strategy may be particularly useful in worksites where data is highly valued.

PREPARING YOUR PROPOSAL

Once you have made key decisions about goal setting, funding and budgeting, and managing WHP programs, it's time to prepare a proposal for management. Presenting the program proposal is a crucial stage in the planning phase. If you present the proposal poorly, the plug may be pulled on the program before it ever has a chance to prove its value.

In preparing a WHP program proposal, it is essential to address a company's specific health-management needs. Although every proposal will vary according to the unique culture and needs of an organization and its workforce, each should include the following sections, at a minimum:

- Problem identification
- Goals

- Environmental assessment
- Worksite strategies
- Resource assessment
- Proposed program
- Expected costs
- Expected benefits
- Overall benefit-cost projection

For example, assume that a company's health care costs are rising faster than projected and that a WHP program is being proposed. When reviewing the company's health care claims data, program planners discover that (1) the most common type of health care claim filed by employees is musculoskeletal and that (2) lower-back injuries are involved in most of these claims. Based on this information, program planners prepare a proposal for a back-injury prevention program (see below).

SAMPLE PROGRAM PROPOSAL

1. Problem Identification
Program planners reviewed the company's health care claims and cost data, which revealed the most common claims to be musculoskeletal:

Type	# of claims	Total cost	Average cost/claim
Back injuries	100	$65,000	$650
Knee injuries	33	$9,174	278
Shoulder injuries	14	$1,400	100

2. Goal
Reduce the number and average cost per claim of musculoskeletal injuries, especially lower-back injuries, within one year.

3. Environmental Assessment
Further analysis and worksite observations by on-site personnel indicated the following:

- Employees most affected: 25- to 45-year-old men working in the shipping department.
- Most common time of occurrence: 75% of all lower-back injuries occurred in the first two hours of the work shift.
- Type of injury: 90% of all back injuries were classified as muscle strains in the lower back.
- Activity at time of injury: 60% of all muscle-strain injuries in the lower back occurred while the employees were lifting, 30% occurred when employees were pulling or pushing, and 10% occurred when employees stood up from a seated position.

(continued)

4. Worksite Strategies

In-house staff members called local employers and reviewed several articles from scientific journals on prevention programs for lower-back injuries. They found numerous companies with successful programs, such as the following:

Company	Program features	Impact
Biltrite Company (Chelsea, MA)	Back education, prework stretching	90% drop in workers' comp costs
Capital Wire (Plano, TX)	Prework stretching, employee education	Fewer back injuries; $180,000 saved
County government (northern California)	Back education, training, fitness activities, ergonomic improvement	179% return on investment within one year
Lockheed Corporation (Sunnyvale, CA)	Prework stretching, employee seminars	67.5% drop in back-injury costs

5. Resource Assessment

What types of on-site resources can be used to develop an effective prevention program for lower-back injuries? Staff members conducted an on-site inventory that indicated available and necessary resources:

- Available Resources

    Facility: Large warehouse area

    Promotional materials: Employee newsletter

    Budget: $1,500 is available in the human resources department's discretionary fund

- Needed Resources

    Equipment: Padded floor mats needed for back and abdominal floor exercises

    Incentives: A quarterly sweepstakes program with prizes!

6. Proposed Program

Based on the health problem identified and available resources, program planners recommend the following program, targeting 50 shipping department employees.

Back Basics: A Worksite Back-Injury Prevention Program

- *Phase 1 (January): Awareness and publicity.* The number of lower-back injuries reported at the worksite will appear in this month's issue of the employee newsletter. They will also be repeated on a quarterly basis. The article will explain the primary reasons for the new program and the specific responsibilities for shipping department supervisors, employees, and the occupational health nurse. This information will also be shared during the next safety meeting (held on the second and fourth Mondays of each month).

- *Phase 2 (February): Training.* The occupational health nurse will conduct training sessions for all shipping department supervisors and employees during bimonthly safety meetings. Topics will include back anatomy, ergonomic factors, and proper techniques for lifting, pulling, and pushing.

- *Phase 3 (March): Incentives.* Worksite posters, newsletter articles, and weekly e-mail messages will describe how to enter the "Back Basics Sweepstakes" program. All shipping department employees reporting no back injuries in the previous quarter can compete for prizes each quarter.

- *Phase 4 (March): Implementation.* Shipping department supervisors will lead their respective employee teams through a mandatory back stretching and strengthening routine during the first five minutes of their work shift. After the first week, individual employees will assume responsibility for leading daily sessions on a rotating basis.
- *Phase 5 (July): Monitoring and evaluation.* The occupational health nurse will review back-injury data every six months to determine the impact of the daily prework routine and the need, if any, to revise the protocol for greater influence in the future.

7. Expected Costs

Based on the identification and needs assessment, program planners estimate that annual operating costs for the proposed program will be as follows:

- Personnel: No additional cost
- Facility: No additional cost (will use existing space)
- Equipment: Padded floor mats; $400 [50 employees × $8.00 per mat]
- Promotions and sweepstakes prizes: $250 per quarter, or $1,000 per year
- Total: $1,400

8. Expected Benefits

Based on a review of other worksite prevention programs for lower-back injuries, the following benefits are expected to occur within 12 months of the program's inception:

Fewer job-related back injuries

Fewer back-injury absences

Reduced costs from lower-back claims

Greater productivity

Improved musculoskeletal flexibility

Less overtime expenses paid to replacement workers

9. Overall Benefit-Cost Projection

The proposed program is modeled after successful worksite programs for back-injury prevention. It is expected to conservatively reduce designated cost outcomes by at least 10%. For example, the proposed program should cut the number of projected back injuries from 90 to 81 (10% drop). Since the average cost of one lower-back strain is about $1,000, a 10% impact would produce cost savings of approximately $9,000. If two or more injuries are averted during the year, anticipated cost savings would exceed programs costs ($1,400), as shown here:

Injuries avoided	Benefit	Program cost	Benefit-cost ratio
1	$1,000	$1,400	[.71:1]
2	$2,000	$1,400	1.43:1
3	$3,000	$1,400	2.14:1
4	$4,000	$1,400	2.85:1
5	$5,000	$1,400	3.57:1
6	$6,000	$1,400	4.28:1
7	$7,000	$1,400	5.00:1
8	$8,000	$1,400	5.63:1
9	$9,000	$1,400	6.23:1

To be effective, every proposal must meet at least three criteria:

1. The identified problem is clearly described and quantified.

2. A practical strategy to address the problem is proposed.

3. Expected benefits are based on real case studies and are likely to exceed programming costs.

While reviewing a proposal, management may want to know when a program or strategy will pay off or break even. For example, assume a company is planning to convert a rarely used conference room into a center with a full-time staff of two certified health coaches. By determining specific costs and estimated usage patterns of the health-coaching center, program planners can factor this information into a **break-even analysis**. A sample break-even analysis follows.

BREAK-EVEN ANALYSIS FOR A HEALTH COACHING CENTER

1. DETERMINE START-UP COSTS FOR CONVERTING AN EXISTING SPACE (YEAR 1 ONLY):

Health center equipment: $50,000

2. DETERMINE ANNUAL FIXED COSTS:

Head health coach: $45,000*

Associate health coach: $40,000*

Maintenance of equipment: $1,000

Depreciation of equipment: $5,000

Program incentives: $3,000

*An annual salary and benefits (compensation) inflation rate of 3% is applied. For example, the head health coach's first-year salary of $45,000 would be $46,350 in year 2, and the associate health coach's first-year salary of $40,000 would be $41,200 in year 2.

3. DETERMINE ANNUAL VARIABLE COSTS:

Utilities, office materials, and so on: $4,000

4. CALCULATE TOTAL START-UP, FIXED, AND VARIABLE COSTS: $148,000

5. DETERMINE PROJECTED USAGE RATE OF FITNESS CENTER:

Size of workforce: 1,000 employees

Percentage of workforce expected to participate: 20% (national average)

Usage rate: 200 employees

Number of weekly visits per participant: 2

Total weekly visits: 400 (200 × 2)

6. DETERMINE FINANCIAL BENEFITS FROM THE FITNESS CENTER VISITS:

The desired outcomes will vary from program to program. The outcome variables classified as corporate benefits (cost savings) in this example are reduced absenteeism and lower medical-care expenses.

Corporate benefit per participant: $6.57**

Number of total weekly participant visits: 400

Total corporate benefit per week: $2,628 ($6.57 × 400)

** ($3.69 + $2.88 = $6.57): Based on research studies showing health-coaching participants (1) are absent at least 1.2 fewer days than nonparticipants: 1.2 days × $320 = $384 per absence, $384 ÷ 52 weeks = $7.38 ÷ 2 (weekly visits) = $3.69 per visit, and (2) incur at least $300 less in annual medical-care expenses than nonparticipants: $300 ÷ 52 weeks = $5.77 ÷ 2 (weekly visits) = $2.88 per visit.

BREAK-EVEN ANALYSIS FOR A HEALTH COACHING CENTER
(continued)

Note: The daily compensation value of $320 is based on the geographic region-based average wage of $20 per hour. Thus, $20 × 8 hours = $160 daily compensation paid to both the absent worker and a replacement worker.

7. DETERMINE BREAK-EVEN POINT BY DIVIDING TOTAL CUMULATIVE COST BY FINANCIAL BENEFIT PER WEEK:

Total cumulative costs: $248,550 (year 1=$148,000; year 2=$100,550)

Corporate benefit per week: $2,628

Time of participation needed to break even: 94.5 weeks (22 months)

[$248,555 ÷ $2,628 = 94.5]

Based on the preceding break-even analysis, the company's health coaching investment is projected to pay for itself (break even) near the end of the second year (between 94 and 95 weeks).

Note that year 2 costs would be approximately $50,000 less than year 1 since all of the coaching equipment was purchased in the first year. Thus, year 2 costs were computed as follows: Projected annual cost ($148,000) minus year 1 equipment cost ($50,000) = $98,000; $98,000 plus $1,350 (year 2 salary increase for head coach) plus $1,200 (year 2 salary increase for associate coach) equals $100,550.

8. PLOT CUMULATIVE COSTS AND BENEFITS ON A TIME FRAME (SEE FIGURE 5.1):

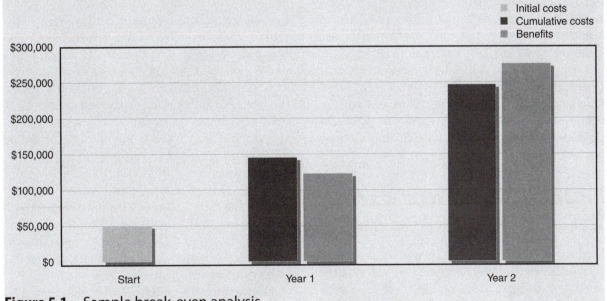

Figure 5.1 Sample break-even analysis.

In using any economic analysis technique, be aware that various factors can jeopardize expected outcomes. In our preceding example, the estimated time frame of 94.5 weeks may be extended by unforeseen or uncontrollable events—if the participation level drops below the expected level, if unexpected programming costs are incurred, or if employee wages and benefits or the company's cost to replace absent workers increase faster than absenteeism costs. On the other hand, if participation levels exceed the expected level, if participant absenteeism drops, or if wages and replacement costs increase more slowly than absenteeism costs, then the break-even point would occur before 94.5 weeks.

Once the program has been proposed and accepted by management, the program planner is nearly ready to implement the program. However, three more steps are necessary before the program can be safely launched: administratively positioning the program to achieve maximum success, conducting appropriate employee-health screenings, and giving the program a trial run. The following section offers strategies for positioning WHP programs. The other steps are described in chapter 7.

Aside from budgeting considerations addressed in previous sections, strategically positioning the WHP program and its personnel is also critical in achieving long-term success. A common denominator of successful WHP programs is the ability of its staff to effectively work as a cohesive team (intradepartmentally) as well as with personnel in other departments (interdepartmentally). WHP programs are far more likely to succeed if they garner and sustain support from various decision makers throughout an organization. Thus, strategically positioning WHP in a broad-based framework of **integrated health management** is strongly recommended, if not required, to gain the political, administrative, and financial support needed for long-term success.

POSITIONING WHP IN AN INTEGRATED FRAMEWORK

Since the mid-1990s, a growing number of worksites have developed an integrated approach to health management to enhance employee health, safety, productivity, and morale. In fact, various studies on the organizational frameworks of many companies have shown a direct relationship between integrated health management and cost control. As a group, companies operating an integrated approach show that the cost of average medical care increases about one-third less than the national average. Essentially, this cost-control advantage enables such progressive-minded companies to make real investments in human capital (e.g., employee training and incentives) as well as business operations (e.g., research and development and equipment upgrades) that are essential for building long-term profitability.

Of course, positioning WHP issues and programs within the integrated teamwork of various decision makers and departments requires both a philosophical and operational transformation in a worksite. Philosophically, decision makers across various departments need to understand the basic foundation of body-mind-spirit wellness (e.g., holistic health) and how important it is for organizations to foster each dimension.

As a valuable catalyst for change, WHP practitioners need to seek, encourage, and foster collaborative relationships with various departments. This often requires a culture change and a commitment to breaking down organizational silos of individual interest. Consequently, WHP personnel can partner with others in human resources, benefits, risk management, safety, and medical services to effectively shift from operating independent cost centers to health and productivity management programs that are more integrated (see figure 5.2). One of the most compelling propositions is that an integrated framework can provide an efficient

What key value proposition can they offer in this effort?

platform for reaching employees at many risk levels at the same time (see figure 4.1 in chapter 4). In addition, a team of allied WHP personnel possesses the leverage to study the impact of health on productivity, safety, and profitability.

Operationally, allied WHP practitioners working within an integrated health-management framework can foster real worksite cases of opportunity and success. For example, consider the following situation, which actually occurred at an insurance company. An employee on disability for a mental-health diagnosis requested a leave of absence as an accommodation. The return-to-work professional identified potential alternatives and requested input from

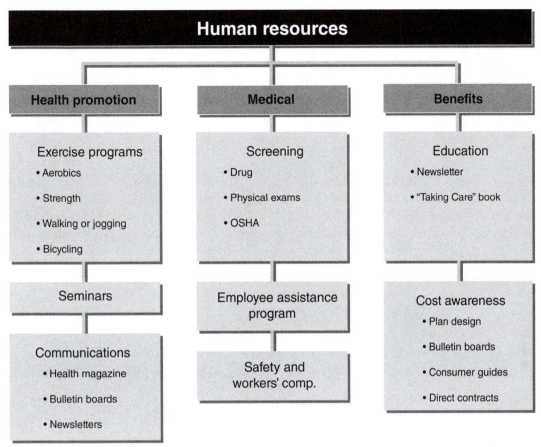

Figure 5.2 A sample framework for integrated health management in a midsized to large organization.

the employee assistance program (EAP). Through that relationship, the employee received counseling and coaching that supported an early return to work. The approach also provided tips on life skills that the employee continues to use to successfully manage the mental-health issues. In another instance, an occupational health nurse conducted a basic health screening on a new employee and detected poor lower-back flexibility. The new employee also reported a history of lower-back injuries during a health-risk appraisal. Since the nurse was working in an integrated health-management framework, she was able to strategically communicate with the following people:

- Human resources to discuss appropriate job tasks within the employee's physical capabilities

- WHP staff members to develop a personalized back-health program to improve flexibility
- Safety personnel to educate the new employee on company policies for proper lifting
- Benefits personnel to inform the new employee on approved health care providers (e.g., back care providers)

Even small employers have shown benefits from an integrated framework of health management. The overall success of this approach depends largely on an organization's ability to do the following:

- Develop realistic health-management goals.
- Employ health-management personnel with the skills to achieve each goal.

- Assign appropriate personnel to specific goals.
- Establish an operational framework that enhances interpersonal and interdepartmental communication and teamwork.

An integrated approach, though increasing in popularity nationwide, also has potential disadvantages as well. The main one involves autonomy. By its nature, an integrated approach depends on teamwork and decision by committee. This can work well, but the decision-making process will likely break down if departmental representatives push their personal agendas. When this occurs, department leaders might become frustrated over the inability to arrive at decisions in a timely manner. In some cases, WHP personnel are discouraged to find out how little clout they have in an integrated approach. In order to minimize reactions that can lead to wide-scale alienation and fallout among personnel, it is important to develop an integrated framework and decision-making protocol that fosters input from all stakeholders. Such efforts obviously require constant monitoring and revisions to factor in changes in personnel, budget, politics, and culture that will occur over time.

ASSESSING YOUR PLANNING EFFORTS

As you proceed from the program planning phase to creating a healthy worksite culture (see chapter 6), check to see whether your planning efforts have created specific standards for success, such as the following:

- A commitment from senior management to dedicate sufficient resources, including funding, personnel time, equipment, and facilities. (Ideally, management also shows support by participating in the program.)
- A clear statement of philosophy, purpose, and goals that declares the organization's commitment to motivate and assist a significant portion of employees to practice healthier lifestyles.
- A process for assessing organizational and individual needs, interests, risks, and costs.
- Leadership from well-qualified, health promotion professionals in the program's design, implementation, and ongoing operations.

- A program design that addresses the most significant health risks, specific risks within the employee population, and needs of the organization.
- High-quality programs and appropriate incentives that motivate participants to achieve lasting behavior changes and a higher quality of life.
- Effective marketing to achieve and maintain high participation rates.
- Efficient systems for program operation and administration.
- Evaluation procedures for assessing program quality and outcomes.
- A system of communication for sharing program results with employees, staff, and senior management.

What Would You Do?

Suppose you work for a company that has never had WHP. Management has asked you to design and implement a new education program for employees on medical self-care. Your research efforts show that the most effective intervention is voluntary. It should consist of self-care books, financial incentives, and quarterly on-site seminars. You learn that this program can yield a monetary benefit as great as $4 for every $1 spent. However, research suggests that a participation rate of 50% for at least a year is necessary to achieve a positive benefit-cost ratio.

Your worksite is currently downsizing, and management expects you to show a positive return within six months. In preparing your proposal for the new program, what should you do to achieve management's goal within the shorter time frame? Should you propose a mandatory program to ensure 100% participation? If not, should you recommend higher financial incentives to motivate a high rate of voluntary participation? Should you offer a higher number of on-site seminars? What would you do?

CHAPTER 5 WRAP-UP

Key Points

- Key facts and information should be presented in a proposal to build a strong business case for WHP programs.

- Allocating appropriate resources requires a careful assessment of employees' needs, interests, and work schedules, as well as in-house budgetary allowances and other factors.

- With the increased advent of outsourcing, decision makers should carefully weigh potential advantages and disadvantages of using external vendors.

- In exploring funding options, WHP personnel should consider specific factors for preparing, presenting, operating, and sustaining a budget.

- A break-even analysis is a good evaluation procedure to determine if, and when, the financial value of positive outcomes (benefits) may equal or exceed the financial cost of a WHP program or policy.

- An integrated framework enables allied WHP personnel to collectively achieve health-management goals.

Glossary

Break-even analysis—An evaluation procedure used to determine if and when the financial value of positive outcomes may equal or exceed the financial cost of a WHP intervention.

business case—Strong evidence used to show why an organization needs and can benefit from strategically aligned WHP programs and policies.

employee assistance program (EAP)—A structured support service offered on-site or off-site designed to help employees with personal needs and concerns.

integrated health management—An organizational framework in which full-time and allied WHP personnel work together to develop and implement programs and policies to enhance employee health.

20 Factor Test—Twenty criteria used by the Internal Revenue Service to determine if a worker is a full-time or a part-time employee.

top-down budgeting—A common budget planning approach in which WHP personnel are given a designated amount of money to run their operation.

zero-based budgeting (ZBB)—Often called *bottom-up budgeting,* in this process a budget is prepared from scratch (with zero funds). It requires justification of all itemized costs.

Bibliography

Health and Wellness Association. 2010. "Annual employer wellness survey." Accessed October 29. www.healthandwellnessassociation.com/index.php.

Kaiser Family Foundation. 2010. "Employer health benefits 2010 annual survey." Accessed October 29. http://ehbs.kff.org/?page=Charts&id=1&sn=11&p=1.

Leutzinger, J. 2009. "The wellness budget." *The Wellness Councils of America.* Accessed December 24. http://infopoint.welcoa.org/blueprints/blueprint1/publications/wi_budget.html.

Meltzer, B. 2009. "Should you outsource wellness?" *HR Benefits Alert.* Accessed: December 28. www.hrbenefitsalert.com/should-you-outsource-wellness.

Miami Dade College Human Resources Department. 2009. "IRS 20 factor test on employment status." Accessed December 18. www.mdc.edu/hr/Operations/AFS/IRSFactorTest.pdf.

Shi, L. 1993. "A cost-benefit analysis of a California county's back injury prevention program." *Public Health Reports* 2: 204-211.

VanWormer, J. and N. Pronk. 2009. *ACSM's worksite health handbook.* 2nd ed. Champaign, IL: Human Kinetics.

Looking Ahead

Now that funding and resource issues have been considered, it's time to establish a worksite environment that will foster a successful WHP program. Chapter 6 provides several strategies for building healthy environmental and cultural norms that will cultivate, enhance, and sustain WHP programming efforts.

Part III

Providing and Evaluating Worksite Health Promotion

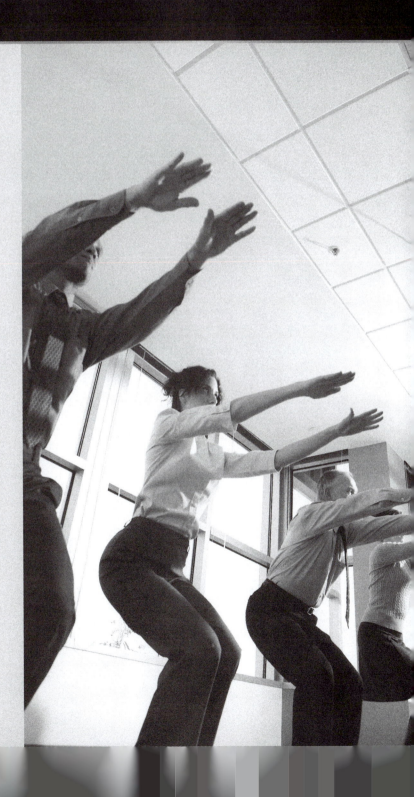

This part of the book includes three interdependent chapters focused on program implementation and evaluation. Chapter 6 highlights how to establish a suitable worksite environment and culture for WHP and provides tips for cultivating a safer, calmer workforce. Chapter 7 presents strategies for actively promoting WHP in today's technology-driven workplaces, engaging employee participation, and assessing and managing employee and organizational risk. Once programs are underway, the evaluation tips presented in chapter 8 can be applied. Evaluation results can then be used in future programming decisions.

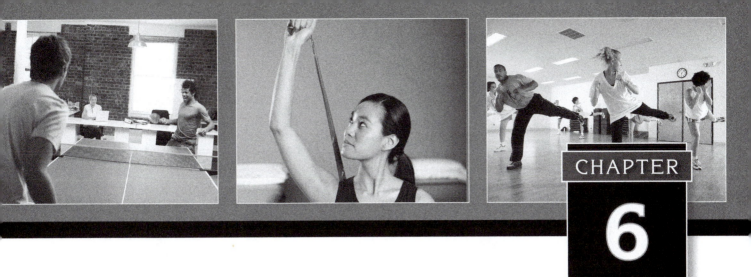

Building a Healthy Worksite Environment

LEARNING OBJECTIVES

After reading this chapter, you will be able to do the following:

✔ Construct a scenario that reflects a worksite with a healthy culture and a worksite with an unhealthy culture.

✔ Describe several ways to build a healthy worksite environment.

✔ Explain why employers should assess the risk of cumulative trauma disorders in the workforce and provide appropriate prevention strategies.

✔ Cite some examples of how WHP initiatives can positively affect rates of occupational accidents, injury, and illness.

✔ Identify several factors that should be considered before establishing an employee assistance program (EAP).

With the information in the preceding chapters addressing goal development, programmatic strategies, and budgetary options, it won't be long until you can launch WHP programs, activities, and policies. However, is your worksite physically, environmentally, politically, and culturally suitable to host, support, and sustain WHP initiatives? This chapter discusses how to deal with work-related issues while creating a healthy worksite environment and culture. (See chapter 2 for an overview of an environmental check sheet, culture audit, and related assessment tools.)

When assessing a worksite's suitability for WHP, there are several dimensions to consider:

• *Physical make-up.* The worksite has an accommodating layout that all employees can easily navigate, essential equipment and resources for high productivity, ergonomically friendly workstations, and so on.

• *Environmental quality.* This includes clean air, proper protection equipment and safe guards, adequate supplies of clean water, and noise control.

• *Employee-centered policies.* These are the policies, standards, and regulations that preserve and promote employee health, privacy, and confidentiality.

• *Health-promoting culture.* Here, pro-health attitudes, beliefs, and norms are commonly reflected by employee and management actions.

As a starting point, consider these two worksites. One has a cafeteria that provides only fried foods and vending machines that carry high-fat, high-sugar snacks and drinks. The second worksite has a cafeteria and vending machines that largely dispense healthy foods, snacks, beverages, and fresh fruit.

Which of these norms would you want at your worksite?

The cultural norm (i.e., expected behavior) in the first company is for employees to consume fried, high-fat, and high-sugar food and drinks. In contrast, the norm in the second company is for employees to eat a healthy diet.

It should come as no surprise that employees are more motivated to lead healthy lifestyles in a worksite that places a high priority on health. Company policies that do not promote healthy lifestyles should be reviewed and changed. In most cases, change should be gradually phased in so employees have time to adjust to new policies. It usually takes a few weeks for a minor change and a few months for a major change (Americans for Nonsmokers' Rights 2010).

Before establishing any major changes in policy, management may take a few months to solicit employees' feedback on the proposed change. In some instances, if management personnel have decided the change is needed, they may choose not to solicit employees' opinions. In both cases, a company will usually spend several months educating employees about the need for the proposed change. Depending on the type of program or policy being proposed, a company may choose to introduce it on a trial basis—say, in certain locations or with a particular group of employees—and then expand it to the remainder of the workforce within a designated time frame. (See chapter 4 for a step-by-step process for phasing in a clean-air policy.)

CULTIVATING A HEALTHY CULTURE

Depending on an organization's culture and goals, top-level management personnel or WHP practitioners can implement various strategies to initiate, promote, and foster healthy behaviors. Unquestionably, implementing health promotion activities and incentives that are built around individual, environmental, cultural, and organizational values is far more effective than focusing on any single dimension. These strategies might be general or more specific, such as taking an ergonomic approach or emphasizing exercise and education.

Ergonomics is a science concerned with arranging objects so that people can interact with them effectively and safely. Fundamentally, *ergonomic strategies* involve designing or placing equipment to make employees' work tasks more efficient or easy. For example, an organization might purchase state-of-the-art office equipment (e.g., custom chairs that adjust to suit each employee's body shape and physical needs) to cut the risk of overuse (cumulative trauma) injuries. Moreover, ergonomic-centric workstations help employees buffer physical and mental stressors, leading to more efficient work patterns and a boost in overall productivity.

Yet, building a healthy workplace culture requires more than ergonomic transformations. It also requires concentrated and integrated efforts that encourage employees and reward them for promoting their health when they are away from their workstations. For example, what can be done to cultivate and foster healthy norms regarding employees' activity during break times, cafeteria and vending machine options, employee assistance services, health-risk assessments, educational advancement, and recreational venues? Exercise, nutrition, stress management, and other incentives that promote personal health play an important role in supporting a healthy worksite culture. In building a healthy worksite, WHP practitioners should partner with other allied health personnel to plan, implement, and sustain important culture-building strategies. Depending on the size and type of worksite, potential partnerships should be explored with human resources and benefits managers, risk managers, occupational health nurses, medical directors, safety managers, and employee assistance directors.

A STANDING DEBATE

In today's computer-centric workplace, more employees spend longer than ever at a desk, using the same limited set of muscles and joints in the same ways. The cumulative damage caused by sitting in a fixed position for eight or more hours is not only a threat to the individual's physical health, but also to productivity. Perhaps the most publicized trend that touches upon ergonomics and health promotion is sit-stand workstations. In an October 2010 Washington Post article, those touting the benefits of standing at raised desks note that they feel focused and awake, while health experts compare the health dangers of extended periods of sitting to the metabolic benefits of standing. Moreover, they contend that workstations with sit-to-stand flexibility provide the widest range of movement and posture for employees, allowing them to alternate from a sitting to a standing position at will. They also feel that standing helps avoid the compression of the spine that can occur from long-term sitting, reducing the risk of back pain. However, other health experts disagree, pointing out that long periods of standing can contribute to back and vascular injuries. While many ergonomic adjustments can be made to improve the comfort of a sit-down workstation, including ergonomic seating and ergonomic keyboarding practices, experts have found that any sustained posture or movement will create stress and strain on the body. However, studies have shown that changing positions throughout the work day can help keep physical stress from accumulating (i.e., repetitive stress injuries).

In realizing the basis of both viewpoints, WHP practitioners may find themselves in the midst of this debate. What should employers who are facing this debate do to clear the air? In gauging the potential value of sit-stand workstations for office-based employees, employers should first carefully assess each worker's health status, type of work, and overall ability to comfortably adopt a sit-and-stand routine. As with any new ergonomic strategy in the workplace, there's no guarantee that all employees will accept or adapt their work style around a new approach. Thus, it's to everyone's benefit—employers and employees alike—to gradually adopt any new ergonomic approach on a trial run basis. Essentially, a phase-in approach allows you to conduct some preliminary trials in gauging employees' feedback and on-the-job performance outcomes. Subsequently, this key information can provide you with a clear perspective on how best to achieve the most reasonable level of ergonomic-driven health and productivity.

Ideas for Initiating Exercise Strategies in the Workplace

• Post prompts at key point-of-decision locations to encourage physical activity (e.g., signs titled "Take a Few Steps to Better Health" in stairwells to encourage stair climbing instead of taking an elevator).

• Offer gentle fitness classes that combine yoga, low-impact aerobics, and relaxation techniques. These may be offered to employees at all fitness levels, but appeal particularly to those who are new exercisers or have special physical needs or limitations (e.g., back pain, arthritis, or muscle stiffness and soreness).

• Develop trails near the worksite and encourage employees to walk or jog during lunch and break times. Trails should be in safe, highly visible areas with established safeguards.

• Provide selected pieces of exercise equipment in suitable locations for use during breaks and lunchtime. Be sure to educate employees and establish guidelines and policies before usage to ensure safety.

• Encourage employees who sit a lot to take a stretch break for better circulation and work efficiency.

• Where feasible, equip a designated break area with basketball hoops, table-tennis equipment, horseshoe pitching stations, boxing bags, and other recreational equipment.

• Offer discounts or subsidies for fitness-club memberships for those who meet minimum guidelines for usage and adherence (e.g., at least 3 sessions per week).

• Provide showers and changing facilities for people who exercise at work.

• Create departmental competitions and reward teams who meet designated exercise levels each month. If the spirit of competition conflicts with the philosophy of the WHP program, sponsor individual participation and reward effort, rather than outcomes.

Ways to Motivate Employees to Eat Healthier

The following list of nutrition-oriented strategies can be used to complement the previously listed exercise tips to improve employee health and productivity:

• Offer lunch-and-learn sessions in the company's cafeteria on a regular basis. Explore the prospect of offering these sessions on paid time or extending the designated lunch break for attendees. Consider videotaping these sessions and making them available for checkout.

• Offer webinars, or presentations for nutrition awareness and education through the company's in-house network. This may be particularly valuable for employees working at distant or multiple locations.

• Work with the vending-machine contractor to place color-coded labels on healthy food and beverage items.

• Organize a healthy potluck, including a recipe exchange.

• Gradually change vending-machine items to healthy foods and snacks.

• Offer fruit and vegetable snacks instead of junk food at meetings, in common areas, and in break rooms.

• Place monthly nutrition tips on cafeteria tables.

• Offer coupons for health-conscious eateries and restaurants to employees who meet certain health-enhancement goals.

• Subsidize or discount the cost of heart-healthy entrée offerings in the company's cafeteria and vending machines.

Informational and Educational Strategies

Some employers offer employees on-the-job educational opportunities to learn about health issues or provide employees with take-home materials. Although it's more likely that employees will take advantage of the first opportunity, many worksites are not practical environments for reading on the job (except during breaks). Here are some informational and educational strategies for reaching employees, which may need to be adapted for your workplace:

• E-mail daily or weekly health tips to all employees.

• Create and maintain bulletin boards with health information and self-development tips in high-density areas.

• If the worksite has an electronic message board in a central location, use it to announce important WHP programs, activities, and policies (e.g., health fairs, annual vaccination, competitions, and incentives).

• Create a library of books, videos, and audio cassettes for employees to check out or peruse on site.

• Stock a cart with health magazines, booklets, and brochures. Periodically move the cart to different locations around the worksite and encourage employees to take complimentary copies home and to share with others.

• Place racks of health magazines in bathroom stalls.

• Include a personal health column in the company newsletter. Check to see if your health plan has a newsletter that can incorporate some news items that are specific to your company.

• Ask WHP-program participants to write personal testimonial and endorsement letters in the company newsletter.

General Strategies

The following is a list of general strategies to consider. Some are very easy to apply, while others will take more time and should be implemented gradually.

• Provide accessible water fountains or water coolers to encourage employees to hydrate at the worksite. Distribute flyers to inform employees of the benefits of hydration and the fact that most people do not drink enough water each day.

• Convert a 10-by-10-foot (3-by-3 meter) area into a personal health kiosk, a self-contained screening and resource module equipped with an automatic blood-pressure cuff, weight scales, health brochures, and other interactive resources.

• Provide a quiet room that is equipped with comfortable seating and soft music for employees to use in stressful times. Establish guidelines to ensure that it is used properly.

• Designate a period of time for employees to participate in company-sponsored health promotion activities. For example, devote the first 5 minutes of the work shift to stretching exercises or add 15 minutes to lunch for employees to take a walk.

• Review the company's absence policy to see if the traditional allowance of sick days can be reclassified to reflect a positive connotation (e.g., *wellness days*).

• Offer employees with excellent attendance a financial bonus or an additional wellness day for each day their absences fall below the company average. Work with human resources personnel to ensure the policy does not discourage employees with real illnesses from seeking necessary health care.

• Establish smoke-free and safety-belt policies in all company vehicles and facilities.

When planning appropriate culture-building strategies for WHP, consider the demographic profile of your workforce. For example, women now make up more than 50% of America's workforce, with considerably higher representation in health care, education, and financial services. In realizing the unique challenges that millions of women face in balancing the demands of work and family, progressive-minded employers have established female-friendly policies, programs, and worksite cultures. One of the most visible examples of this cultural awakening is seen in the growth of worksite lactation services and programs for working mothers.

First National Bank (FNB) in Omaha, Nebraska, is a national leader in providing lactation services to its nursing employees. FNB's worksite setting includes a lactation suite composed of six private nursing rooms,

a refrigerator, a sink, and pumping supplies. Each suite is furnished with a glider rocker, a table, a clock radio, and other amenities to make working mothers feel right at home. Security and privacy are protected in the lactation suite—only those with current clearance gain entry. Each nursing mother is issued an access card that allows her to enter the suite. Additionally, two outsourced lactation specialists staff the suite, coordinating registration, scheduling, and training. It's a good thing—the service is becoming more popular with new mothers each year. Best of all, nursing mothers need not worry about losing work time to spend time with their babies. Management at FNB decided that time spent in the lactation suite is well spent, and it does not have to be made up. Working mothers appreciate it.

Building a health-promoting culture at the worksite cannot be done in a day—or even in a few days or weeks. The development will take some time, and is best done gradually. Programs implemented too quickly often vanish as fast as they appear. Gradual change is much more reliable. Large-scale or new programs should not be sprung on employees all at once. Small, gradual changes can effectively alter a culture's values, whereas big, sweeping changes are usually met with resistance.

REDUCING OCCUPATIONAL INJURY

Along with developing a work culture that values each person's health and overall well-being, an organization must regularly monitor the worksite to ensure that the facility and equipment are structurally and operationally safe. The risk of accidents always exists, but if all stakeholders respond properly to the mishap, the same accident should never occur twice.

In 1970, the **Occupational Safety and Health Act (OSHA)** was signed into law to establish comprehensive health and safety standards in the workplace. Since then, the incidence of occupational illnesses and injuries and the number of lost workdays have dropped (see figure 6.1). Yet, overall costs continue to climb because declining

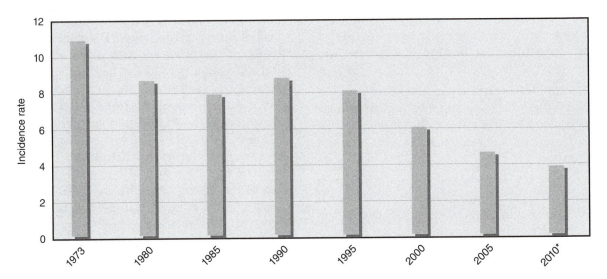

Figure 6.1 Number of nonfatal injuries and illnesses per 100 full-time workers.

*Projected.

U.S. Department of Labor 2008.

incidence rates—albeit a positive trend—do not offset higher year-to-year *percentage-cost inflation rates* for costs related to medical care, absenteeism, disability, and workers' compensation that are associated with occupational illnesses and injuries.

Nearly half of all on-the-job ailments lead to serious work restrictions or lost work time (U.S. Department of Labor 2008). Moreover, the Social Security Administration predicts that over the next 10 years, the aging of the baby-boomer generation will lead to a 37% increase in the incidence of disability. The most common worksite injuries are **cumulative trauma disorders (CTD)**, such as lower-back strain and carpal tunnel syndrome. These repetitive stress injuries occur over time, usually as a result of performing movements repeatedly day after day.

Cumulative trauma disorders affect approximately 19 million U.S. workers annually. About 2.5 million of them suffer some degree of carpal tunnel syndrome, 4.5 million get tendonitis, and about 9 million have CTD-related lower-back pain. In fact, since 1980, the incidence of CTDs has risen nearly 600%. They now account for more than 40% of all workplace injuries (see figure 6.2). No indication exists that this percentage will decrease in the near future (U.S. Department of Labor 2008).

What causes CTDs? Contributing factors include poorly designed equipment, fast-paced work, few or no rest breaks, stress, poor posture, force and repetition, and poor physical fitness. Research suggests that employers are becoming more aware of the high cost of CTDs, prompting more companies to invest in ergonomic equipment.

Many studies show the positive effect that specific types of WHP programs and policies can have on occupational injuries, including CTDs. In general, the bulk of these studies demonstrate that when employees increase both their exercise level and their musculoskeletal flexibility, their personal risk of sustaining a repetitive-motion injury or other CTDs is markedly decreased. Moreover, the overall injury risk is reduced even further when the preceding enhancements are supplemented with ergonomic improvements to workstations.

There appears to be a direct relationship between an employee's fitness status and injury risk. For example, a study by Canadian researchers investigated the effect of a physical fitness program on job-related injuries and associated costs at a municipal worksite (Shore, G., P. Prasad. and M. Zroback, 1989). Each of the 134 participants was tested for back fitness, strength, aerobic power, flexibility, weight, body-fat

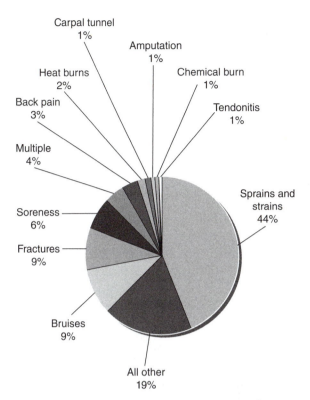

Carpal tunnel
1%

Amputation
1%

Heat burns
2%

Chemical burn
1%

Back pain
3%

Tendonitis
1%

Multiple
4%

Sprains and
strains
44%

Soreness
6%

Fractures
9%

Bruises
9%

All other
19%

Figure 6.2 Percentage distribution of injuries and illnesses in private industry

U.S. Department of Labor 2008.

percentage, blood pressure, lifestyle, and productivity. Participants were given an exercise prescription based on their overall fitness level. After six months of exercising, participants who were retested exhibited a 14.2% increase in their overall level of back fitness. Moreover, injury-related absences dropped one-fourth of a day (while nonparticipants' absences increased approximately 3.1 days), producing an estimated savings of nearly $63,000 in less than a year.

These results resemble those of another study conducted to determine the effect of physical fitness on back injuries in firefighters. To ensure high fitness levels, the program provided participants with three hours of exercise each week and periodically assessed them for the duration of the study. Overall, the study indicated that physical fitness and conditioning prevented back injuries. Moreover, it showed a statistically significant drop in the number of injuries sustained and a corresponding gain in

physical fitness. A follow-up study spanning a period of 14 years showed enhanced fitness levels strongly corresponded to lower injury rates and associated costs. The fittest employees had only one-eighth as many injuries as the least-fit employees, and unfit workers incurred twice as many costs due to lower-back injuries as fit workers. In addition, workers' compensation claims dropped by half for the entire department in the final 8 years of the study and disability costs declined 25%. (It should be noted that these improvements are probably the result of both the physical fitness program and changes in the administration of a return-to-work program.) These and other studies that categorize exercise or fitness status as an independent variable suggest that workers who regularly engage in appropriate exercise may be at less risk of sustaining musculoskeletal injuries than people with little or no exercise habits.

Another study looked at the effect of two five-minute exercise breaks on musculoskeletal strain among data-entry operators (Saulter 1990). The exercises, which relieved strain on cervicobrachial posture, included arm, wrist, and lower-leg manipulation. In the two years before the introduction of the exercise program, at any one time, 7 to 12 active workers' compensation claims were filed on behalf of operators with CTD injuries. In the year following the introduction of the program, no new claims were filed. There was also an immediate 25% climb in productivity and a savings in overtime reported in other areas.

A study of manufacturing workers included a protocol in which employees were broken into 35 teams of 6 to 12 employees. Employees started each day with a 10-minute safety meeting that integrated flexibility and strength exercises and included safety training with a flipbook system. The flipbook provided a safety message on a single topic and prompted leaders to solicit any employee safety concerns. Supervisors and teams were audited at monthly intervals. At the one-year mark, employees' flexibility improved approximately 89%, employees incurred no musculoskeletal injuries, and the worksite moved to the top one-third of the 40 company plants in safety performance. (Prior to the program, the worksite's injury rate was the fourth highest in the entire organization.)

Historically, many CTD-based studies have focused on back injuries, since back strains and sprains make up the highest portion of occupational injuries. Yet, as the burgeoning service economy requires many workers to do manual-intensive jobs involving repetitive hand, wrist, arm, and shoulder movements, industry watchers expect that worksite-based research on carpal tunnel syndrome and other repetitive motion injuries will undoubtedly grow in the coming years. Interestingly, some research suggests that workers who regularly engage in whole-body exercise, such as swimming, are at a lower risk for carpal tunnel syndrome and other types of CTDs. Yet, since many factors—modifiable and nonmodifiable—are associated with occupational injuries, WHP practitioners should continue to identify the influences in their particular worksites that can be addressed with environmental, ergonomic, and health-improvement strategies.

Some strategies for CTD prevention are relatively inexpensive and simple to implement, such as adjusting workstations to fit individual needs (see figure 6.3). Others (e.g.,

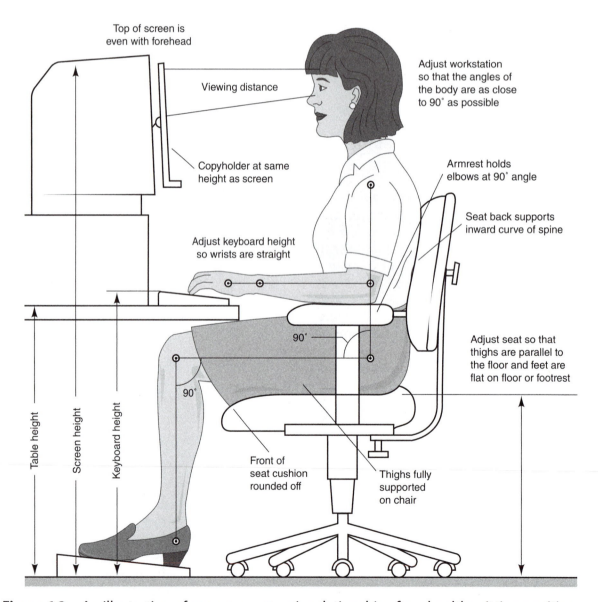

Figure 6.3 An illustration of proper ergonomic relationships for a healthy sitting position.

providing indirect light to minimize glare, providing adjustable chairs with armrests and good lower-back support, supplying monitor screens, and supplying resting pads for hands and wrists) may require additional costs, but are relatively easy to implement and will reduce CTDs. Finally, some strategies require more effort to initiate than simply purchasing new equipment or modifying workstations (e.g., education and training sessions, scheduling employees' work breaks to prevent or mitigate cumulative trauma, and monitoring employees to make sure their work practices are not predisposing them for CTDs), yet could prove to be as beneficial as ergonomic-based strategies in the long run, if not more so.

PERSONALIZING DISABILITY MANAGEMENT

While safety experts believe that most injuries are preventable, they realize that some simply cannot be avoided. Fortunately, most injuries are minor and don't impair the injured worker from returning to work in a timely manner. However, a small percentage of occupational accidents result in serious bodily injury that prevents the affected worker from working, leading to placement on *short-term disability (STD)* or *long-term disability (LTD)*. In such cases, an employer needs to have a good **disability management (DM)** program in place to provide personalized services to employees in need. As an important component of a comprehensive health-management program (see figure 4.1 in chapter 4), personnel, programs, and policies for disease management are crafted into an integrated, team-oriented approach to assist injured and disabled employees in regaining a reasonable amount of work function. In doing so, DM efforts focus on creating and establishing cultural, environmental, and occupational incentives and services, such as the following:

• Open and regular communication among key on-site and off-site decision makers (e.g., occupational health nurse, health planner, and case manager)

• An absence-management program with financial incentives for good attendance

• An organizational culture that returns workers on STD to employment at the earliest possible time

• An organizational culture that discourages the progression from STD to LTD

• More vocational rehabilitation programs for employee retraining

• Tuition reimbursement, as necessary

• Maximized use of transitional employment on a time-limited basis for workers with temporary medical restrictions, including a wage-loss provision

• Implementation of reasonable accommodations, especially job restructuring and job modification, to comply with the guidelines of the Americans With Disabilities Act (ADA)

Since many employers have a self-administered workers' compensation program, they should develop and maintain aggressive efforts at work return for employees on disability and should establish modified positions utilizing reasonable accommodation as quickly as possible. Essentially, disability management is an interactive procedure that is set in motion once the disability has been identified. It is common for several of the personnel interviewed to be involved in a particular case with a supervisor and an employee. Job analyses are provided to employees with a disability that involve physical, cognitive, and behavioral demands of their positions, and those that might be used or modified to keep them working. Meetings include disability management as required with a benefits manager or a specialist in long-term disability or the Family Medical Leave Act. Disability cases can then be reviewed monthly by members of the preceding team. In addition, certified rehabilitation counselors and nurses outside the team can be contracted as needed. Of course, these external consultants must be matched to the worker on disability in terms of background and communication style.

IMPLEMENTING EMPLOYEE ASSISTANCE PROGRAMS

Considering the stresses of balancing the demands of home and work, initiatives for quality of work life are making inroads at the workplace. According to several surveys, more employers are recognizing that employees need flexible human resource and benefit programs to help them deal with health-related changes throughout their working years. For example, more employers are offering programs for life-cycle benefits that include health promotion incentives for employees and dependents. These programs allow employees to tailor their benefits package according to their greatest needs at the time. Employees can choose from a varied menu of benefit offerings, including those listed in table 6.1.

Many life-cycle benefits programs have evolved from employee assistance programs, or EAPs. Currently, more than 10,000 U.S. employers provide EAPs, compared to only 50 in the early 1970s (EAP and Counseling Associates 2010). Although the original EAPs—established in the early 1950s—primarily focused on helping alcoholic workers and dependents, most of today's EAPs provide a full spectrum of services, including financial counseling, substance abuse treatment, assistance with eldercare and child care, and retirement planning. The most common problems currently addressed are tied to problems with jobs, personal relationships, and emotional issues (see figure 6.4).

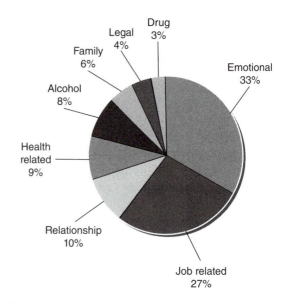

Figure 6.4 The most common problems reported by a randomly selected group of worksite EAPs.

Reprinted, by permission, from Chenoweth & Associates, Inc.

Developing and operating effective life-cycle benefits and EAP programs involves various administrative issues. For example, employers should select the physical location of an EAP to ensure that it can serve the target population in a timely and effective manner. In addition, the EAP operational model is an important consideration. Some employers opt to integrate an EAP within a comprehensive health-management program because they feel such an arrangement does the following:

Table 6.1 Components of a Life-Cycle Benefits Program

Covered expense	Areas of reimbursement	Annual maximum
Healthy lifestyle	Health club membership, smoking cessation, weight loss	$400
Child care, eldercare, or adoption	Services of a nonfamily child-care or eldercare provider, adoption referral service	$250
Financial planning	Financial planning by a qualified professional or the purchase of a financial-planning software program	$250
Legal assistance	Legal assistance in connection with wills, estates, and adoption	$200
Housing assistance	After 4 years of service, for the purchase of a primary residence only	$1,000

• Maximizes resources, especially for smaller companies with limited finances.

• Makes the working environment healthier as more staff members work toward a common goal.

• Reduces the stigma associated with getting personal help—as part of a comprehensive program, workers are more likely to view EAP services the way they consider other health promotion programs.

• Helps meet the holistic needs of high-risk workers because programs can be tailored to help people with psychological problems related to alcoholism or other drug abuse, eating disorders, stress, recent heart attacks, and other personal health crises.

However, potential drawbacks of an integrated approach do exist. Sharing resources may limit allocations and jeopardize the potential impact of an EAP. EAP services may be underrepresented if another health promotion component (a fitness center, for example) becomes too visible. Employees may also underestimate the importance of an EAP and fail to seek help. Finally, other health promotion programs may inadvertently try to address EAP-related issues. Other programs must complement EAP services rather than try to replace them.

Since the various issues and problems typically referred to EAP personnel are complex, staffing guidelines should be followed as closely as possible. First of all, staff members should be professionally trained and certified in the areas of mental health and substance abuse, family relations, financial counseling, preretirement planning and other disciplines relevant to the scope and specificity of employee needs.

Each staff member should be evaluated once a year. Managers and union representatives should be kept informed of any changes to EAP staffing and how these changes affect responsibilities. To minimize the chance of malpractice and liability claims, employers should conduct a legal review of the EAP and keep thorough files of all associated activity. Finally, an outside firm should evaluate the overall effect of the program every 2 to 4 years to ensure that operating standards are properly followed and that designated goals are achieved.

EAP Location

Each on-site and off-site EAP has its own advantages and drawbacks. An on-site EAP may give a company greater opportunity to perform quality control measures, but workers may wonder whether their identities can be protected if others are aware of their EAP usage. In contrast, some workers may find it inconvenient or indiscreet to visit an off-site EAP. The format that would suit your situation better may also depend on financial considerations. Larger employers are usually more likely to staff and fund an in-house EAP. However, companies of all sizes have opted to use an alternative arrangement, such as an off-site consortium or an internal referral system.

In a typical consortium arrangement, a group of employers pays a local EAP organization—for example, a local mental-health center—to provide specific services to employees and dependents. Usually the fee for these services depends on the size of a workforce. For example, if an employer has a workforce of 100 employees, the employer may pay $10 for each employee ($1,000) plus a base rate of $1,000, for a total cost of $2,000 a year. Employers with a larger group of employees may pay the same per-employee rate but a proportionately higher base rate.

In an *internal referral arrangement*, supervisors trained in EAP issues identify employees with personal problems that may be affecting their attendance, productivity, or morale. The troubled employees may be referred to an on-site EAP coordinator or to a designated EAP provider in the community for counseling. In the early 1980s, Union Pacific Railroad introduced Operation Red Block, one of the first programs in the industry to advocate peer intervention to reduce alcohol and other drug use (American College of Occupational and Environmental Medicine 2010). (The program is named for the signal that stops traffic at railroad crossings.) If employees either refer themselves or are referred by a peer for treatment, they are exempt from the company's disciplinary process for drug use if they cooperate with their treatment plans and they return to work after successful treatment. However, a second episode results in termination. Operation Red Block works in tandem with a very active EAP, in which confidential treatment plans are tailored to the needs of each person. This coordinated effort is provided at no cost and is responsible for the program's low recidivism rate of less than 10%.

Substance Abuse Prevention and Treatment

A common goal of life-cycle and EAP programs is to prevent and treat employee substance abuse. Historically, strategies for preventing and treating substance abuse centered on alcohol. However, today, abuse of prescription medications and illegal drugs are also emphasized. The Department of Health and Human Services (DHHS) estimates the incidence of illegal drug and heavy alcohol use among workers in specific industries, as shown in table 6.2.

Substance abuse has a formidable economic impact on businesses. Consider these statistics:

• Lost productivity and quality defects related to substance abuse cost businesses worldwide several hundred billion dollars each year.

• Each substance abuser costs his or her employer more than $7,500 a year in lost productivity, increased medical care, and damaged property.

• At least 10% of health care cost is because of substance abuse.

Table 6.2 Percentage of Workers by Industry Who Use Illegal Drugs or Drink Heavily

Industry	Illegal drug use (% workers)	Heavy drinking (% workers)
All industries average	8.2%	8.8%
Accommodations and food service	16.9%	12.0%
Agriculture/forestry/fish/hunting	6.2%	9.7%
Arts/entertainment/recreation	11.6%	13.6%
Construction	13.7%	15.9%
Educational services	4.0%	4.0%
Finance and insurance	6.8%	6.9%
Health care and social assistance	6.1%	4.3%
Information	11.0%	10.4%
Administrative support, waste management and remediation	10.9%	10.4%
Manufacturing	6.5%	9.5%
Mining	7.3%	13.3%
Other services (except public admin.)	8.8%	9.9%
Professional, scientific, technical services	8.0%	7.1%
Public administration	4.1%	5.9%
Real estate, rental, and leasing	7.5%	9.8%
Retail trade	9.4%	8.8%
Transportation and warehousing	6.2%	8.6%
Utilities	3.8%	10.1%
Wholesale trade	8.5%	11.5%

Data from DHHS 2007.

• Approximately 10% of workers abuse alcohol or other drugs.

• Nearly 50% of all industrial accidents involve alcohol.

• 40% of all worksite deaths can be traced to alcohol abuse.

The following are some strategies for employers to use in dealing with substance abuse:

• Publicize a written statement on the costs and health risks associated with substance abuse and other problems covered by the EAP. The chief executive and union representatives should sign this document when appropriate. The statement should reflect management and labor philosophies and agreements that coincide with EAP objectives.

• Develop written guidelines that specify how and for how long records will be maintained, who will have access to them, what information will be released to whom and under what conditions, and what use (if any) can be made of records for purposes of research, evaluation, and reports.

• Establish written procedures to inform employees about the actions management and union representatives will take at each phase of the program.

• Operate the EAP within the standards and practices established by one or more of the following associations:

1. Employee Assistance Professionals Association (EAPA)

2. Employee Assistance Society of North America (EASNA)

3. National Institute on Alcohol Abuse and Alcoholism (NIAAA)

4. National Council on Alcoholism and Drug Dependence (NCADD)

When a company decides to conduct drug testing, it is wise to include goals that clearly specify provisions for protecting employees' identities and preserving all facets of the program at all times. Sound ethical procedures need to be established to protect employees' rights and minimize litigation. For example,

you should hire laboratories certified by the College of American Pathologists, the National Institute of American Pathologists, or the National Institute on Drug Abuse to do the testing. To maximize accuracy, if a urine sample tests positive for drug use, it should undergo radioimmunoassay, gas chromatography, or, preferably, GC-mass spectrometry. These advanced tests (which cost between $30 and $50) break drugs into single molecules, thus confirming or contradicting the presence of even small amounts of a particular drug.

Daily stressors can compound risk factors that predispose people toward alcohol or substance abuse. Recovery rates for substance abusers entering treatment through worksite interventions are the highest of any referral source. Approximately 60% to 80% are successfully rehabilitated, producing substantial savings tied to lower absenteeism, fewer on-the-job accidents and injuries, reduced medical care costs, and higher on-the-job productivity (Alander 2006).

CREATING A LESS STRESSFUL WORKSITE

According to several employee-based surveys, job stress is the most common risk factor in today's worksites. Yet, less than 1 of every 5 worksites provide programs for employee stress management. These programs are in great need, considering the following:

• 1 of 4 employees views work as the greatest stressor in his or her life.

• 8 of 10 employees feel stress on the job, and half of them express a need for help in managing their stress.

• 4 of 10 employees say their job is very or extremely stressful.

• Nearly 1 of 3 employees feel quite or extremely stressed at work.

• 1 of 4 employees indicate being often or very often burned out or stressed by work.

Some industry insiders contend that U.S. workers are more stressed than their European counterparts because of longer working hours and less vacation time. However, the work culture and vacation allotment in Europe is starting to mimic American patterns. Stress-related disorders at the workplace continue to increase in Japan, forcing employers to address the problem. For example, a report on Japanese companies shows the following (Tsutsumi et al. 2001):

- Nearly 86% of companies replied that depression is the most frequent stress-related disorder among employees.

- In nearly 70% of the companies, some workers took more than a month's leave of absence from work because of an emotional disorder.

- Many companies are working to address mental health through a health and safety committee.

Why is worksite stress a problem for employees and employers? Distressed employees have higher rates of absenteeism, accidents, illnesses, and productivity errors than their less-stressed counterparts. They also file the majority of stress-related workers' compensation claims, which have climbed to an all-time high in recent years.

More worksites are moving away from a strong emphasis on controlling symptoms of stress. Instead, they realize the value of helping people identify the origin of stress and understand the relationship between daily stress and the development of illness and pain.

Many employers have responded by integrating stress-management counseling services within their EAPs. Additional ways to monitor and reduce employee stress include reviewing health care claims data to determine whether stress is, in fact, a problem at the worksite (e.g., monitoring medical claims, especially those classified as *mental, nervous,* and *ill-defined*), e-mailing stress-management tips at designated time intervals to all employees, converting an unused employee lounge into a quiet, dimly lit room where employees can relax, printing monthly newsletter articles on how to identify and manage various kinds of stress, establishing a humor room or playing comedy videotapes for employees during lunch and break times, and replacing the traditional label for stress-management programs with one that is more relevant to individual needs.

What Would You Do?

Suppose you have been hired as a health promotion specialist by a midsized company. Despite the worksite's clean exterior and neat appearance, your environmental assessment reveals that the work environment is very unhealthy because of wide-scale smoking, vending machines filled with junk food, and cramped work areas. Your supervisor asks you to recommend specific changes to improve the work environment. Considering that you are the newest (and probably youngest) employee, which of the three challenges would you tackle first? Why? Describe your step-by-step process, justifying your decisions.

CHAPTER 6 WRAP-UP

Key Points

- Creating a healthy worksite culture requires strategic improvements in an organization's policies, programs, employee workstations, and physical environment.

- Cumulative trauma disorders (CTDs) are the most common occupational injury in many worksites, especially those with jobs that require repetitive motion.

- Disability management programs provide injured or ill employees with the resources to regain essential capabilities for job function.

- Today's employee assistance programs (EAPs) and life-cycle benefit programs provide an ever-expanding array of services for employees with certain needs and interests.

- Reducing stress at the worksite is essential for reducing the prevalence of stress-related conditions among employees that increase an organization's costs in health care, workers' compensation, and lost productivity.

Glossary

cumulative trauma disorder (CTD)—A disorder that can affect the bones, muscles, tendons, nerves and other tissues due to repetitive motion or trauma.

disability management—A form of case management designed to rehabilitate and enhance the health status and work performance of employees with an identified physical or mental disability.

occupational Safety and Health Act (OSHA)—The primary federal law establishing health and safety standards in the workplace.

Bibliography

Alander, R., and T. Campbell. 2006. "An evaluative study of an alcohol and drug recovery program." *Human Resource Management* 14: 14-18.

American College of Occupational and Environmental Medicine. 2010. "Corporate health achievement award." Accessed November 11. www.chaa.org.

Americans for Nonsmokers' Rights. 2010. "Corporate smoke-free policies." Accessed November 11. www.no-smoke.org/goingsmokefree.php?id=452.

Boyce, R. 2005. "Ergonomics and exercise program to improve employee comfort and productivity while reducing repetitive illness." *Medicine & Science in Sports & Exercise* 37: S405.

Deyo, R., and J. Weinstein. 2001. "Low back pain." *New England Journal of Medicine* 344: 363-370.

EAP and Counseling Associates. 2010. "Workforce prevention research: Employee assistance programs fact sheet." Accessed November 11. www.eapc.org/EAP-FactSheetResearch.htm.

Ferrucci, L., and D. Alley. 2007. "Obesity, disability, and mortality: A puzzling link." *Archives of Internal Medicine* 167: 750-751.

Gable, A., and A, Forsht. 2000. "Stretching for safety's sake." *ISHN*. Accessed January 28, 2010. www.ishn.com/Articles/Feature_Article/17f4afadc9fb7010 VgnVCM100000f932a8c0.

Hu, H.Y., Y.J. Chou, P. Chou, L.K. Chen, and N. Huang. 2009. "Association between obesity and injury among Taiwanese adults." *International Journal of Obesity* 33: 878-884.

Kalina, C. 1999. "Strategies in disability management." *Annals New York Academy of Sciences* 880: 343-355.

May, D. and C. Schwoerer. 2009. "Employee health by design: Using employee involvement teams in ergonomic job redesign." *Personnel Psychology* 47: 861-876.

Melhorn, M. 1998. "Cumulative trauma disorders and repetitive strain injuries: The future." *Current Orthopaedic Practice*. Accessed December 31, 2009. http://journals.lww.com/corr/Abstract/1998/06000/Cumulative_Trauma_Disorders_and_Repetitive_Strain.15.aspx.

Mills, S. 2009. "Workplace lactation programs: A critical element for breastfeeding mothers' success." *American Association of Occupational Health Nurses Journal* 57: 239-250.

Minter, S. 2005. "ASSE: Integrating fitness into safety." *EHS Today*. Accessed January 28, 2010. http://ehstoday.com/news/ehs_imp_37647/index.html.

Ostbye, T., J. Dement, and K. Krause. 2007. "Obesity and workers' compensation: Results from the Duke health and safety surveillance system." *Archives of Internal Medicine* 167: 766-773.

Rosenwald, Michael S. "Those with a desk job, please stand up." *Washington Post*. Oct 17, 2010.

Saulter, S. 1990. *Promoting health and productivity in the computerized office.* London: Taylor and Francis.

Schulte, P., et al. 2007. "Work, obesity, and occupational safety and health." *American Journal of Public Health* 97: 428-436.

Shore, G., P. Prasad, and M. Zroback. 1989. "Metrofit: a cost-effective fitness program." *Fitness in Business, 3: 147-153.*

Tsutsumi, A., et al. 2001. "Association between job stress and depression among Japanese employees threatened by job loss in a comparison between two complementary job-stress models." *Scandinavian Journal of Work Environment and Health* 27(2): 146-153.

U.S. Department of Health & Human Services (DHHS). *Worker Substance Use and Workplace Policies and Programs* (DHHS Publication No. SMA 07-4273.) 2007, Rockville, MD.

U.S. Department of Labor. 2008. *Number of non-fatal injuries and illnesses per 100 full-time workers.* Washington, D.C: Author.

Looking Ahead

Now that we've identified ways to enhance the worksite environment and culture, it's time to promote and implement employee-centered programs. Chapter 7 presents how to develop a marketing strategy, use promotional techniques, and create appropriate incentives for employees with different levels of motivation. It also discusses the value of doing a trial run of the new WHP program.

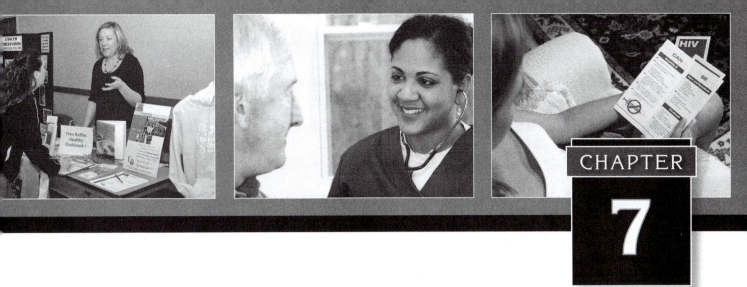

Promoting and Launching Worksite Programs

LEARNING OBJECTIVES

After reading this chapter, you will be able to do the following:

✔ Assess a worksite and determine if its WHP program possesses sufficient attributes for success.
✔ List the four Ps of the marketing mix and give examples of each one.
✔ Describe the difference between intrinsic and extrinsic rewards.
✔ Distinguish between the various segments of a workforce in terms of their willingness to participate.
✔ Explain the rationale for establishing policies for risk and liability management in a WHP program.

Some of the most successful WHP programs do not have expensive facilities, a large staff, or a hefty budget. However, an ingredient that most of these programs do share is WHP personnel who are committed to identifying needs, coordinating responsibilities, and applying appropriate resources toward achieving reasonable, well-defined goals. The checklist on the next page includes a dozen features typically found in successful WHP programs. Program planners may wish to copy and use the checklist to see how well their programs meet the criteria.

Developing a program that includes all of these features requires careful planning before implementing the program, as well as regular maintenance once the program is under way. Worksites vary tremendously, so no guarantees exist. However, if WHP program directors possess at least 10 of the 12 items on the checklist, they can rest assured that their programs should appeal to employees. If you check fewer than 10 of the items, your program may need to be modified to better resemble programs that have been proven successful. For example, if a WHP program lacks a clearly established budget, decision makers should work to establish a protocol to ensure a dedicated budget for the program (see chapter 5 for budgeting tips).

CHECKLIST FOR A SUCCESSFUL PROGRAM

Choose the items that are true for your program. If you check fewer than 10 items, you may have more work to do.

_____ 1. Top management supports the program.

_____ 2. The company has a designated budget for health promotion.

_____ 3. The program is free or inexpensive to employees.

_____ 4. Qualified personnel operate the program.

_____ 5. The program staff seeks regular input from both management and employees.

_____ 6. Opportunities to participate in the program are convenient for all employees.

_____ 7. Health screenings and staff surveys are conducted regularly to assess employees' needs and interests.

_____ 8. Attractive and informative program materials are available for employees to use at work and at home.

_____ 9. When possible, health promotion activities are open to dependents and retirees.

_____ 10. The company's mission statement cites a healthy workforce among its top priorities.

_____ 11. The program provides both general and customized health promotion activities for employees at all work locations.

_____ 12. The company gets involved in local health promotion programs to show its commitment to improving the community's health status.

If a program contains 10 or more of the dozen features, it is probably ready to be implemented at the worksite.

Plans for launching a successful WHP program include (1) developing a marketing strategy to make the program appealing to employees, (2) preparing employees to take action, (3) developing a health fair, (4) conducting employee health screenings, (5) **managing risk and liability,** (6) giving the program a trial run, and (7) determining appropriate **rewards** to build long-term employee participation.

DEVELOPING A MARKETING STRATEGY

Marketing is defined as an aggregate of functions involved in moving goods from producer to consumer. Depending on the goods involved, these functions might include describing the product to those who have never heard of it, explaining what the product is and how to use it, advertising the product so that consumers know it exists, monitoring the product at the developmental site to check for consistent quality, distrib-uting the product in various quantities to match the needs of different consumer segments, transporting the product to places where the consumer can easily get to it, seeking feedback about the product from the consumer to learn ways to improve the product's future marketability, and again monitoring the product at the distributor, wholesaler, or retailer to ensure consistent quality. When people talk about goods, we tend to think of tangible items. However, the marketing principles that apply to tangibles also apply to intangibles, such as WHP. As the producer, the job of WHP staff is to make the product (WHP) available and appealing to the consumer.

Organizations with successful WHP programs usually focus their marketing efforts on the four Ps—product, price, placement, and promotion—also called the **marketing mix**.

Product

When your product is health promotion—helping people to feel better, reduce health risks, and be more productive—you might think the product would sell itself, but unfortunately it doesn't. As with all other products or services, a health promotion program must be marketed so that consumers consider it attractive and advantageous. As summarized in table 7.1, you should ask some important questions about the program: What is our service? Is it tangible, visible, and measurable? Why is the worksite version better than the commercialized,

off-site version? What is the need for this service?

Employees need to know precisely what they are being offered. Does the WHP program require a commitment of an hour a day or only an hour a week? Does the program offer customized options for personalized services or a one-size-fits-all approach? How much flexibility is allowed for employees

Table 7.1 The Four Ps of Marketing

	Questions to Address	Considerations

Product	1. What is our product, program, or service?
	2. Is it tangible, visible, and measurable?
	3. What is the employee's or client's need for the product, program, or service:
	  - To look better?
	  - To feel better?
	  - To be more productive?
	  - To lower health risk?
	  - To socialize with others?
		Define the product, program, or service in precise, easy-to-understand terms.

Price	1. Should participants be charged? 2. Can the employee/company reasonably afford the product, program, or service? 3. Does the product, program, or service produce a greater benefit than cost?	Cost may be an extremely important factor in small businesses and other organizations with tight budgets. Thus, variably priced options of the product, program, or service may be necessary. Determine the probable cost savings of the product, program, or service with cost-effectiveness analysis or benefit-cost analysis (see chapter 8).

Placement	1. Who will receive the product, program, or service:
	  - All employees?
	  - Employees with specific risk factors?
	  - Only high-risk employees?
	  - Only men or only women?
	2. Which employees are likely to benefit from the program, product, or service?
		Consider breaking the workforce into segments based on specific attributes:
		• Age
		• Family size
		• Education level
		• Work shift
		• Past participation status

Promotion	1. What types of incentives can be used to make the product, program, or service appealing?	A demonstrated benefit must be shown for consumers (employees) to use the program, product, or service. Use tangible incentives to create a unique selling point. Some examples include the following: • Freebies (T-shirts, on-site day care, health screenings) • Discounts (health insurance premium, health club membership) • Personal coaching and training.
	2. What is the best time to promote the product, program, or service?	Periods of layoffs, sluggish business, or merger talks may preoccupy or compel some employees to work overtime. Thus, they may not respond to a promotion.
	3. Where should promotional efforts be directed?	Promotions can be targeted on site (employee workstations, time clocks, cafeteria, break areas, health clinic, safety meetings) and off site (mailings to employees' homes)
	4. What promotional techniques should be used?	Promotional options include e-mail, company website, newsletters, paycheck stuffers, voice mail messaging, bulletin boards, on-site television channel, benefits updates, health-plan enrollment week, and direct mailing to employees' homes.

with busy schedules outside of work? Can employees participate during work hours? What exactly can they gain by participating in a program that promotes health? Will the benefits be financial, tangible, practical, or otherwise directly applicable to their current situation, or will they be more abstract and hard to measure? These questions and possibly others must be answered to employees' satisfaction if they are going to be enticed to try the program.

Price

No matter how the program's expenses are covered—100% by the employer, 100% by the employee, or somewhere in between—if employees do not perceive that the benefits of the program outweigh their own personal costs, they will not participate. Even if a program is free of charge, some employees may find it too expensive in terms of time, location, special clothing, or equipment. Whether the costs are in dollars, hours, or ounces of sweat, the employees' perception must be that they have more to gain than they have to lose.

Price considerations exist from the employer's perspective as well. Some employers will find that a program is not financially feasible unless it is partly funded by the participants or unless participation occurs only on employees' time. Will this compromise employee participation? Will employees resent paying even a small percentage and consequently choose not to participate? Or, if employees are charged a modicum up-front fee to participate, can they qualify for a full refund if they participate in a designated number of programming sessions? Such questions need answers before the program is launched.

Placement

Another consideration for WHP practitioners is which employees to focus on when starting the program. Should the program target all employees equally, or should only particular groups be targeted? Keep in mind that success or failure is often determined in the early stages of any endeavor. If the program is to receive a trial run, it might be

best to include only some employees rather than all of them. This way, if the trial fails, the program can be adjusted and restarted without losing credibility with everyone. If all employees are targeted and the first run of the program fails, it will be more difficult to create enthusiasm again.

Some WHP programs (e.g., disease management and case management) aim at only high-risk employees because the services are designed to meet specific needs. However, it is also true that some high-risk employees are less likely to participate in a WHP program than employees at moderate or low risk. Why is this? Part of the reason is explained in the preceding section: Some workers simply feel that their cost in time or exertion is not worth the benefits they may receive from the program. The same factors that have led to their high-risk status make them less likely to sacrifice time and effort for health improvements. Conversely, employees whose healthier lifestyles keep them at relatively low risk may be more likely to participate in a WHP program because the program is aligned with their current values. Such considerations, although potentially disheartening for WHP practitioners, need to be acknowledged and dealt with if the program is to have realistic goals and successfully counter potential pitfalls.

It can be worthwhile to vary aspects of a WHP program for different groups of employees. If possible, an employer might consider offering a cafeteria-style program in which employees choose portions of the program that they perceive best suits them. For instance, instead of focusing on nutrition or stress management for all employees in a given week, a program might give employees the option to forego that week's designated activity and spend an additional week in another program instead.

Sometimes it can be advantageous to target employees by stratified groupings based on age, gender, type of occupation, or other factors. This allows employees to focus on the areas they are most concerned about. For example, 20- to 30-year-old men might be more interested in weight training based in fitness centers than older employees, who are probably more interested in a financial-wellness seminar or program on medical self-care.

Promotion

The fourth dimension of the marketing mix, promotion, is focused on the tools and techniques used to the reach the target population. Appropriate tools should be used to effectively reach as many employees as possible. In a single worksite where all employees work in a common setting, promotional displays in heavily traveled areas may be sufficient to reach most employees (see figure 7.1). However, in worksites where

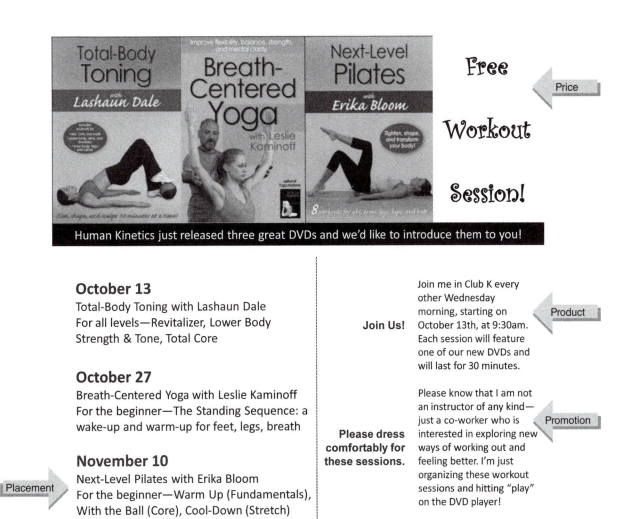

Figure 7.1 A sample poster for promoting exercise programs highlighting the four Ps of the marketing mix.

employees work in different buildings, point-of-contact tools, such as e-mail, paycheck stuffers, company website postings, and weekly safety meetings, are generally used to reach dispersed groups of employees.

USING E-HEALTH TECHNOLOGY

Today, more people are turning to the Internet for health information. According to a nationwide randomized telephone survey of adults, of the hundreds of millions of people who surf the Internet daily, more than 70% use the resource for personal health information. This number is expected to increase as much as 5% a year in this population, commonly referred to by pollsters as *cyberchondriacs* (Mearian 2010). With the advent of the Internet and related communication options that continuously appear in our daily lives, many WHP professionals are using these new technologies for education and information. This evolving phenomenon, classified as **e-health technology,** is defined as the application of Internet and other related technologies to improve the access, effectiveness, and quality of clinical and business practices used by organizations, practitioners, and consumers to improve and maintain the health status of workers and organizations.

Many worksites have on-site access to Internet and related technologies for employee use in various WHP activities. In particular, numerous worksites have expanded their capabilities for e-health technology beyond the Internet by building their own intranet system composed of integrated, company-specific databases. An intranet system gives employees one-stop access to information and resources from various departments. In many companies, employees can use this integrated system to quickly inquire about WHP program schedules, schedule a personal coaching session, log in exercise points, trace their readiness-to-change progress, learn new techniques for stress management, access a smoking cessation hotline, and acquire a host of other self-help news bits and resources. Commercial vendors are also offering these programs, which typically include a virtual fitness center, nursing hotline, disease-management services, and an e-health website.

Health promotion professionals can use e-health management tools to effectively launch and implement WHP programs, events, and activities in a timely and cost-effective manner. However, in doing so, they need to use some time-tested techniques to maximize the influence of their e-health efforts. First, they should take the time to get in-house communications experts involved in the marketing plan and related goal-setting initiatives. It is also important to provide regular updates to senior managers to secure their continued support for the program by helping them to see how e-health management resources relate to the company's goals and financial health. Although communication tools vary from worksite to worksite, a few communication channels appear to work well in most organizations, such as the following:

- Broadcast e-mail messaging
- Internet mailings
- Home mailings
- Intranet feature postings
- Announcements during company meetings, events, and activities
- Promotional posters and table tents in highly visible locations at the worksite

Second, an integrated multidisciplinary team is required to implement and maintain a highly successful e-health initiative. The most successful teams are led by key individuals who take on the sole responsibility of coordinating team action and delegating responsibilities to the necessary players. A common approach is to form teams made up of diverse departments, including communications, risk management, benefits, human resources, health and safety, information services, and any other human-capital interest groups. In organizations with multisite operations, establish a key contact at each location to spearhead and coordinate these functions.

Third, it is important to realize that e-health management is a platform, not a program. According to industry experts, if e-health is to be fully optimized, organizations need to recognize this approach as a company-wide, web-based platform that addresses human capital. It is not simply the next health-improvement program.

Fourth, in building an integrated e-health platform, it is necessary to take inventory of your company's resources in terms of employee health (departments, events, programs, and incentives). Once these resources have been identified, it will be more evident to decision makers that they should establish integrative opportunities.

Finally, e-health efforts must be positioned to reach as many people in as many ways as possible. Before any of the preceding four principles can be institutionalized, the overall infrastructure must be seen as moving—or, better yet, transforming—the organization's culture in a new and positive direction. Perhaps the most relevant example is the ability of an e-health platform to synchronize with the newest business trend of electronic self-service. This feature saves money and time by eliminating administrative tasks. It also includes venues, such as online enrollment in health benefits, financial planning, and office procurement.

PREPARING EMPLOYEES TO TAKE ACTION

In realizing how difficult it is to motivate employees to participate in WHP programs on a consistent basis, many worksite health and fitness professionals have incorporated a model for stages of change in their programming efforts. James Prochaska and Carlo DiClemente created this model to describe the various levels of a person's readiness or motivation to act (Prochaska, Norcross, and DiClemente 2004). It is composed of the following five stages:

1. *Precontemplation.* The person has not considered doing any health-enhancement action.

2. *Contemplation.* The person is considering action but has not yet acted.
3. *Preparation.* The person has intentions to act soon and is planning a course of action.
4. *Action.* The person is actively participating.
5. *Maintenance.* The person has been participating for at least six months and has been working to prevent a relapse.

Because the bulk of your WHP marketing efforts may focus on persons in stages 1, 2, and 3, it is important to structure your resources around all employees, including those in stages 4 and 5. Far too often, WHP staff members assume that persons in the action and maintenance stages will automatically continue to be loyal participants in their programs, only to be surprised when these die-hard workers end up on the sidelines because of an injury, work-related changes, greater family demands, boredom, or other unforeseen circumstances that take them out of action.

Realizing the need to tailor their motivational efforts around the diverse needs and interests of employees, many WHP providers are using different technological strategies to reach more workers. In our high-tech society, one of the fastest-growing motivational strategies used by health and fitness professionals is actually a low-tech phenomenon called coaching.

Personal and group coaching, long used by executives and elite athletes to boost performance, has now moved into the realm of health, fitness, and wellness. The International Coach Federation (ICF) defines *coaching* as an ongoing professional relationship that helps people produce extraordinary results in their lives, careers, businesses, or organization. Through the process of coaching, clients deepen their learning, improve their performance, and enhance their quality of life. Coaching accelerates the client's progress by providing greater focus and awareness of choice. The interaction creates clarity and moves the client into action. Major features of **health coaching** include the following:

- *Health assessment.* A health-risk appraisal or health screening is used to establish a baseline on the client.

- *Review of assessment data.* During this process, the coach uses the data to establish an outline of procedures to use in guiding the initial sessions with the client. The coach may or may not share the outline with the client.

- *Initial coaching session.* In this session, the coach and client discuss and assess the client's readiness to act and ways to proceed.

- *Follow-up coaching sessions.* These regularly scheduled sessions are held to assess the client's current status, recent progress, and ways to continuously improve.

The most common venue for health coaching is the personal, face-to-face approach. However, telephonic services, while unique in their challenges, provide a convenient way for some organizations to offer accessible health-coaching services. For instance, telephonic-based health coaching is growing in organizations with (1) worksites in multiple locations, (2) a small number of employees in a single location, or (3) employees who do not have access to suitable face-to-face coaching interactions. Table 7.2 describes various

Table 7.2 Coaching Strategies Tailored to Specific Stages of Readiness

Stage	Coaching strategies
1. Precontemplation	• Assess personal health status of client. • Assess priorities related to personal health with client. • Assess client's level of readiness to act. • Inform client that taking action is (1) important, (2) personally beneficial, and (3) achievable.
2. Contemplation	• Ask open-ended questions to assess client's intentions and readiness to act. • Avoid giving action-oriented instructions, such as joining a fitness class or adopting a particular diet plan. • Help client understand that the advantages of acting outweigh disadvantages of not being able to live a high-quality lifestyle (e.g., "Acting now will help you feel better, sleep better, reduce your health care usage, save health care dollars.") • Use reflective listening to build client's self-confidence to take action (e.g., "It seems as if you see a connection between a lack of regular exercise and being overweight, lacking energy, not sleeping well."). • Help clients identify positive role models that will support their actions. • Ask clients to set a personal goal that is achievable and can be incorporated into their current schedule without much inconvenience.
3. Preparation	• Ask clients to set a realistic goal, if they haven't already done so. • Help clients identify an incentive that would motivate them to take action. • Ask clients to identify potential barriers to action and ways to overcome them. • Encourage clients to act on their goals in progressive steps.
4. Action	• Reinforce clients' good actions. • Encourage clients to track personal progress and tell others. • Ask clients to identify potential barriers to action and ways to overcome them. • Encourage clients to act on their goals in progressive steps. • In subsequent coaching sessions, encourage clients to move beyond the initial goal (e.g., exercise 2 more min. per session than before).
5. Maintenance	• Reinforce clients' good actions. • Encourage clients to review personal progress and revise goals, if necessary. • Encourage clients to track personal progress and tell others. • Ask clients to identify potential barriers to action and ways to keep them from causing a relapse. • Provide clients with handouts, articles, testimonials from others, and personal screening and progress results to reinforce the benefits of sustaining/maintaining. • In subsequent coaching sessions, encourage clients to personally set a new goal or to add some variety to their personal health plan.

complementary coaching strategies that can be integrated with WHP programs.

Incentives and Rewards

In today's downsized worksites, more employees are required to do more work in shorter time frames. Therefore, many workers find it increasingly difficult to engage in WHP programs and activities. It's not surprising to find more employers offering **incentives** to boost employee participation in such offerings. What's behind this movement? Much of it is based on mounting evidence clearly showing that levels of employee participation influence the prevalence of major risk factors that, in turn, affect employees' health status, productivity, health care utilization, and health care costs.

Although health promotion has its own rewards, sometimes these rewards take too long for the impatient beginner. For instance, many newcomers in fitness programs quit before they have invested enough time to accrue any exercise-related benefits. Understanding this, astute WHP staff members offer tangible rewards to those with consistent participation, especially in the first few weeks of the program. After that, external rewards may be less necessary. Participants begin to enjoy the more intrinsic rewards of increased well-being and energy, reduced stress, and an enhanced quality of life. Early in the program, staff members need to decide what kind of external rewards work best. This information can be learned from trial and error, of course, but a simpler way to discover what employees prefer is to use an incentive survey (see chapter 2).

For maximum effect, employer-driven incentives and rewards must be matched with employees' interests. They must also be administratively efficient, strategically integrated at appropriate times, and, of course, financially scaled within a company's budget. Although employers may offer many types of incentives and rewards to boost employee participation, some are more powerful than others. For example, recent surveys indicate that the four incentives that generated the highest level of employee participation among the surveyed

worksites were (1) cash bonuses, (2) reductions in health insurance premiums, (3) gift cards, and (4) health account contributions (National Association of Manufacturers 2007). Since no one particular incentive is a universal catalyst at all worksites, it's important to customize incentives and rewards around the unique physical, demographic, social, political, and financial composition of each organization. Table 7.3 provides a general overview of options and factors to consider when planning and administering incentives and rewards.

Nothing promotes a program better than employees who see, feel, and internalize the benefits of their efforts. For example, if an on-site walking program helps workers feel better, chances are good they will return for as long as the program provides these benefits. On the other hand, if employees do not see or feel the benefits they are gaining in the program, they will need external incentives to boost and maintain personal adherence until they experience the intrinsic benefits of their actions.

Program Adherence

Once a program has been successfully promoted and is under way, program planners need strategies for motivating employees to stick with the program. Many employees get excited at the beginning, but lose interest if they don't see immediate results for their efforts. Because perceptible changes in a person's health status and fitness level are usually gradual, it may be necessary to offer external rewards until an intrinsic reward—such as feeling better—becomes a self-perpetuating force. The following suggestions may help employees stay with a program:

- Help employees set realistic goals. Break a long-term goal into short-term goals (e.g., split a proposed 10% weight loss into six monthly goals of losing 5 pounds, or 2 kg, a month).
- Stress the need to begin slowly, especially in exercise and weight-loss efforts.
- Give regular verbal support and written feedback to all participants while assessing their progress.

Table 7.3 A General Framework of Options and Factors to Consider in Offering Incentives and Rewards

	Tangible (extrinsic)	Intangible
Types	Merchandise	Recognition
	Discounts on health-plan premium	Sense of belonging
	Wellness days off	Competition
	Lottery for free trip	Participating on company time
	Health club membership	
	Lifestyle/health coaching	
Best time to administer	An incentive is offered prior to participation; a reward is offered when certain goals are achieved.	
	Note: Tangible incentives should be aggressively offered early on to boost enough participation to produce intrinsic (internal) rewards. Tangible incentives may be necessary at certain intervals to maintain participation.	
Promotion techniques	Several weeks prior to a program:	
	E-mail	Table tent cards
	Printed mailings to employees' residences	Newsletters
	Worksite posters	
Suggested financial investment	HRA participation rates increase about 10% for every $50 increase.	
	For each $100 increase, program participation is likely to increase 5%-10%.	
	Incentives ranging from $350-$550 typically generate program participation levels of 60% to 80%	
	Note: Select a financial value that can be affordably sustained over a long period of time.	
Evaluation methods	Aggregate HRA data*	Medical claims data
	Participants' self-report*	Biometric screenings
	Corporate medical care costs	
Legal considerations (HIPPA)	Avoid incentivizing a test result.	
	Financial incentives can't exceed 20% (30% in 2014) of the annual cost of an employee's health plan.	
	Note: Offer reasonable alternatives as incentive criteria based on health status or activities.[1]	
Legal considerations (GINA)	If using an HRA, exclude any questions relevant to family history, personal medical history, or genetics.	

*Relying solely on these may not reflect actual changes to behavior and risk factors. When possible, incorporate actual claims data and biometric screening data.

[1]For example, if rewarding nonusers of tobacco, a reasonable alternative for tobacco users must be established, such as participating in a smoking cessation program.

- Establish a point system in which participants can redeem wellness bucks for mugs, T-shirts, self-care books, and other prizes.
- Use a map to signify the distance walked, biked, or swum by participants in a coast-to-coast cross-country challenge. Give awards at certain landmarks or cities.
- Feature a participant of the month for outstanding attendance or performance.
- Sponsor a fun run and walk with participants predicting their finish times.

- Reward those with the closest actual times.
- Use an honor system to reward employees who promote their health at home or away because they work on the road.

For example, create check sheets for personal health promotion on specific topics (e.g., exercise, nutrition, weight loss, smoking cessation). Have employees check off their weekly accomplishments and submit them at regular intervals for prizes (see the sample check sheet below).

SAMPLE EXERCISE-BASED CHECK SHEET

Instructions: Please calculate points earned each week for the entire month. Turn the check sheet in to your personal health coach on the first day of each month. Point credits are as follows:

15 minutes of nonstop activity = 2 points
20 minutes of nonstop activity = 3 points
25 minutes of nonstop activity = 4 points
30 minutes of nonstop activity = 5 points
35+ minutes of nonstop activity = 6 points

Personal Health Promotion Check Sheet

	Type of exercise completed					Total points
	Walk	Bike	Swim	Jog/Run	Other (list)	**Total points**
Week #1	2	3				
	2	3				
	2	3				15
Week #2		3				
			3			
	2					
	2					10
Week #3	3					
	3					
		2				
		4				12
Week #4		4				
		4				
		4				
		3				15
					Monthly total	52

One of the most popular incentive campaigns used at many worksites is offering points for participation. Many program directors think it allows employees more flexibility to select what they consider valuable—cash, prizes, or even time off work. When setting up a point program, some program directors stack the deck by offering fewer points for popular programs and more points for programs that are valuable but less popular.

When offering incentive-based programs, it's essential to reward employees within the stipulations established by the Health Insurance Portability and Accountability Act (HIPAA). For example, employers may offer rewards within a bona fide wellness program, also called a disease-prevention or health promotion program, as long as all of the following criteria are met:

1. Any reward or discount cannot exceed 20% (30% in 2014) of the cost of an employee's annual health plan.

2. The program must be designed to promote health and prevent disease.

3. The program must give workers eligible to participate the opportunity to qualify for the reward at least once a year.

4. The rewards must be available to similarly situated employees. For example, you may legally allow full-time employees to participate but exclude part-time employees. You may also classify by length of service and disallow new (probationary) employees from participating. However, when it comes to something like a smoking cessation program, you must have an alternative standard of success for people who cannot comply with your behavioral objectives because of a medical or physical condition. For example, smoking is considered an addiction. As such, if you offer an incentive to quit smoking, you must offer an alternative standard of success so that smokers can have access to the reward on an equivalent basis.

5. Finally, the alternative standard of success must be disclosed to the same extent as the general standard of success.

Since financial incentives are believed to be one of the strongest incentives, more employers are offering financial-wellness banks or health care accounts to employees who complete an annual health assessment or who participate in specific WHP programs. Employees who meet specified criteria can access a personal account of company-funded dollars (generally $250 to $750 a year), which they can apply toward their medical insurance premium, deductible, or copayment, or for reimbursement for approved medical services.

Nonparticipants and High-Risk Employees

While incentives and rewards work well at many worksites, all companies have their share of nonparticipants. These no-show employees are costly, since they often have greater health risks that can lead to premature illnesses and productivity impairments that are paid, in large part, by their employers. For example, three large-scale studies conducted on employees at Ceridian Corporation, Steelcase, Inc., and DaimlerChrysler Corporation show that workers with potentially modifiable risk factors (e.g., smoking, obesity, and physical inactivity) miss more work days and incur greater health care expenses than lower-risk employees (Healthcare Intelligence Network 2009). Presumably, these employees could benefit from WHP activities, but less than 5% of all high-risk employees actually participate in such programs. Due to these lackluster participation rates among high-risk employees, more companies are customizing their incentive programs to reach this challenging population. Yet, to be successful, incentive planners first need to identify a group's values, interests, and readiness to act.

As more employers become aware of the strong correlation between employees' health status and health care costs, they offer customized incentives and rewards to this hard-to-reach sector. However, to be successful, decision makers first need to identify their workers' specific values, interests, and readiness to act. In any workforce, you can probably identify at least four (perhaps more) different types of employees by their interest, or lack thereof, in their personal health. For instance, the first group is often called the *die-hard workers* because of their strong interest and regular participation in health-enhancement activities. These employees are the easiest to recruit. They are often willing to assist WHP staff in various capacities (e.g., promoting WHP programs to coworkers).

The second segment, perhaps best called *the dependers*, are those employees who express an interest in their health, but often need tangible incentives and regular encouragement from family members, coworkers, and staff members to regularly participate in health-enhancement activities.

A third segment, perhaps best called *the conditionals*, might participate if the conditions are personally appealing, such as a free program on company time. They are also more likely to prefer participating with a buddy or in a group with their immediate coworkers.

A fourth segment, *the resisters*, is the toughest group to motivate. These employees, who have little interest in their personal health, often delay lifestyle changes until a major crisis has occurred, such as a heart attack. Unfortunately, since many resisters have never had a healthy lifestyle, they cannot appreciate the many benefits of good health.

No secret recipe exists for motivating the resisters. However, this doesn't mean that program planners should not continue to try to get these employees involved. Doing so requires more creativity and perseverance in developing, marketing, and implementing WHP programs for this challenging audience. Interest surveys and other assessment tools (see chapter 2) can help staff members design appealing programs. Fortunately, a WHP program can be successful without engaging every employee. In most cases, the success or failure of a program depends on the extent to which customized promotional campaigns and programs can be

GENETIC INFORMATION NONDISCRIMINATION ACT (GINA)

Many employers offer workers cash incentives or insurance premium discounts to complete personal surveys for health-risk assessment. Some use that information to provide at-risk employees with targeted advice or to direct them to risk-reduction (e.g., disease-management) programs. Surveys for health-risk assessment have traditionally included questions about medical history or family history. Yet, this is quickly changing due to the Genetic Information Nondiscrimination Act (GINA). GINA, which became federal law in 2008, restricts employers and health insurers from collecting and disclosing any information related to genetics.

Understandably, many WHP practitioners feel that by forbidding use of critical information to help at-risk employees, GINA has compromised their ability to expand the scope of wellness efforts. Recent surveys indicate that most employers have complied with the law by dropping any genetics-related questions from their health-assessment tools. Nonetheless, some employers have decided to use a two-option approach to health-risk assessment, especially in face-to-face screening encounters. For instance, a few employers reported that their screening personnel fill out two forms of a health-risk assessment on employees. One version includes family medical questions and the other version doesn't. Health screeners give employees the first form for submission to their personal health care provider, but use the second form (without family history and genetic questions) in their wellness programming (e.g., personal coaching and program planning).

offered in sync with employees' likes and capabilities. The greatest potential lies in carefully targeted incentives and rewards that fit individual and group preferences. In addition, whenever possible, it is best to use promotional strategies that include awareness and hands-on activities, such as a health fair.

DEVELOPING A HEALTH FAIR

A good way to generate employee health awareness and program participation is to sponsor a worksite health fair, especially one that includes colorful exhibits, audiovisual displays, interactive kiosks, educational materials, and various health screenings. To minimize the labor-intensive nature of planning a comprehensive health fair, WHP staff may choose to recruit selected employees (e.g., die-hard participants) to assist them in preparing the location, setting up exhibits, and distributing promotional materials. Since the quality of a worksite health fair largely depends on the quality of its exhibitors and vendors, it pays to carefully screen and select appropriate personnel. In doing so, consider the following organizations or people:

- County health department
- Fire, rescue, and police
- Local health care or hospital organizations
- Local health clubs
- Local physicians and dentists
- Registered dietitians and nutritionists
- Licensed massage therapists, physical therapists, optometrists, and chiropractors
- Community health associations (e.g., heart, cancer, lung, diabetes, asthma)
- College or university faculty and students in health-related disciplines

In the initial planning, the company sponsoring an employee health fair should take several precautionary steps to comply with specific HIPAA guidelines. Examples include the following:

- Offer events only at on-site locations. Prepare and distribute communication materials explaining that on-site health fairs and similar events are not part of any company health insurance plan.
- Clearly state that health-risk assessments are not a benefit under the plan. Individual results will be shared only with the employees.
- Meet with vendors and staff to ensure that only deidentified, aggregate (group) information will be sent from the on-site health fair to the health plan or the company. Vendors may also obtain requests from participants to send the results on their behalf to the health plan.
- Educate and train company employees who might provide medical care to other employees to never use electronic media to perform a transaction for which there is a HIPAA electronic standard.

After receiving a verbal agreement from the preceding personnel or organization, it is important to follow up in writing with a tangible agreement. This agreement will also serve as a notice to all who participate that the health fair is a nonprofit event and that the company holding the fair will not accept responsibility for any losses or damages incurred. To avoid any possible legal problems, the sponsoring worksite should receive a signed copy of the agreement from all participants. The company holding the health fair can use a modified version of the sample agreement, shown on the next page, to suit its circumstances.

Planning Framework

When preparing a worksite health fair, program planners need to consider their compiled data on employee needs and interests (collected though various techniques discussed in chapter 2). This information is helpful in progressing through the three phases of building a health fair: preliminary planning, development, and implementation.

SAMPLE LETTER TO HEALTH FAIR EXHIBITORS

Dear _____ *(health promotion exhibitor/vendor)* _____:

Thank you for expressing interest in our health fair, to be held on___*(date)*___from *(time)* to *(time)*. We expect that your participation will help make our health fair a huge success. This letter confirms our arrangement for your participation in the _____ *(event name)* _____. Your participation at the health fair *(describe service, such as giving a presentation, presenting an exhibit, conducting a health screening, and so on)* will be as an independent contractor of and not as an agent for or an employee of *(worksite sponsoring health fair)*.

[If vendor will be doing an invasive, diagnostic, or potentially risky procedure, include the next paragraph.]

(Contractor name) shall indemnify and hold *(worksite sponsoring health fair)* and their respective agents and employees harmless from any and all manner of loss whatsoever, including reasonable costs of litigation and attorneys' fees, which *(worksite sponsoring health fair)* may hereafter incur, become responsible for, or pay out as a result of (1) death or bodily injury to any person, (2) destruction or damage to any property arising out of negligence by *(worksite sponsoring health fair)* or their respective agents and employees, or (3) in connection with the services provided by contractor, except to the proportionate extent that such loss, liability, damage, or claim was due to the willful misconduct of *(worksite sponsoring health fair)*, its respective agents, and its employees.

[If the contractor will be doing an invasive, diagnostic, or potentially risky procedure or will be providing a piece of equipment for trial use, include the next paragraph.]

As an independent contractor, you are responsible for having current general and professional **[also include product liability if the contractor is an equipment seller who is bringing in equipment for employee use]** liability coverage (minimum of $1,000,000). Please return copies of the appropriate certificates of insurance with this letter.

[If the contractor is a sole proprietor or is not affiliated with an established and reputable organization, such as a local hospital, and if the service is an invasive, diagnostic, or potentially risky procedure, include the following paragraph.]

Please prepare a form for informed consent and release of liability to be signed before participation in your service. *(Worksite sponsoring health fair)* should be released from all liabilities associated with your service. Enclose a copy of the form with your confirmation. Your services will be provided at no charge to *(worksite sponsoring health fair)*. **[If those who desire (health fair host company) service will pay, note fee schedule.]** We appreciate your participation in making the health fair a success. If you understand and agree to these arrangements and requirements, sign in the space provided. To participate in the health fair, the exhibitor must sign and return the original copy of this letter, along with any required documents named above by *(date)*. If you have any questions about these requests, please call me at ___*(phone number)*___.

Sincerely, _____

Acknowledged and agreed to by, _____

Name (please print) _____ Date _____

Phase I: Preliminary Planning

1. Determine primary goals for the health fair.

2. Review and rank employees' health needs using company health records (group accident forms, medical claims, and workers' compensation data).

3. Identify and assess on-site and community health resources.

4. Develop and distribute a survey to local health-related professionals and organizations to determine their interest in participating.

5. Compile survey information into a database showing names, services or products, and contact information for prospective vendors and exhibitors.

Phase II: Developing the Health Fair

1. Choose an on-site coordinator for the health fair.
2. Develop a theme and logo (see table 7.4 for ideas).
3. Set locations, dates, and times for the event.
4. Prepare a working budget.
5. Confirm participation details with prospective vendors and exhibitors.
6. Share the health-fair layout and setup requirements with all vendors and exhibitors.
7. Design and prepare publicity materials (e.g., newsletter articles, flyers, and posters).
8. Use various media venues to encourage employee participation.

Phase III: Program Implementation

1. Contact and inform all vendors, exhibitors, and on-site personnel about final arrangements, including setup procedures, dismantling times, and procedures.
2. Conduct a mock walk-through to check traffic flow, spacing, and supervision needs.
3. Open the fair!

Promotion

Organizers can use posters, bulletin boards, newsletters, e-mail, and other internal resources to advertise the health fair and subsequent events to employees. For greatest exposure, promotional materials should be displayed at key locations at least two weeks before the fair. Targeting promotional efforts to specific employee groups can also enhance participation. Groups can be classified by various characteristics, such as age, gender, race, specific risk factors, and previous participation. Timing is obviously an important factor in promoting new programs. Numerous worksites launch their health fairs in January, in sync with employees' New Year's resolutions. Also, consider promoting specific programs around various state and national campaigns for health and fitness, such as the National Employee Health and Fitness Day in mid-May (see table 7.4).

Table 7.4 Themes and Occasions for Promoting Health Fairs

Program	Health fair theme	Occasions	Month
Physical fitness	Physical fitness	Physical fitness and sports month	May
		Family health and fitness day USA	September
		Women's health and fitness day	September
Nutrition and weight control	Healthy weight	Healthy weight week	January
		Nutrition month	March
		5-a-day month	September
		Diabetes month	November
	Healthy heart	Heart month	February
		Women's heart day	February
		High blood pressure education month	May
		Stroke awareness month	May
Back health	Healthy joints	Correct posture month	May
		Arthritis month	May
		Osteoporosis awareness and prevention month	May

Program	Health fair theme	Occasions	Month
Prenatal health	Healthy moms, healthy babies	March of Dimes walk	April
		World health day	April
Smoking control	Healthy breathing	Clean air month	May
		Healthy lung month	October
		Great Smoke Out	November
		Lung cancer awareness month	November
		Asthma and allergy awareness month	May
AIDS education and HIV disease prevention	Facts for life	National black HIV/AIDS awareness day	February
		World AIDS day	December
Medical self-care and health care consumerism	Cancer prevention and awareness	Cervical cancer screening month	January
		Colorectal cancer awareness month	March
		Cancer control month	April
		Skin cancer awareness month	May
		Ovarian cancer awareness month	September
		Prostate cancer awareness month	September
		Breast cancer awareness month	October
		Mammography day	October
	Healthy awareness	Wise health consumer month	February
		Kidney month	March
		Healthy vision month	May
		Immunization awareness month	August
		Cholesterol education month	September
		Liver awareness month	October
		Talk about prescriptions month	October
		Healthy skin month	November
	Personal wellness	Better sleep month	May
		Mental health month	May
		Headache awareness week	June
		International massage week	July
		Men's health week	July
		Depression screening day	October
Occupational injury	Safety	Safety month	July
		Workplace eye health and safety month	March
		Drive safely at work week	October
Employee assistance program (EAP) and quality of work life (QWL)	Substance abuse, child care, eldercare, financial and retirement planning	Drunk and drugged driving prevention month	December
		Child care awareness days	June
		Family caregiver week	May
		Financial awareness week	July
		National retirement week	November
Stress management	Workplace stress	National stress awareness day	November

To encourage a good turnout, choose an appropriate number of vendors that can provide employee-focused participation opportunities. For instance, as employees enter the health fair, give each person a personal health card (e.g., large index card) with specific instructions. Ask them to read and follow the instructions listed on the card to qualify for a healthy reward and a grand prize (to be awarded at the end of the health fair). Have each vendor with a participating event stamp the cards after employees have fully participated in the activity (e.g., employees have a blood pressure screening at the appropriate booth).

CONDUCTING EMPLOYEE HEALTH SCREENINGS

Any time employees participate in company-sponsored health fairs and other types of WHP events, an employer assumes some degree of risk. Legally, an employer may be held liable for an employee's injury in the following scenarios:

- An employee is injured while participating in an employer-mandated program or activity.
- The employer benefits from the employee's attendance or participation in the program in which the injury occurred.
- The employee is injured on the job.

Although WHP-related lawsuits are rare, worksites should naturally take steps to minimize any liability risk. For example, many companies have positioned their programs so that workers' compensation insurance or private liability insurance covers any program-related or on-the-job injuries. Another strategy is to develop a screening program that effectively identifies high-risk employees for appropriate referral to specific programs that are in tune with their capabilities and needs.

If employers offer programs or facilities with policies for admission or participation that exclude or limit certain people, they should carefully review the requirements of Great Britain's Disability Discrimination Act (DDA) or the Americans with Disabilities Act

(ADA). For example, using safety-screening criteria is probably permissible under the acts, provided that the criteria are based on actual risks, not stereotypical ones. The ADA stipulates that employers cannot discriminate on the basis of a person's disability, so it is essential to know what types of conditions are considered legitimate disabilities. Under the ADA, a person with a disability possesses at least one of the following characteristics:

- Has a physical or mental impairment that substantially limits one or more major life activities
- Has a record of such an impairment
- Is regarded as having such an impairment

Specifically, the ADA defines a physical impairment as follows:

[A]ny physiological disorder or condition, cosmetic disfigurement, or anatomical loss affecting one or more of the following body systems: neurological, musculoskeletal, special sense organs, respiratory (including speech organs), cardiorespiratory, reproductive, digestive, genitourinary, hemic and lymphatic, skin, and endocrine.

The ADA defines a mental impairment as follows:

[a]ny mental or psychological disorder, such as mental retardation, organic brain syndrome, emotional or mental illness, and specific learning disabilities.

Worksites that use a screening system to admit or exclude employees from exercise or recreation programs may have to modify their policies to accommodate the provisions of the law. If so, they should seek legal advice for guidance in reviewing current policies. Also, health-screening personnel should comply with the following standards:

- Screening techniques should be medically warranted and should be conducted only by authorized, competent professionals.
- Before employees are screened, they should be informed of the purpose of

the screening and any other pertinent information.

- A postscreening follow-up meeting should occur in which authorized personnel interpret screening results for employees on an individual, confidential basis.
- Employee health screening should not rely solely on a physical exam to evaluate a person's total health status. A physical examination should identify organic signs and symptoms, such as high blood pressure or a heart murmur. However, a health assessment should also review lifestyle habits and other relevant information.

Virtually all employees have some level of measurable health risk. For example, researchers at Michigan State University found that only 3% of the 153,000 American adults randomly sampled achieved low-risk status on four targeted lifestyle characteristics: (1) nonsmoker, (2) healthy body weight, (3) healthy diet (ate at least five servings of fruits and vegetables a day), and (4) regular exercise (Reeves and Rafferty 2005).

Because risk factors vary in type and prevalence from worksite to worksite, screening procedures must detect risk factors for all possible participants. In particular, any selected procedure should factor in age, gender, current health status, activity level, and occupation.

In many worksites, on-site fitness screenings are conducted to determine employee health status, fitness level, and exercise capabilities. Unfortunately, some employees fail to show up for this important screening, which is often time-consuming and labor-intensive. One way to minimize no shows is to first ask employees to complete an appropriate questionnaire, omitting the biomedical section (blood pressure, cholesterol, blood glucose, and so on). Screening personnel then review the questionnaires to identify employees who are not high risk and permit them to enter the program. After participating in several sessions, employees are called in individually for their personal biomedical measurement. Employees failing to attend a minimum number of exercise sessions do not receive the biomedical screening until they do so and, likewise, are not permitted to exercise in the program.

Before employees enter an exercise, fitness, or recreational program, they should be physically screened and cleared for participation. A preexercise screening protocol based on age and known risk factors is illustrated in figure 7.2.

Diagnostic laboratory testing is indicated if risk factors for coronary heart disease (CHD) include hyperlipidemia (high blood fats), hyperglycemia (high blood sugar), or hyperuricemia (blood in urine).

In developing a preexercise screening protocol, health professionals should remember that exercise stress testing in a symptom-free population may detect more false positives than true positives. A false positive means that the test result indicates that something is wrong when, in fact, nothing is wrong. Moreover, an exercise electrocardiogram (ECG) has limited value in detecting or predicting coronary artery disease in asymptomatic persons with no known risk factors.

Two types of preexercise tests exist: (1) symptom-limited, ECG-monitored, *graded exercise tests (GXT)* and (2) *submaximal tests.*

GXTs should be conducted in a clinical setting by trained personnel, under a physician's direct supervision. The GXT protocol, administered to the subject on a motorized treadmill, is specifically designed to detect coronary ischemia (when the heart muscle receives inadequate oxygen because of diseased or blocked coronary arteries) and to determine functional capacity and safety of exercise for at-risk and symptomatic persons. People at such risk who may be in need of the GXT protocol include those who exhibit one or more of the following risk factors:

- Cigarette smoking
- Diabetes mellitus
- Family history of high blood cholesterol or heart disease
- Obesity
- High blood pressure (systolic over 140, diastolic over 90)
- Other high-risk condition as defined by a physician

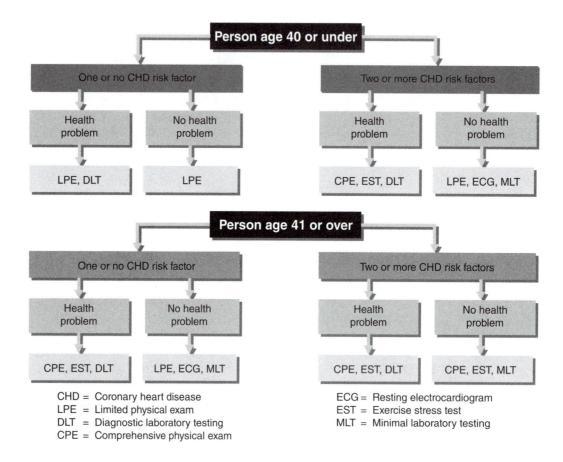

Figure 7.2 A sample preexercise screening protocol.

Submaximal testing is used to determine an employee's fitness level and to assist in prescribing the right type and amount of exercise. A submaximal test can be administered with a bicycle ergometer, which is considerably less expensive than a motorized treadmill. To determine the appropriate testing protocol for each employee, follow screening guidelines established by the American College of Sports Medicine (2010). In all cases, the selected protocol should be scientifically based and tailored to each employee's overall health status. For example, a common approach is to group employees into the following classes for preexercise screening:

- Class I: Healthy, conditioned workers of all ages
- Class II: Healthy, inactive workers under age 35

- Class III: Healthy, inactive workers over age 35
- Class IV: Conditioned people of all ages with major coronary risk factors, cardiorespiratory disease, or both
- Class V: Inactive people of all ages with major coronary risk factors
- Class VI: Inactive people of all ages with either acute or chronic cardiorespiratory disease
- Class VII: People for whom exercise is contraindicated

Employees in classes I, II, or III should have the submaximal test. Those in all other classes should have the symptom-limited GXT. Employees in class VII may not be tested at all.

SAMPLE QUESTIONNAIRE FOR CARDIORESPIRATORY SCREENING

CONDITION	YES	NO
1. Have you ever had a heart attack?	___	___
2. Have you ever had a heart problem?	___	___
3. Have you ever had *angina* (chest pain)?	___	___
4. Were you born with a heart condition?	___	___
5. Have you ever had high blood pressure?	___	___
6. Have you ever had diabetes?	___	___
7. Do you smoke?	___	___
8. Have you ever had a thyroid condition?	___	___
9. Have you ever had surgery?	___	___
10. Are you currently taking any medication?	___	___
11. If you are female, are you pregnant?	___	___

MANAGING RISK AND LIABILITY

Employers are ultimately responsible for the safety of their WHP programs. Therefore, they must minimize the prospect of participant injuries. Before they enter any type of employer-sponsored exercise program, employees should be informed in writing of their personal responsibility in meeting all preexercise clearance requirements. Most companies require employees to complete an informed consent form before participating. However, for maximum protection, employers should develop clear and concise policies requiring participants to read such releases in the presence of a staff member and to acknowledge their understanding in writing. Without such documentation, employees may claim that they signed the release unwittingly. It is a good idea to consult legal counsel in developing and reviewing all forms for informed consent and liability release.

A sample informed consent form on the next page can be modified for your needs. Additional risk-management guidelines include the following:

- Make sure all exercise instructors and other staff are properly certified by a reputable organization.

- Require participants in high-risk activities to wear appropriate clothing and use appropriate equipment at all times.

- Make sure all equipment and facilities (e.g, spas, whirlpools, and steam rooms) feature clear, easy-to-see instructions with precautionary warnings.

- Explain the possibility of injuries associated with aerobics, racquetball, weightlifting, and other activities to all participants before they begin.

- Require employees to sign an informed consent form before participating.

- Use only nationally recognized screening tests and procedures.

- Develop and follow a reliable system of injury reporting.

- Have a clearly established system and support personnel in place to handle any injuries or emergencies (e.g., first-responders, AEDs).

- Develop a hierarchy of supervision to ensure accountability for all phases of program and facility operations.
- Designate specific duties and chain of command (who is responsible for what and to whom).

Many smaller worksites do not have adequate personnel, facilities, and equipment to conduct appropriate preexercise screening. In such settings, a questionnaire can be helpful in assessing a person's cardiorespiratory health. Employees with any positive responses on the questionnaire should meet with their personal physician for further consultation and permission to exercise. You may use the questionnaire shown in the sidebar on this page or modify it as necessary.

Because health screening is both labor and time intensive, efficiency is particularly important for small businesses. Although most small businesses do not have in-house screening personnel, they can consider networking with local agencies by doing the following:

- Negotiating with the local health department to conduct a basic health screening for employees at little or no cost.
- Arranging with a local health club for employees to receive a complimentary health screening in exchange for allowing the club to display its literature at the worksite.
- Sponsoring an annual health fair and asking exhibitors to provide health screenings for employees.
- Asking faculty members (exercise physiologists, nurses, physical therapists, and health educators) at a local university to conduct employee health screenings in exchange for using their worksite as a possible research site.

SAMPLE INFORMED CONSENT FORM

In consideration of my voluntary participation in (company's name)'s health promotion program or any other activities sponsored by (company's name) conducted on or off company property, I hereby release and discharge (company's name) from any and all claims for damages suffered by me as a result of my participation in these activities. I specifically release and discharge (company's name) and its health promotion staff from all injuries or damages arising from or contributing to any physical impairment or defect I may have, whether latent or patent, and agree that (company's name) is under no obligation to provide physical examination or other evidence of my fitness to participate in such activities, the same being my sole responsibility. Further, I understand that participation is not a condition of employment at (company's name).

Date_____   Signature _____

Printed name _____

Preactivity screenings

Date	Staff member	Type	Results
_____	_____	_____	_____
_____	_____	_____	_____
_____	_____	_____	_____

Employee health status

_____ Excellent
_____ Good
_____ Fair
_____ Poor
_____ Very Poor

Activity recommendation

_____ Approved for participation
_____ Approved, conditional
_____ Unapproved, further screening needed

Date_____   Program director _____

GIVING THE PROGRAM A TRIAL RUN

As the planning process winds down and implementation nears, it's a good idea to conduct a trial run to identify potential problems and make necessary adjustments. It is especially helpful to assess traffic flow, space, equipment, facilities, and employee interest when planning a health fair or a new exercise program. You can conduct a trial run in four steps:

1. Recruit the number of employees you expect to participate at one time.
2. Explain the physical environment in which the program or event will occur to the employees (e.g., layout of health fair or program site, equipment functions, exhibits, technical aspects, participation flow, and operations).
3. Have each person occupy a specific piece of equipment or station so that the entire facility is occupied.
4. Instruct all participants to proceed from station to station at designated intervals.

As employees engage in a mock run-through, check to see if the time allotted is sufficient for employees to successfully complete each routine. Is the transition smooth or is it choppy? If you notice a delay or congestion, identify possible reasons for it and consider revising the facility layout or instructions for better efficiency.

In completing final preparations before launching the actual WHP program or activity, take some time to review your over-all implementation strategy. In reviewing your approach, check to see if you've adequately considered key issues, such as the following:

- Offer programs at or near normal working hours and on days and times preferred by employees, when possible.
- Make programs and activities available to workers on all shifts.
- Use positive and catchy titles when promoting certain programs and activities. For instance, instead of referring to a nutrition program as a weight-loss program, consider using an action-oriented title such as "Eating to Energize Your Life" or "Eating for the Good Life." Other examples include "Taking Charge!" (exercise program), "Smooth Transitions" (stress-management program), and "Kicking Butts" (smoking cessation program).
- Use personal testimonies from past and current participants to highlight the benefits of your new program. To be the most inspirational, testimonies should be short and to the point.
- Charge participants a small fee (e.g., $5) that can be pooled into a reward bank to purchase awards for employees who reach their personal goals.

END-OF-PROGRAM REWARDS

As a program or activity nears completion, WHP planners should think ahead to the next program. Part of this involves motivating employees who have finished one program to pursue other programs that may benefit them. Consider giving employees who complete a program the following rewards:

- Enter the employee in a company-wide sweepstakes or lottery. Draw one or more winners for prizes.
- Highlight employees with notable achievements in the company's newsletter.
- Designate a wall of fame to highlight employees who consistently set a good example for others.
- Offer employees with noteworthy improvements designated parking spaces at work for the month.
- Provide T-shirts that convey a specific theme or accomplishment at designated times (e.g., "I kicked butts" at the end of the smoking cessation program).
- Ask management to send a congratulatory letter to employees who complete a program.

- Explore the feasibility of providing employees with at least one hour of paid release time each week to participate in on-site health programs.
- Offer small-group (interdepartmental) competitions to boost motivation and fun for participants.
- Offer financial rewards to employees who participate in WHP programs.

Of course, some WHP practitioners select end-of-the-program rewards when they select their front-end incentives. Whatever approach you use, it's important to (1) consistently inform employees of the company's commitment in their health and overall well-being and (2) adapt the types and timing of incentives and rewards to keep employees fully engaged in your programs.

What Would You Do?

Read the following four real worksite case studies. Then, choose one case study to which you can apply the strategies described in this chapter in terms of the following three components.

1. *Client research.* How will you identify employee needs and interests?
2. *Marketing.* Create a marketing mix.
3. *Development and implementation.* Describe how you will develop and implement your program.

Case study 1. A coal mine in New Mexico employs 85% Navajo American Indians. The total employee population is 375 people (90% men and 10% women). The mine is unionized and works three rotating 8-hour shifts. The mine has three different sites with separate entrances. The union participates in a nationwide health plan negotiated specifically for coal miners, which includes little preventive care. Management will only participate and pay for preventive activities if employees drive the program.

Case study 2. A refinery employs 90% men and 10% women. The total employee population is 1,200 and the average age is 42. The nonunion workforce requires 70% heavy labor done in two rotating 12-hour shifts. A health promotion program has been in place for two years with an on-site fitness facility of 10,000 square feet (3,048 square m). The top employee risk factors are poor eating habits, stress, back injuries, high blood cholesterol, and lack of daily aerobic exercise.

Case study 3. In a large city, a cellular phone company has five worksites with a total of 1,500 white-collar employees. The population is 50% male and 50% female, and the average employee age is 34. The majority of employees have a college education, and the company is nonunion. Access to health promotion and risk-reduction programs is limited to the choice of two managed care programs.

Case study 4. Located on the East Coast are 55 offshore oil platforms, which house 15 to 40 employees at each bunkhouse. Each facility has a catered food arrangement, and 17 have functioning fitness facilities. The population is nonunion and is 90% blue-collar males. The employees belong to a traditional indemnity (fee-for-service) plan and emergency care is the most common claim.

CHAPTER 7 WRAP-UP

Key Points

- A well-planned marketing effort greatly enhances the probability for successful WHP programming.

- More worksites are adopting *e-health methods,* or technological tools and applications to reach employees in a more timely and cost-efficient manner.

- Creating employee-oriented incentives and rewards is essential for boosting participation among at-risk and hard-to-reach employees.

- Federal laws, such as ADA, GINA, and HIPAA, present some unique challenges for WHP practitioners. However, these can be overcome with innovative planning.

- Establishing appropriate protocols for risk and liability management for all aspects of your WHP programs and activities is in the best interests of all stakeholders.

Glossary

e-health technology—The application of Internet and other related technologies to reach targeted populations with health information and resources.

health coaching—A confidential one-on-one communication between a trained health practitioner and a client to enhance well-being.

incentive—An inducement or stimulus to do something; something offered before an effort is performed.

marketing mix—Four distinct, yet interrelated, dimensions that reflect a strategic effort to promote a product or service to a targeted population.

reward—Something that is given during or after the performance of a desired action.

risk and liability management—The identification, assessment, and prioritization of risks, followed by a coordinated application of resources to minimize, monitor, and control the probability or impact of unfortunate events.

Bibliography

ACSM. 2010. *ACSM's guidelines for exercise testing and prescription.* 8th ed. Baltimore: Lippincott, Williams and Wilkins.

Chapman, L. 2008. "Understanding wellness incentives." *WELCOA's Absolute Advantage* 7: 5, 40-48.

Healthcare Intelligence Network. 2009. *Benchmarks in health and wellness incentives: Utilization and effectiveness data to drive health promotion, compliance and ROI.* Wall Township, NJ: Author.

Incent One. 2009. "The science of health incentives: Impact of incentive values on participation on comprehensive wellness and health risk assessment interventions." Accessed January 15, 2010. http://65.51.196.73/joomla/index.php?option=com_content&view=article&id=193%3Athe-science-of-health-incentives&catid=60&Itemid=160.

Lewis, S. 2007. "Integrated, flexible incentive programs encourage change." *Managed Healthcare Executive*, March 1.

Mearian, L. 2010. "'Cyberchondriacs' jump to almost one-third of all adults." *Computer World*. Accessed November 11, 2010. www.computerworld.com/s/article/9180147/_Cyberchondriacs_jump_to_almost_one-third_of_all_adults.

National Association of Manufacturers. 2007. "Employee health and productivity management programs. The use of incentives: A survey of major U.S. employers." Accessed November 11, 2010. www.nam.org.

Palmer, S., I. Tubbs, and A. Whybrow. 2003. "Health coaching to facilitate the promotion of healthy behaviour and achievement of health-related goals." *International Journal of Health Promotion and Education* 41(3): 91-93.

Prochaska, J., J. Norcross, and C. DiClemente. 2004. *Changing for good*. New York: William Morrow and Company.

Reeves, M., and A. Rafferty. 2005. "Healthy lifestyle characteristics among adults in the United States, 2000." *Archives of Internal Medicine* 165: 854-857.

Society of Human Resource Management. 2010. "Wellness programs get a boost in health reform law." Accessed November 11. www.shrm.org/publications/HRNews/Pages/WellnessReformBoast.aspx.

Sullivan, N. 2002. "5 factors for success: Byte size advice for e-health management." *WELCOA's Absolute Advantage* 2(1): 14-17.

Tuna, C. 2010. "Wellness efforts face hurdle." *The Wall Street Journal*, February 1.

Wojcik, J. 2009. "Health risk assessments face bias hurdle." *Workforce Management*. Accessed February 1, 2010. www.workforce.com.

Looking Ahead

Now that we've covered important promotional and implementation strategies, it's time to consider a plan to evaluate the WHP program. Chapter 8 presents a step-by-step process for preparing a customized program evaluation. Particular emphasis is placed on identifying factors that can jeopardize an evaluation, tailoring an evaluation around stakeholders' expectations, preparing basic and advanced evaluation designs, and applying economic-based evaluations in WHP settings.

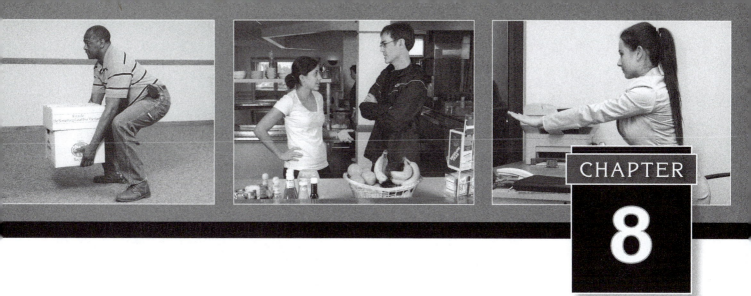

Evaluating Health Promotion Efforts

LEARNING OBJECTIVES

After reading this chapter, you will be able to do the following:

✔ List several pitfalls that can compromise an evaluation.

✔ Identify typical WHP program stakeholders by title and rationale for their interest in evaluation.

✔ Distinguish between goals and objectives.

✔ Give examples of process, impact, and outcome evaluation.

✔ Explain the primary differences between nonexperimental, quasi-experimental, and experimental evaluation designs.

✔ Distinguish between cost-effectiveness analysis, benefit-cost analysis, and break-even analysis.

Early supporters of WHP activities, particularly in the worksite, based their personal commitment to efforts in health promotion and disease prevention largely on intuitive reasoning. However, the time for blind acceptance of WHP's presumed effectiveness has passed. Some programs that have forgone evaluation in favor of investing those dollars in other endeavors are now in trouble or have ceased operations. Moreover, the traditionally heavy emphasis on programs based on exercise and fitness centers is no longer sufficient. By and large, most current multifaceted WHP programs are designed to reach the entire workforce population, not just fitness enthusiasts.

Thus, they warrant a broader continuum of evaluations that are oriented toward process, impact, and financial outcome. This chapter describes this three-tiered evaluation approach.

Today's business leaders are asking for data-driven results to support the continuation of longstanding and, in some cases, expensive programs. Other organizations that are just establishing new programs are setting clear expectations for measurable outcomes.

With greater challenges to produce more results using limited resources, how can an organization know whether its WHP program is on the right track? How do you show tangible proof that something is working? In large part, this depends on how decision makers approach program evaluation and on their ability to avoid common pitfalls that compromise the integrity of any evaluation. Some of the most common pitfalls include the following:

- *Lack of goal or vision for doing an evaluation.* You must have a clearly delineated concept of why an evaluation is needed, what components will constitute an evaluation, and who can benefit from the results.

- *Unrealistic expectations.* For example, decision makers expect that a single evaluation will tell them exactly what they need to do to turn an underachieving program into a successful program overnight.

- *Lack of interdepartmental consensus on the scope and specificity of an evaluation.* For example, program managers may disagree about what to evaluate, when to evaluate, where to evaluate, how to conduct an evaluation, and how they will use the results.

- *Inadequate financial resources.* Although 5% to 10% of a program budget is generally acceptable to devote to an evaluation, many organizations grossly underfund this important component of program accountability.

- *Inaccessibility to essential data or inability to obtain it.* For example, the benefits director may have not established a good rapport with the third-party administrator and, thus, is unable to obtain aggregate medical-claims data in a timely manner.

- *Evaluating a program before its time.* For example, a **break-even analysis** is conducted on a new injury-rehabilitation center only several months after it opens.

- *Lack of adequate resources in place.* For instance, no one makes a plan to secure appropriate data tools, equipment, and personnel in a timely manner.

- *Improper scope and specificity in an evaluation.* For example, evaluators fail to incorporate the appropriate types of variables to measure or lack the degree of sensitivity needed to yield objective results.

- *Inappropriate evaluation design.* For example, no one makes an effort to include a matched group of nonparticipants to minimize the potential (unexpected) effect of external factors.

- *Failure to identify the needs and interests of evaluation stakeholders.* For example, someone conducts an evaluation without considering the goals and interests of all decision makers.

Most of these pitfalls relate to factors that decision makers consider in the preliminary planning (preevaluation) phase. Let's investigate how specific factors affect decisions when planning and conducting an evaluation. To cut this huge task down to size, it is important to approach an evaluation through decision points. A simple way to envision a decision point is to look at the questions listed in table 8.1.

IDENTIFYING PROGRAM STAKEHOLDERS

Several decades ago, Edward Suchman, one of America's great social researchers, said this about program evaluation:

> *All social institutions or subsystems— whether medical, educational, religious, economic, or political—are required to provide proof of their legitimacy and effectiveness in order to justify society's continued support. Both the demand for and type of acceptable proof will depend largely on the nature of the relationship between the social institution and the public. In general, a balance will be struck between faith and fact, reflecting the degree of man's respect for authority and tradition within the particular system versus his skepticism and desire for tangible proof of work.*

Perhaps Suchman's insightful message can serve to remind us that any program, service, or commodity rendered needs substantiation. To evaluate anything, you have to know what it is you are evaluating and why. Thus, one of the first things to do when

Table 8.1 Sample Decision Points in a Socratic-Based Evaluation Plan

	Evaluation goals	Evaluation design	Evaluation objectives	Scope and specificity	Financial and budgeting	Reporting
What	What are the goals of this evaluation?	What target population will be evaluated?	What actions need to be taken to complete an evaluation?	What type(s) of evaluation (process, impact, or outcome) is appropriate?	What type of benefit and cost variables are appropriate?	What stakeholders should receive the evaluation results? In what format?
Why	Why are we evaluating this program?	Why are we using this particular design?		Why is a specific type of evaluation appropriate for this setting?		
How	How were the goals established?	How long is the evaluation time frame? How will data be collected?		How precise (sensitive) should the measurement be?	How much will the evaluation cost?	How much detail should be reported to selected stakeholders?
When		When will measurements be performed?	When should each objective be completed?	When will we know if the evaluation is proceeding as originally planned?	When is a reasonable time frame to compare costs and benefits?	When is the best time to report results?
Where		Where will we conduct the evaluation?			Where can we obtain funding for an evaluation?	Where is the best venue to report results?
Who	Who constructed the evaluation goals?	Who will conduct the evaluation? Who will analyze data?	Who is responsible for each objective?	Who should decide which type of evaluation to use?	Who can assess the cost of an evaluation?	Who should officially be responsible for reporting the evaluation results?

Reprinted, by permission, from Chenoweth & Associates, Inc.

planning an evaluation is to identify everyone who has a stake in knowing about the influence and results of the program you are proposing to evaluate. Next, find out what they want to know. Once you understand what they are interested in, you can proceed with the task of developing appropriate evaluation goals. However, take this precaution: If you are either inexperienced or simply new to an organization, it may be very useful to do a quick, informal survey of available resources before developing goals. By doing so, you can get some idea of which resources are likely to be available to guide your goal planning. Moreover, it will keep you from being overly optimistic about what can be done or from underestimating the possibilities.

You cannot effectively design an evaluation unless you include input from the *program stakeholders,* or those people who have something to gain or lose from the evaluation results. Thus, you must establish who the program stakeholders are and then enlist their cooperation. For example, corporate financial officers, relevant program managers (e.g., benefits, safety, medical, risk management, loss prevention, and so on) health promotion staff members, program participants, and sponsors (if a funding source is involved) will probably all have questions about the program. You will find that different stakeholders have different interests. Be sure to include evaluation goals that address all of their questions.

How can you be sure you have identified all the stakeholders? It will help to take these four factors into account:

1. The administrative structure of an organization's decision-making style.

2. The rationale for doing an evaluation.

3. The history and maturity of the program being evaluated.

4. The political realities surrounding the evaluation.

Each of these factors is important to consider. For example, suppose a WHP program director approached an outside consulting firm to do an analysis of medical claims data. The primary reason for doing the data analysis was to identify the percentage of employees' claim costs linked to smoking, physical inactivity, obesity, and other potentially modifiable risk factors. Based on the risk-factor cost distributions from the analysis, appropriate programming and risk-reduction interventions were then established by the WHP staff. Although the director only requested that the analysis be prepared for her, the consultants suggested the report also be prepared for and shared with the benefits director, occupational health nurse, and other allied health representatives throughout the company.

Here is how the four factors that identify stakeholders affect this recommendation:

1. *The administrative structure of an organization's decision-making style.* Through discussions with the WHP program director, the consultants discovered that she had requested that an evaluation address several employee health issues initially identified initially by her boss, the benefits director. Clearly, the benefits director was a key decision maker in the program.

2. *The rationale for doing an evaluation.* Because the evaluation centered initially around risk factors, the consultants recognized that various health-management personnel (e.g., occupational health, workers' compensation, safety, loss prevention, risk management, and so on) who were responsible for implementing specific risk-reduction

programs might also have wished to receive the evaluation results.

3. *The history and maturity of the program being evaluated.* The consultants learned that the WHP program was relatively new and that the program director was trying to expand it to reach a larger share of the workforce. This suggested that they should apprise various stakeholder groups of the program's current and future value, thereby creating support throughout the company for the WHP program director's goal.

4. *The political realities surrounding the evaluation.* By recognizing that the benefits director and others had been very influential in establishing past and present program policies, it was clear to the consultants that without their support, the expansion of the WHP program could not evolve.

When the consultants shared their concerns about tailoring the report to the benefits director and other targeted people, the program director quickly understood that expanding the audience for the report and addressing the concerns of major stakeholders would significantly enhance her ability to expand the breadth of the WHP program.

What kinds of questions will stakeholders have? In many cases, they are as numerous and varied as the people involved. Program administrators may want to know what percentage of the program budget is spent on operational costs within the program. Health promotion staff members may want to know whether the newly enacted financial incentives are motivating high-risk employees to participate. Funding sponsors may want to know whether their money produced some positive outcomes. Finding out all of these questions may take some ingenuity. Based on an organization's culture and decision-making style, it may be appropriate to call a meeting of key decision makers. Brainstorm, distribute a written survey, or quiz them by phone or e-mail. Some companies hold an annual WHP planning retreat in which stakeholders are invited to brainstorm with the staff about programs and program evaluations they would like to see in the future.

QUESTIONS ADDRESSED BY EVALUATION

- Can a WHP program provide measurable, tangible benefits to employees and an organization?
- To what extent do all participants benefit from a WHP program?
- How can we tell whether a program has a greater effect on direct benefits or indirect benefits?
- Can these programs really affect productivity measures, such as absenteeism, presenteeism, on-the-job injury, and short-term disability?
- What types of programs are most cost-effective in a company with a demographic profile similar to that of our workforce?
- How long does it take for a program to break even?

ESTABLISHING GOALS FOR EVALUATION

Goals of greatest interest to stakeholders are of two primary types: health related and financial. If you neglect to include both categories of goals, you also neglect to plan for the evaluation types, designs, and instruments necessary to measure them. Evaluation helps determine whether health program goals and objectives are met. It also answers questions about the program as it is being implemented. Thus, evaluation planning should be tied closely to the development of a program's goals and objectives.

Assessments can be made easily during the course of the program, enabling staff members to improve the program as it progresses. For example, if ongoing evaluations are scheduled, WHP personnel might discover that the low enrollment in a stress-management workshop reflects an inadequate location, inconvenient hours, ineffective marketing, or lack of publicity. These problems, once identified, could be addressed and eliminated. Unequivocally, clearly defined goals can help program presenters and participants keep on track through ongoing mini evaluations.

Yet, if the evaluation is not designed until the program has ended, neither of these benefits is possible. Moreover, carefully designed goals will let you focus on what the intervention can reasonably be expected to achieve, clarifying the effect of the intervention on its target.

Laudable as health-related goals may be, they cannot be pursued apart from financial goals. If money is not available to run WHP programs, the health-related goals can never be achieved. Thus, it is crucial that these goals be addressed within the limitations imposed by financial necessity. These limitations vary from organization to organization, depending on financial resources as well as on the values of those who control the purse strings. Key decision makers are usually interested in financial goals. They want to address questions that can be answered by using econometric-based evaluation tools, such as break-even analysis, cost-effectiveness analysis, forecasting, and **benefit-cost analysis**.

DEVELOPING INTERVENTION GOALS

After you have clearly delineated goals for doing an evaluation, you can develop goals for your program interventions. For example, what is the goal for your back-health program? Because you are developing your evaluation goals in connection with specific programs, you must think not only about goals that are tied to evaluation, but also about the general goals of the programs. If these are properly developed, it makes your program intervention goals that much easier to develop as well. (Note that the following terms are used interchangeably: *outcome variable, dependent variable, outcome,* and *goal.*) Evaluation is greatly enhanced when the targeted program contains goals with these characteristics:

1. Compatible with stakeholders' personal health and values.
2. Measurable.
3. Quantifiable.
4. Incorporated around a sufficient time frame.
5. Realistically achievable.

See chapter 3, pages 44 through 48, for a discussion on setting appropriate goals, goal criteria, and establishing measurable objectives.

DEVELOPING YOUR EVALUATION APPROACH

Some evaluators make the mistake of planning an evaluation after a WHP program is under way, rather than in the planning phase. In these cases, evaluation procedures are often rushed and off base, creating unreliable results. Good planning gives evaluators enough time to properly lay out important elements of an evaluation, such as the following:

- Which variables to measure
- Which subjects to target
- Who conducts the evaluation
- How much financial support is needed
- When the evaluation should be conducted
- Where the evaluation should be conducted
- Which evaluation equipment and instruments are needed
- What type of evaluation design is most appropriate
- How to use the results
- Who should have access to the results

As an evaluator, you should incorporate six basic guidelines in addressing each of these elements:

1. Have some idea of what type of outcome you are looking for. Decide which factors and outcomes are most important to track.

2. Be in a position to act on the results. Secure management support and form alliances with specific departments in order to obtain essential data (safety, medical, benefits, and human resources, in particular).

3. Follow scientifically sound statistical procedures that are appropriate for the scope and specificity of your evaluation.

For example, will a T-test be sufficient to compare pre- and postprogram results? What type of regression analysis is necessary to properly identify the relationships between several variables at the same time? Were previous cost savings adjusted to reflect today's market value?

4. Differentiate between normal and abnormal results. A slight drop in absenteeism among program participants may be normal, but a quitting rate of 50% or higher among smokers would be unrealistic.

5. Closely monitor each variable being measured. Are participants as satisfied with their personal coach now as they were on the first day? How many participants are losing body weight at a healthy rate? What types of health care claims have changed the most by ranking in the past year?

6. Convert data-driven effects and outcomes into valuable information when possible. Identify and record any evolving trends by age, gender, risk-factor level, and so on. What implications can you extract from the results for future WHP programs, marketing strategies, health plan benefits, financial incentives, and so on?

Impact Evaluation Categories

As you establish your evaluation framework, consider how the results of your evaluation will be used. An initial step in development should involve a technique to categorize your overall evaluation. It is common to find proponents of the *process-impact-outcome approach,* while others advocate the *formative and summative approach.* While both of these approaches can be applied in WHP evaluations, the author prefers the former approach, primarily because it has a three-tiered evaluation time frame that provides evaluators with more opportunities to scrutinize an intervention on an on-going basis (see figure 8.1)

Process evaluation focuses on what happens during a program and specific aspects

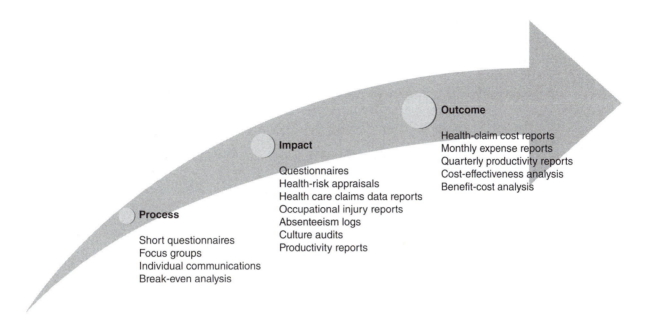

Process

Short questionnaires
Focus groups
Individual communications
Break-even analysis

Impact

Questionnaires
Health-risk appraisals
Health care claims data reports
Occupational injury reports
Absenteeism logs
Culture audits
Productivity reports

Outcome

Health-claim cost reports
Monthly expense reports
Quarterly productivity reports
Cost-effectiveness analysis
Benefit-cost analysis

Figure 8.1 A suggested timeline for conducting process, impact, and outcome evaluations.

of the intervention that may need attention. It can focus on either qualitative or quantitative questions.

Qualitative issues include aspects of program delivery, such as program registration, educational content, and instructor effectiveness. For example, by looking at the age, gender, and job classification of employees who have participated in various program offerings, the evaluator can see whether one delivery mode, teaching method, instructor, or incentive appears to appeal to certain segments of the workforce more effectively than another. Reactions from participants about programming schedules, health-screening procedures, fitness center hours, or workshop speakers could show program administrators which changes might improve participation rates. The tools of qualitative analysis include short questionnaires, personal solicitation, focus groups, suggestion boxes, e-mail communications, and other on-site media.

Process evaluation can also address financial problems and other quantitative issues. For example, using a break-even analysis to determine when defined benefits may offset a program's cost can tell administrators whether they should scale down, maintain, or expand their original plans.

As an intermediate strategy, *impact evaluation* assesses the overall effectiveness of a program in producing desirable levels of knowledge, attitudes, behaviors, health status, and skills among participants. Sample questions include the following: How many people stopped smoking? How many employees meet or exceed the recommended daily intake of fruits and vegetables? How many people currently practice medical self-care compared with six months ago? Essentially, impact evaluation measures changes in participants' behaviors and attitudes and in organizational culture, using one or more survey techniques to compare pre- and postprogram status.

Common tools for impact evaluation include the following:

- Surveys or questionnaires
- Health-risk appraisals
- Health care claims
- Data reports
- Occupational injury reports
- Absenteeism logs
- Culture audits (i.e., observing the worksite environment)
- Productivity or quality reports

Considered the back-end or bottom-line strategy along the evaluation continuum, *outcome evaluation* quantifies the financial consequences that may occur when an intervention affects absenteeism, productivity, health care utilization, and the like. Outcome evaluation addresses the question: *Did the intervention influence the changes that occurred and, if so, was the cost justifiable?* For example, did a particular intervention do the following?

- Reduce employees' hypertension enough to lower their medication costs.
- Decrease the level of workplace stress enough to reduce to cost of mental-health claims
- Decrease the incidence of lower-back injuries enough to lower workers' compensation costs.
- Reduce presenteeism in enough employees to increase an organization's productivity.

Commonly used instruments of outcome evaluation include health-claim cost reports, monthly expense reports, quarterly productivity reports, cost-effectiveness analysis, and benefit-cost analysis.

While process, impact, and outcome evaluation options are being considered in planning an evaluation, it is a good time to consider the rigor of an evaluation expected by the stakeholders. In today's budget-minded economy, many WHP program directors have to constantly justify their programs. Consequently, the scope of an evaluation must show that any changes are primarily influenced by a WHP intervention, while minimizing the potential effect that outside factors, such as the media, corporate policies, demographic changes, and societal forces, may have on the actual outcome. Although it is impossible to completely eliminate the influence of media and societal forces on employees' behavioral and health-status changes, WHP evaluators should use appropriate designs to establish a reasonable level of rigor and objectivity. Let's take a look at several options for WHP personnel to consider when selecting an evaluation design.

Scope and Specificity

The structure of your evaluation plan is influenced largely by the scope and specificity of your evaluation needs. *Scope* refers to the range of variables and the time frame of the evaluation. For example, an evaluation consisting of several outcome variables that are measured over a one-year time frame has a broader scope than an evaluation involving one or two variables spanning six months. In contrast, *specificity* refers to the level or degree of precision that evaluators use in measuring selected variables within an evaluation.

The number of variables you choose to look at and the time frame in which you do so will define the scope of your evaluation. For example, the scope of an evaluation for a back-injury prevention program will probably be smaller than that for a medical self-care program. Why? Because the back-program evaluation is more likely to focus on a single variable (number of back injuries) that can be influenced in a relatively short time, whereas the medical self-care program is likely to include several variables (e.g., employee's confidence in doing self-care, past and present self-care actions, outpatient encounters, out-of-pocket medical care costs) that usually take longer both to monitor and to change in response to the intervention.

In addition to establishing the scope of your evaluation, consider the specificity, or level of precision, that is appropriate for defining outcome variables. For example, an outcome variable that is referred to generically as *absenteeism* has virtually no level of specificity because it does not delineate specific types of (or reasons for) the phenomenon. In contrast, when absenteeism is defined as *lower-back-injury absenteeism,* it has some level of specificity because it specifies the primary cause. Programs that include outcome variables with a high level of specificity are generally preferred because they give evaluators greater opportunities to closely study the real impact of an intervention on a specific outcome variable (table 8.2).

Table 8.2 Sample Variables with Low and High Levels of Specificity

Variable	Less specificity	More specificity
Absenteeism	All causes, combined	Caused by sick leave alone
Health care claims	Total number	Number by type of claim (e.g., major diagnostic category, diagnostic-related group, International Classification of Diseases)
High-risk employees	Total number	Incidence rate (per 100) of employees in 10-year age intervals with at least 3 targeted risk factors
Injuries	Total number and cost	Incidence rate (per 100) of top 5 most common and top 5 most costly by type
Participation	Total number of weekly encounters	Average number of weekly encounters per participant

Defining highly specific variables is only possible if problems and needs are carefully analyzed early in the evaluation process. The sidebar on page 167 ("Simplify!") shows how one company wrote a dependent variable with a high degree of specificity based on a careful examination of various factors affecting their rising health care costs. When considering scope and specificity issues, evaluators should also consider the feasibility of doing an economic-based evaluation.

CHOOSING AN EVALUATION DESIGN

An evaluation design includes the following essential components:

- **Experimental group (E):** The group of employees that participate in the program.

- **Control** or **comparison group (C):** A control group consists of employees who are similarly matched to the experimental group of employees participating in the intervention. In contrast, a comparison group consists of persons who are not matched (nonequivalent) to the experimental group.

- **Observation (O):** When a measurement is performed.

- **Independent variable (X):** The program intervention designed to produce a positive outcome.

Evaluation designs vary significantly in their scope, specificity, and strength. Thus, you will need to tailor your evaluation plans and selected design to the specific WHP culture of your worksite. For example, if you have a WHP program in a small business with little or no budget, you may be limited to using a basic, nonexperimental evaluation design. However, if your WHP program is on a larger scale, with additional budgetary or staffing resources, you may want to consider an intermediate-level, quasiexperimental evaluation design. Finally, if you have a well-established program, plenty of resources, and programming features that allow you to do some *randomization*, you may wish to consider a high-end, truly experimental evaluation design.

The rigor (power) of a particular evaluation design depends largely on the degree to which evaluators can (1) randomly select subjects for experimental, control, or comparison groups and (2) randomly assign subjects to participate or not participate in a specific WHP program or activity. Essentially, the more randomization that evaluators can exert within a particular design, the more powerful it is.

Several examples of designs for program evaluation follow.

Nonexperimental

Nonexperimental designs (table 8.3) represent basic and relatively weak designs that, in real worksite settings, may be the only viable option when evaluators cannot assign participants to an experimental or control group, or when a comparison group cannot be established. The most basic example is the one-group pretest and posttest design. This design consists of a

Table 8.3 Two Common Nonexperimental Evaluation Designs

Design	Diagram						
Pretest and posttest	E	O_1	X	O_2			
Time series	E	O_1	O_2	O_3	X	O_4	O_5 O_6

single measurement before a program is implemented and a second evaluation at the end of the program. This design is easy to conduct in worksite settings, but has two major drawbacks:

1. Because no measurement is taken during the program, evaluators have to wait until the end of the program to determine whether the program made an impact.

2. Without a control or comparison group, it is difficult to determine whether observed changes in outcomes are the result of the intervention. For example, changes in weather conditions, company policies, work responsibilities, or personal health status could actually influence employees' weight loss more than their participation in a weight management program.

Essentially, in these types of situations, we have to ask whether the results were influenced by the following factors:

- Extraneous events, such as a television program or public information campaign that occurred between O_1 and O_2 that may have influenced the subjects' behavior

- The growth and development of subjects that occur with the mere passage of time between O_1 and O_2

- The effect of O_1 on O_2 (that is, the pretest could have sensitized the subjects to what to expect in the posttest)

- Changes in the measurement tools or procedures between O_1 and O_2

- Interaction between the pretest and the program intervention (For example, the pretest itself may influence behavior by making participants aware of things they should or should not do.)

Because outside forces can interfere with an intervention, evaluators should try to add a comparison group in their evaluation efforts. This would expand the scope of the nonexperimental design to that of a quasi-experimental design.

Presumably, the comparison group and the experimental group would have exercised the same amount outside of work, on average, and so would have experienced equal or similar benefits from any additional exercise they did on their own. Thus, the difference between the two groups in the amount of weight lost could be directly attributed to the worksite weight-management program.

Despite their inherent drawbacks, nonexperimental designs are commonly used at many worksites, especially in programs with very limited resources or small numbers of participants. In some cases, logistical constraints prevail, and a shorter-than-usual intervention makes it impractical to recruit a comparison group. Regardless, the point is that an evaluation generally has more credibility when a comparison group can be included.

Quasi-Experimental

Another type of evaluation commonly used in WHP settings is the **quasi-experimental design** (see table 8.4). The prefix *quasi* means almost or nearly. Thus, a quasi-experimental design is similar to, but not as strong as, a true experimental design because of limitations in the random selection and assignment of subjects to specific interventions. Although these designs can be used to show evidence of a program's effectiveness, they cannot control all the factors that influence the actual outcome of a WHP intervention. Most quasi-experimental evaluation designs are similar to experimental evaluation designs, except that the subjects are not randomly assigned to either the

Table 8.4 Two Common Quasi-Experimental Evaluation Designs

Design	Diagram							
Pretest and posttest	E	O_1	X	O_2				
	C	O_1		O_2				
Time series	E	O_1	O_2	O_3	X	O_4	O_5	O_6
	C	O_1	O_2	O_3		O_4	O_5	O_6

experimental or non-experimental groups. Evaluators also cannot control which group will get the treatment (program).

The pretest and posttest quasi-experimental design is often used when a control group cannot be formed by random assignment. In such cases, a comparison group (a nonequivalent control group) is identified, and both groups are measured before and after the program. For example, you could use a pre- and postprogram fitness test to evaluate a fitness program. Employees volunteering to participate in the program would make up the experimental group, while the remaining employees could serve as the comparison group. Since it is quite likely that volunteers already are more physically active and fitter than nonvolunteers, we can assume an initial difference between the groups on their pretest fitness tests. Thus, in order to achieve more equality between the two groups, it is necessary to identify nonparticipants with similar baseline levels of fitness as the participants. You can identify them through matching (see the following section for an example of matching).

One of the strongest frameworks for quasi-experimental evaluation is the *multiple time series (MTS)* design. It is structured as a true experimental time-series design, but it uses a nonequivalent comparison group. This design can be extended in the same way a staggered evaluation design is: by (1) adding more posttests for the two groups, (2) adding experimental groups to examine variations in the program, or (3) adding both.

This design is especially suited for evaluators who have access to past (retrospective) and future (prospective) data, or who can conduct measurements on a regular basis. For example, suppose a company has established a voluntary stretching program to reduce the prevalence and cost of back injuries. Various types of MTS designs can be used to evaluate the program, assuming that evaluators can measure the number of lower-back injuries that occurred before, during, and after the program. Measurements are taken before the program to determine whether one group is noticeably different from the other group. By comparing any change in the number of back injuries among participants (O_1 to O_2) to any change in the number of back injuries among nonparticipants (O_1 to O_2), evaluators can compare injury rates between the two groups before the program begins. In addition, they can compare injury data for both groups a second time (O_2 to O_3) to give evaluators greater insight about any possible preprogram differences between the groups. If one group shows noticeably fewer back injuries than the other group before the program begins, evaluators can select a second group of nonparticipants for comparison. Ideally, this comparison group should have a similar number of back injuries to the participant group. If not, evaluators can choose a third group of nonparticipants, and so on, until a comparison group with back-injury risks similar to those of the experimental group is identified. Table 8.5 illustrates several comparative methods used to establish varying levels of control and comparison groups.

Random assignment is not required in MTS designs, so it is possible for participants to be inherently different from nonparticipants. For example, suppose a benefits manager suspects that a high percentage of employees are inappropriately using a local hospital's emergency department for nonemergency conditions. A review of health care claims shows 75% of suspected emergency department abuses were incurred by

Table 8.5 Control and Comparison Group Methods for WHP Program Evaluation

Method to develop a comparison group	Randomized control	Nonrandomized matched control	Nonrandomized unmatched control	Comparison group: Book of business	Comparison group: Comparable employee population	Own control
General description of method	Intervened population compared with people randomly selected for withheld services	Intervened population compared with nonparticipants matched to have similar demographic, clinical and behavioral characteristics	Intervened population compared with nonparticipants	Intervened population compared with book-of-business population in same program	Intervened population compared with similar employee group in same program	Pre and post comparison of intervened population
Competition time frame	Concurrent with intervention	Concurrent with intervention	Concurrent with intervention	Prior period	Prior period	Concurrent with intervention
Primary outcome measures	Modifiable risk factors; biometric variables	Modifiable risk factors; biometric variables	Modifiable risk factors; biometric variables	Modifiable risk factors; biometric variables	Modifiable risk factors; biometric variables	Modifiable risk factors; biometric variables
Population selection bias	None	Somewhat significant	Significant	None	None	
Source of comparison group	Population for whom program was implemented; randomly selected group withheld from program	Population for whom program was implemented; purchaser decision to not participate	Population for whom program was implemented; purchaser decision to not participate	Vendor data	Vendor data	Intervened population
Credibility of causal statements	Extremely strong	Moderate	Poor	Very poor	Very poor	Very poor
Control of confounding variables	Controls known and unknown, measured and unmeasured confounding variables	Controls known and measured confounding variables	Does not control confounding variables	Does not control confounding variables	Does not control confounding variables	Does not control confounding variables
Program sponsor resistance to approach	High	Moderately high	Moderate	None	None	None
Ease of implementation	Very difficult	Difficult	Somewhat difficult	Easy	Easy	Easy
Clarity of method to lay audience	Very clear	Very unclear	Somewhat unclear	Clear	Clear	Clear
Multiyear application vs. single-year application	Much harder	Much harder	Somewhat harder	Same	Same	Same
Method availability	Rarely possible	Occasionally possible	Occasionally possible	Always possible	Usually possible	Always possible
Blend of interventions to comparison population	Control group may get provider-based interventions, other vendor interventions, secular interventions, and self-care	Control group may get provider-based interventions, other vendor interventions, secular interventions, and self-care	Control group may get provider-based interventions, other vendor interventions, secular interventions, and self-care	Comparison population already intervened	Comparison population already intervened	Not applicable

Method to develop a comparison group	Randomized control	Nonrandomized matched control	Nonrandomized unmatched control	Comparison group: Book of business	Comparison group: Comparable employee population	Own control
Key strengths	Gold-standard evaluation method	Possible to infer reasonable level of causality without experimental design	Least costly and easiest method of comparing intervened to nonintervened population	Low cost, availability of data, ability to answer question asked: How does my group compare to other groups that have been in the program?	Low cost, availability of data, ability to answer question asked: How does my group compare to other groups that have been in the program?	Low cost, availability of data, ability to answer question asked: Did the intervened group change over time?
Key problems/biases	Cost, sponsor resistance, IRB imperative, low generalizability	Cost, availability of control group HRA data	Limited ability to make causal inferences	No inferences on causality are possible	No inferences on causality are possible	No inferences on causality are possible; no information on relative performance of intervened group

employees under 40 years of age. During the process of planning a new medical self-care program to address this problem, the company distributed surveys on three preprogram occasions (O_1, O_2, and O_3) to assess employee interest in a self-care program. Suppose employees who expressed the highest interest in the program on the first occasion (O_1) also reported the most visits to the emergency department over the past year. Yet, on the second (O_2) and third (O_3) occasions, responding employees reportedly had the lowest rate of emergency department visits. By assessing employee interest on three separate occasions before implementing a self-care program, program planners were able to see that employees interested in the self-care program actually represented a broad cross section of employees. They could then use this information to determine whether a self-care program should be offered to the entire workforce or directed primarily toward employees under 40.

To minimize the possibility of significant preprogram differences, evaluators should try to match participants and nonparticipants as closely as possible, especially on attributes linked with the outcome variable being measured. For example, various worksite studies suggest that an employee's risk of experiencing a back injury is influenced by these factors:

- Age
- Type of job
- Body weight
- Exercise habits
- History of back injury
- Job rotation opportunities
- Prework stretching
- Lifting habits
- Abdominal strength
- Hamstring and lower-back flexibility
- Work satisfaction
- Stress level

An effective matching technique is to select (randomly, if possible) nonparticipating employees to form a comparison group that resembles participants. For example, if a new program for back-injury prevention is being implemented, consider matching the groups on as many predisposing factors tied to back-injury risk as possible. Because it is highly unlikely that you can choose nonparticipants that will closely match participants on all relevant criteria, you can establish a legitimate comparison group if it has some overall resemblance to participants. In essence, it is usually necessary to establish an acceptable range for specific criteria (table 8.6).

Once you develop acceptable ranges for each criterion, you must decide on a minimum number of acceptable criteria in selecting nonparticipants for the comparison group.

Another way to equate various groups is to randomly assign participants to different versions of a program. Random assignment is feasible when a new program has been added to an existing program or when a new program has two or more versions offered

simultaneously. Say, for example, you have 50 employees sign up for a smoking cessation program. You can randomly divide the volunteers into two subgroups of 25 each, then assign one group to the self-help video intervention and the other group to the on-site professional seminar (see table 8.7). Since both groups are selected from the same (single) pool of volunteers, it's likely that most of the subjects have a similar level of motivation to quit smoking. This design also allows evaluators to compare one particular intervention with another intervention to determine which is most cost-effective.

Experimental

The most powerful type of evaluation design is the **experimental design**, in which participants are (a) randomly selected and (b) randomly assigned to experimental and control groups. An experimental design offers the greatest control over outside factors that may interfere with the intervention. Potential

Table 8.6 Sample Acceptable Ranges of Targeted Criteria Relevant to Risk of Back Injury

Criteria	Participants	Nonparticipants
Work location	Warehouse	Warehouse
Average age	37 years	35-40 years
Average body weight	195 lbs. (88 kg)	185-205 lbs. (84-94 kg)
Daily exercise level	10 min. of moderate intensity	5-15 min. of moderate intensity
Previous back injuries	1.5 per person	1 or 2 per person
Jobs rotated	No	No
Prework stretch performed	No	No
Lifting habits at work	15 lifts per day	10-20 lifts per day
Abdominal fitness	25 sit-ups in 1 min.	20-30 sit-ups in 1 min.
Work satisfaction	80% of time	>70% of time
High stress level	50% of time	>40% of time

Table 8.7 An Experimental Multiple Time Series Design with Two Randomly Assigned Groups

Group	Diagram								
E_1 (self-help video)	R	E_1	0_1	0_2	0_3	X	0_4	0_5	0_6
E_2 (on-site seminars)	R	E_2	0_1	0_2	0_3	X	0_4	0_5	0_6

disadvantages of the experimental design are that they require a relatively large number of subjects and that the intervention may have to be delayed for those in the control group. Moreover, experimental designs typically have time- and labor-intensive protocols. They may also require informed consent from participants. Perhaps the main challenge for evaluators is that such designs have to be applied under highly controlled conditions in which the behavioral circumstances may be unnatural or unusual. For example, people who participate in a program that encourages a change in behavior (e.g., exercising more, eating less fat, or reducing television viewing) may experience greater stress and, thus, behave differently than they normally do. Therefore, evaluation outcomes cultivated in a worksite setting may not always be transferred to or maintained in an employee's home setting. Simply put, the rigorous nature of an experimental design may increase the validity of the results in a particular worksite, but may have limited feasibility and generalization to other worksites that lack such controlled conditions.

Table 8.8 illustrates various experimental designs. Because evaluation designs vary significantly in their rigor and utility, you need to tailor your design to the specific needs and interests of your worksite. As you do so, take time to check that you are addressing all of the Socratic elements listed in table 8.1. As you prepare your evaluation and select an appropriate design, consider the scope and specificity of your evaluation needs and plan accordingly.

EMPHASIZING ECONOMIC-BASED EVALUATIONS

In today's cost-conscious environment, decision makers are placing greater emphasis on getting the biggest bang for their buck. Thus, we're seeing that many WHP programs are expanding the scope of traditionally heavy process and impact evaluations to include those based on financial outcomes.

Three of the most versatile economic-based evaluations used in various WHP settings are (1) break-even analysis, (2) cost-effectiveness analysis, and (3) and benefit-cost analysis. Break-even analysis (BEA) can be used as both a preintervention and intermediate protocol to measure when a program's anticipated or real benefits will offset its costs. The remaining evaluation protocols are used primarily at designated intervals or at the conclusion of a WHP intervention. Of the three evaluation methods, BEA is more of a front-end protocol. Thus, it should be presented first.

Break-Even Analysis

Various measurement tools are available for measuring the financial value or liability of a WHP intervention, but some evaluators

Table 8.8 Several Experimental Designs

Design	Diagram							
Pretest and posttest	R	E	O_1	X	O_2			
	R	C	O_1		O_2			
Posttest only	R	E	X	O_1				
	R	C	O_1					
Time series	R	E	O_1	O_2	O_3	X	O_4	O_5	O_6
	R	C	O_1	O_2	O_3		O_4	O_5	O_6
Staggered treatment	R	E_1	X	O_1	O_2	O_3		
	R	E_2	O_1	X	O_2	O_3		
	R	E_3	O_1	O_2	X	O_3		
	R	E_4	O_1	O_2	O_3	X	O_4	

believe that none is more powerful than break-even analysis (BEA). Sometimes referred to as *cost-volume-profit analysis* or a *contribution analysis,* BEA is a specific application that can be an effective pre-intervention planning or forecasting tool to guide decision makers in allocating appropriate levels of resources. For example, when used as a prospective guide, decision makers can integrate what-if scenarios into a BEA framework to determine which level of benefits (e.g., cost savings) will need to be achieved to offset the cost of a particular WHP program. This up-front approach can help decision makers answer key questions, such as the following:

- If we attract 25 employees into our fatigue-management program and 20 of them reduce their personal on-the-job injury rates by 15% from the previous year, how much can we spend on a per-capita basis and still break even?

- How many cases of hypertension do we need to eliminate within a year to offset the cost of a program for multisite stress management and antihypertensive medication provided by our health plan?

- If we conduct a designated number of health-risk screenings, how many significant findings (cases) do we need to identify to justify the expense?

In addition to serving as a prospective planning or forecasting tool, BEA can also serve as an intermediary tool to indicate if a particular program is on the right track. When used in this fashion, BEA can answer questions, such as the following:

- Since the new self-care program is generating emergency department costs that are 10% lower every three months, when will cumulative savings reach programming costs?

- Since we're seeing a 5% drop in migraine-related absences, when can we expect to see productivity gains offset the costs of migraine treatment?

- Since our overhead costs are dropping 3% per month, 5% more chronic condition cases are being recruited each month in

our disease-management program, and per-capita outpatient medical-claim costs have dropped by $250 within six months, are we on the verge of achieving a positive break-even point?

As the demand for greater accountability and tighter budgets intensify, WHP practitioners need to know the operating status of their programs and services. There should be a clear understanding of which interventions are profitable and which are not. As new or expanded programs are considered, well-informed decisions can be made only after determining the potential impact of these offerings. Certainly, not all programs and services are established to generate a direct monetary profit. Nonetheless, program directors and decision makers should understand where the break-even point is and which factors influence how quickly or slowly it occurs. A sample break-even graph is shown in figure 8.2.

Preliminary Steps

The first step in conducting a BEA is to identify, measure, and calculate the monetary value of all cost items. A simple form, such as the one shown in table 8.9, provides a good structure for listing the monthly totals of key cost categories you may need to add once you begin the BEA.

The second step is to add fixed and variable costs to calculate total costs, as shown in table 8.9, using the following formula:

Total costs = fixed costs + variable costs

The third step actually involves two procedures. The first is to determine a *baseline* so you will have a reference (starting point) against which to project future costs and benefits. The second procedure is to determine a *benefit variable* to compare against fixed and variable costs identified earlier.

Since BEA generally involves some degree of forecasting, it is important to establish a valid baseline or reference point on which to base your projections. For example, if employees' average body mass index (BMI) readings over the past three years

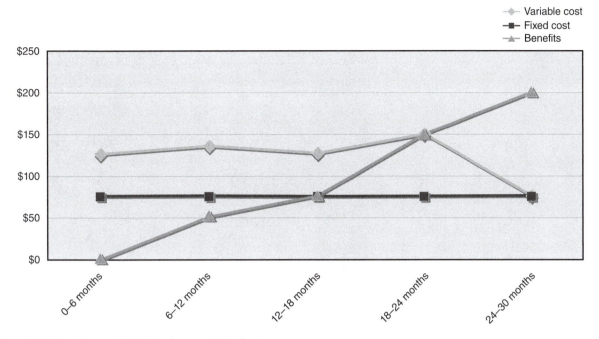

Figure 8.2 A sample break-even analysis.

Table 8.9 A Sample Six-Month Expense Record Form

	January	February	March	April	May	June	Total
Fixed							
Salaries							
Rent							
Insurance							
Property tax							
Depreciation							
Other:							
Variable							
Staff wages							
Utilities							
Phone/fax							
HRAs							
Equipment							
Other:							

were 29, 29.3, and 29.9, you have several options to use in selecting a representative baseline:

1. Use the most recent BMI: 29.9.
2. Use the average of the three readings: [29 + 29.3 + 29.9] ÷ 3 = 29.4.
3. Use the median of the actual three readings: 29.3.
4. Use the median of the lowest and highest readings: 29.45.

Conventional reasoning suggests that the most recent BMI (29.9) should be used as the baseline. However, some circumstances or factors may compel you to use another value, which should be justified.

Once you have an established baseline value to serve as your reference point, you need to decide how to properly calculate a benefit variable. The benefit value should reflect one or more of the primary goals of a particular intervention. For example, the main goals of your prevention program for lower-back injuries may be as follows:

- Reduce the number of lower-back injuries.
- Reduce the average cost of a lower-back injury.

In this case, your corresponding benefit variables would be as follows:

- Number of lower-back injuries
- Average cost of a lower-back injury

The best way to calculate a benefit variable for a BEA is to compute and compare future injuries and costs without the intervention (based on past trends) versus future injuries and costs with an intervention. The latter is based on the initial impact of the intervention being evaluated.

To proceed with our example, let's assume that costs for lower-back injuries have risen 5% every three months for the past year. Your intervention has been underway for three months, and it has reduced medical-care costs related to lower-back injuries by 20% during that time. Projecting the future is, of course, an iffy proposition. But, even while acknowledging that the unexpected may happen, you can make reasonable assumptions by looking carefully at factors that could influence the outcome, such as the following:

- The figures quoted in the preceding section
- The fact that more employees will be brought into the program over time
- The expectation that employees in the program will report their lower-back injuries earlier than they did before they were in the program, resulting in less severe injuries that are less costly to treat than previous injuries.

The evaluator feels safe in assuming that the 20% savings will be repeated every quarter for the 21 months. She projects how the trend established during the three-month intervention will play out during that time period (see table 8.10).

Every forecasting scenario, no matter how meticulously prepared, is subject to many factors that will influence its accuracy. Note that the evaluator of table 8.10 has done more than take the data into account. She has included other factors, such as more employees being brought in and injuries being reported earlier. Like this evaluator, you should conceptualize about factors beyond the data. For example, is the program already covering the departments where lower-back injuries are most common, or are these departments yet to be included? Are you including publicity about positive results, expecting that it will bring more employees into the program? Is the nature of the intervention such that its benefits will level off for participants after, say, one year of supervised exercise? If so, how will this affect the bottom line? In any case, because uncertainty characterizes most forecasting situations, short-term projects carry less risk for evaluators than long-term (multi-year) projections do.

Table 8.10 A Comparison of Lower-Back Injury Claims and Costs

Interval	With intervention*		Without intervention**	
	Cost ($)	Claims (#)	Cost ($)	Claims (#)
Baseline	$100,000	200	$100,000	200
0-3 months	$80,000	180	$105,000	210
4-6 months	$64,000	160	$110,250	220
7-9 months	$51,200	150	$115,762	220
10-12 months	$40,960	130	$121,550	230
13-15 months	$32,760	120	$127,628	240
16-18 months	$26,210	110	$134,009	240
19-21 months	$20,970	100	$140,710	250

* Based on initial 20% influence

** Based on past trend of 5% increase per year

Calculate the Current and Projected Benefits

The fourth step is to calculate projected benefits (in dollars) based on any cost reduction. For example, using the comparative cost data for lower-back injuries (LBI) in table 8.10, you can see that cost savings per quarter with the intervention would be as shown in table 8.11. If the annual cost of operating the LBI prevention program is $45,000, you can see from table 8.11 that, if the projected benefits are correct, the cost-reduction value would offset the program costs—or break even—early in the second quarter. Even if there were little or no continuing impact from the program, it will pay for itself before midyear. Now suppose that annual program costs were $100,000 and that the intervention impact could be sustained throughout the entire year. How long would it take for savings to offset the cost of the program in

that case? At the sustained 20% impact, cost savings would offset the program costs at approximately the eighth month, or about midway through the third quarter.

If your initial impact is not as dramatic as those in our LBI example, you should use actual cost differences over two or more consecutive time frames to verify any assumption before making your break-even prediction. Note the significant differences between the quarterly and cumulative costs. It is important to decide the best way to use and illustrate these cost-differences in your BEA report. You have at least two viable options to consider:

- Treat cost-differences on an interval basis (e.g., quarterly, semiannually, annually), listing costs per year.
- Treat cost-differences on a cumulative basis, adding interval-to-interval differences.

Table 8.11 Program-Generated Savings

Time frame	LBI costs with intervention	LBI costs without intervention	Program savings quarterly	Program savings cumulative
0-3 months	$80,000	$105,000	$25,000	$25,000
4-6 months	$64,000	$110,250	$46,250	$71,250
7-9 months	$51,200	$115,762	$64,562	$135,812
10-12 months	$40,960	$121,550	$80,590	$216,402

Calculate the Break-Even Point

The fifth step is to illustrate the break-even point. This can be done in several ways. One way is to construct a graph in which the intervention-cost line intersects the cost-savings (benefit) line at the break-even point, as shown in figure 8.3. Of course, bar charts and linear grids may also be used to illustrate this relationship.

Cost-Effectiveness Analysis

What if you want to compare one program with another to decide which one produces the greatest benefit for the least expense? When properly designed and implemented, *cost-effectiveness analysis (CEA)* can answer that question. Rather than assigning monetary values to a single outcome of a program, as is done in some analyses, CEA compares only the costs of similar programs for achieving a specific outcome. For example, if you wanted to know which type of smoking-cessation program was the most cost-effective, you could implement the CEA framework shown in table 8.12. Conducting a CEA in a worksite setting involves several key steps:

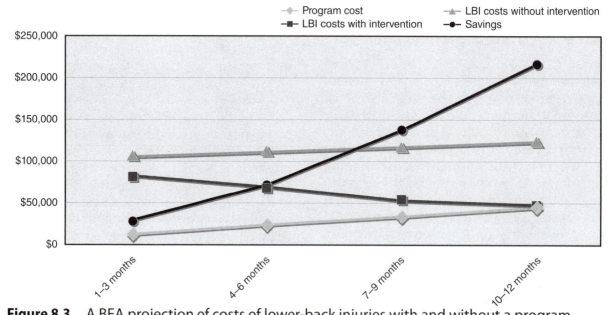

Figure 8.3   A BEA projection of costs of lower-back injuries with and without a program intervention, and cumulative cost savings at quarterly intervals. Note that the program costs $45,000 per year, not per quarter.

Table 8.12   A Cost-Effectiveness Analysis Framework Used in Comparing Four Different Smoking Cessation Interventions

Strategy	Cost of program	Participants (#)	Cost per participant	Successful quitters (#)	Cost per person*
Cold turkey with self-help guide	$500	100	$5.00	3	$166.00
Nicotine patch	$1,500	75	$20.00	8	$187.00
Nicotine gum	$1,100	50	$22.00	6	$183.00
Bupropion	$900	25	$36.00	12	$75.00

*Cost of program divided by number of successful quitters.

1. *Plan your evaluation as you design your interventions.*

• Determine your program goals and objectives. Ask yourself what your interventions are supposed to do for employees and the organization. For example, the goal of your back program may be to prevent lower-back injuries. Objectives listed in table 8.13 represent several activities that must be accomplished to achieve that goal. For example, the first and second objectives include screening as many employees as possible in the yearlong program. The third objective is to recruit and involve as many at-risk employees as possible in the yearlong program. The fourth and final objective is to obtain feedback from participants as to whether or not they incurred a lower-back injury during the intervention. The final objective listed in a CEA framework should reflect the main goal (desired outcome) of the intervention.

• Set up thorough record-keeping procedures. Consider major cost items, such as personnel, facilities, and equipment, and minor cost items, such as photocopying, printing, and record keeping.

• Determine the time frame in which you will compare the interventions.

2. *Calculate total costs for each intervention.* During the trial period, keep careful records following the procedures that you established in step 1. At the end of the trial period, add up all expenses to calculate the total cost for each intervention during that period.

3. *Determine the cost per outcome for each program intervention.* Divide the cost of the program intervention by the number of quantitative units (impacts) listed within each objective.

SIMPLIFY!

A midsized utility company had been experiencing double-digit inflation in health care costs over the past few years. Health managers reviewed several years of claims data and noticed that emergency department (ED) utilization was the fastest-growing claim during this time frame and that 35- to 45-year-old women had the highest ED usage, followed closely by 25- to 35-year-old men. The identified group of women worked primarily in the customer service department, while the targeted group of men worked in the line repair division. Small-group sessions were conducted to identify which factors were causing higher ED usage.

Both groups indicated similar reasons for their ED usage: Many customer complaints reported in the late afternoon required customer-service representatives to stay on the job beyond their scheduled 5 p.m. quitting time. This prevented them from seeking care from their health care providers, whose offices closed at 6 p.m. Many line repairmen used the ED because they often worked overtime during late-afternoon power failures. A final review of the individual ED claims by the occupational health nurse indicated that virtually all of the health problems prompting ED visits were not emergencies, but rather minor ailments, such as colds, sore muscles, and skin rashes.

Realizing they could do little to influence the timing of customer complaints and power shortages, health managers decided to try reducing ED visits by teaching and motivating employees to treat minor ailments through a medical self-care (MSC) program. The health-management staff established a program goal of reducing the number of ED visits associated with minor ailments by 25% within one year, based on their review of MSC program results reported in professional literature. The MSC program included weekly small-group seminars during an expanded lunch period. By taking into consideration each target group's work schedule and health problems, staff members were able to establish an appropriate *scope* (selecting the fastest-growing claims and allowing ample time for the MSC program to have an effect before evaluating it) and *specificity* (targeting only nonemergency ailments) for the program-dependent variables, ensuring that the program could reasonably be evaluated.

Table 8.13 A Cost-Effectiveness Analysis of Two Worksite Programs for Back Health

Criteria	Monthly back seminar	Daily prework stretch
Annual cost	$5,000	$1,000
Objective	Cost per impact	
Provide lower-back screening	100 screenings = $50 per screen	100 screenings = $10 per screen
Identify high-risk workers	50 identified = $100 per finding	80 identified = $12.50 per finding
Full program participation	40 participants = $125 per impact	75 participants = $13.33 per impact
Achieve injury-free status for 12 consecutive months	37 without injury = $135 per impact	50 without injury = $20 per impact

4. *Compare the final cost per outcome value for each program intervention and determine which is most cost-effective.* Although the seminar-based program initially costs five times as much as the daily stretching intervention, the stretching routine produced a higher return on investment. The daily stretch protected employees against a back injury at nearly one-seventh ($20/$135) of the cost of the seminar intervention.

Although a CEA may show one program having a greater return on investment than another, the decision to eliminate a particular program should not be based solely on this comparison. After all, a program with a moderate return on investment may produce benefits that are not easily quantified (e.g., improved employee morale, fewer quality-control issues, and better management-labor relations).

Benefit-Cost Analysis

The primary purpose of a benefit-cost analysis (BCA) is to determine whether a program is worth its cost. Because the BCA method compares program benefits to program costs, it might be most effective to measure both variables in monetary terms. However, some experts caution that quantification should not be the sole basis for performing a benefit-cost analysis, contending that important factors should not be neglected just because they cannot be tangibly measured. For example, how would we quantify the suffering of people with severe back pain or chronic depression? Benefit-cost analysis doesn't purport

to introduce rigor and quantification when the data are imprecise or when quantification is not feasible. However, when benefit and cost can be quantified, a BCA is a relatively simple and efficient way to evaluate a program's success or value.

Because benefit-cost analysis provides meaningful data only to the extent that current or future benefits and costs can be accurately measured or projected, the first step in executing a BCA is to identify and measure benefits and costs as precisely as possible.

The cost side of a benefit-cost analysis involves calculating the price of all resources, such as personnel, equipment, and facilities used in planning and implementing an intervention. Table 8.14 shows various direct and indirect cost entities that are used, in varying degrees, in WHP settings.

The benefit side of the equation involves calculating the monetary value of any positive outcomes that can be quantified. As with costs, it is necessary to take both direct and secondary benefits into account. Direct benefits reflect positive outcomes incurred immediately or within a short time frame by employees and an organization. Secondary benefits reflect positive, often unexpected, outcomes that may eventually accrue for employees and an organization (see table 8.14).

The effects of direct benefits can usually be measured using standard accounting reports and conventional financial analysis. Before calculating any benefit, evaluators must identify an outcome (dependent) variable that can be treated as a tangible ben-

Table 8.14 Examples of Direct and Indirect Cost and Benefit Units.

Direct cost unit	Direct benefit unit	Indirect cost unit	Indirect benefit unit
Medical care costs (e.g., services, supplies, medications)	Reduced or contained medical care costs	Absenteeism and presenteeism	Reduced costs (e.g., fewer replacement workers and overtime pay)
Rehabilitation costs	Reduced or contained rehabilitation costs	Administration (e.g., claims processing)	Lower third-party administrative costs
Compliance with OSHA	Fewer costs related to OSHA violations	Drug testing	Reduced drug-testing costs and off-the-job production
ADA accommodations	Fewer costs related to ADA violations; increased on-the-job performance	Replacement training costs	Reduced training costs
Health-risk assessments	Fewer assessments required in the future	Short-term disability and long-term disability costs	Reduced STD and LTD costs
Workers' compensation premium cost	Reduced or contained premium cost	Workers' compensation indemnity payments	Reduced indemnity payments

efit. In doing so, remember that a variable must be both measurable and relevant to the intervention.

After measuring all cost items and the value of all benefits, you can compare the two categories. To do this comparison, you may use either the *net benefit* method or the *benefit-cost-ratio* method.

In the first method, the evaluator determines the net benefit of a particular intervention and compares it with its cost. If the difference is positive, the analysis reveals that the intervention is financially worth the effort. The net benefit of any intervention may be calculated as follows:

Net benefit = [L$ + GP + PI] – C

The symbols represent the following:

- *L$* (sometimes called the direct benefit) stands, for instance, for a reduction in medical-care expenses tied to reduced risk, disease, or disability. For example, if the number of lower-back injuries decline, then fewer health care services and associated costs will be required.
- *GP* stands for the increase in general productivity, leading to greater output and income. For example, if we reduce the incidence of lower-back injury, we also increase the performance capabilities of employees who are prone to such injuries so they may continue to produce at desirable levels.

Therefore, we enhance the odds of earning more compensation.

- *PI* stands for the gain in working income because of reduced injury and illness and their effects on absenteeism. GP and PI are secondary (indirect) benefits.
- *C* stands for the cost of the intervention.

For example, suppose an organization is experiencing a significant increase in costs related to lower-back injuries. It responds by establishing an appropriate prevention program. After six months, evaluators conduct a benefit-cost analysis. To use the preceding formula, they need to determine the value of reduced medical-care expenses related to lower-back injuries, the increase in general productivity, and the drop in the cost of absenteeism that was initially traced to lower-back injury. Here is what they find:

- Medical care expenses for back injuries have dropped from $125,000 to $35,000, so L$ = $90,000.
- Production output (as measured by the financial value or goods produced by employees) has increased by $35,000, so GP = $35,000.
- Employees' absenteeism due to lower-back injuries declined 2%, resulting in a drop of $20,000 [20 employees with a history of LBI multiplied by $50,000 (annual salary)] multiplied by 2%. Therefore, PI = $20,000.

• The cumulative program-intervention cost for operating the program is $35,000, so C = $35,000.

If we apply the preceding data to the net-benefit equation, it is as follows:

Net benefit = [$90,000 + $35,000 + $20,000] − $35,000 = $110,000

When one considers that the program has generated savings at almost three times its cost, the intervention clearly seems worth it.

Another method that can be used to econometrically evaluate WHP programs is the benefit-cost ratio (BCR). BCR is calculated by dividing the sum of all program-related benefits by the sum of all program costs:

$$BCR = \frac{Benefit}{Cost}$$

For example, consider a program for migraine-headache reduction that generated cost-avoidance savings of $50,000 through reduced medical care and absenteeism costs. Comparing these cost savings against annual program-intervention costs of $20,000:

$$\frac{Benefit}{Cost} = \frac{\$50,000}{\$20,000} = \frac{\$2.50}{\$1.00}$$

Note that the final step is to divide both the upper and lower figures by the lower number. This calculation will always result in $1.00 as the denominating unit of cost. Thus, in our example, a preliminary benefit-cost ratio of $50,000 to $20,000 would apply. Dividing both figures by $20,000 reveals that for every $1 of costs, $2.50 of benefits was achieved. Evaluators can compare the preceding ratio to that of another program if they want to determine how two or more programs compare in terms of cost-effectiveness. By doing so, a BCA can be used as a prerequisite for a cost-effectiveness analysis. For example, suppose the preceding program's benefit-cost ratio is compared with that of a lower-back-injury prevention program that yields the following ratio:

$$\frac{Benefit}{Cost} = \frac{\$20,000}{\$3,000} = \frac{\$6.66}{\$1.00}$$

Although both programs are econometrically successful, the lower-back program produced a better benefit-cost ratio. From an econometric viewpoint, it is as important to the workforce as the migraine-control program.

Whatever BCA approach is used, it is important to realize that the *validity* (accuracy) and *reliability* (consistency) of any formula depends largely on the accuracy of the data used to quantify benefit and cost variables. The benefit-cost approach is typically used when one or two general categories of benefits and costs can be monetarily quantified. The net-benefit approach is typically used when only one or two types of benefit and cost data are available. In contrast, the BCR approach is commonly used when several types of benefit and cost data are available.

Determining Present Versus Future Value

Even when monetary values have been assigned to benefits and to direct and indirect costs, they are not usually directly comparable. This is because they occur over a period of time during which the *value of dollars* will most likely change.

Because dollars available today may be worth more or less than dollars available tomorrow, the present value of future dollars needs to be calculated to make reasonable comparisons across different time periods. Although this adjustment can be made in various ways, one of most common approaches involves choosing a discount rate that will be used in the formula for reducing future costs and benefits to make them comparable to the present value of money. Unfortunately, there are no standardized guidelines to follow in choosing a discount rate to be used in present value calculations. Many economists prefer to tie discount rates to the inflation rates associated with major cost items that are calculated. For example, if wages are rising annually by 4%, a discount rate of 4% would apply to personnel costs. Because present value calculations—as well as benefit-cost ratios and net gain or loss figures—are very sensitive to the discount rate chosen, an evaluator should conduct several analyses using different discount rates to determine how an intervention would fare under each rate.

For example, a range of low-end to high-end discount rates may be used to represent possible best- and worst-case scenarios. Suppose an organization is in the midst of trying to determine what its current health care budget can purchase in the next 3 to 5 years. It has been told by various benefits consultants that health care inflation is expected to rise 9% to 12% per year during this time frame. In an attempt to determine the full spectrum of potentially good or bad outcomes, the organization elects to consider various discount rates, ranging from the low end at 9% to 15%, on the premise that health care inflation rates may actually exceed the consultants' estimates.

Once you have chosen the discount rate, you can use the following formula for **present-value adjustment (PVA)** for calculating future costs:

$$PV_C = C_1 + C_2 + C_3$$

PV_C refers to the cost for the entire program figured in current dollar values, C_y refers to the program costs for each year in which they occur, r refers to the discount rate, and y refers to the year. For example, if an organization were to invest $40,000 per year for three consecutive years in a WHP program in which the discount rate was 10%, the present value of the year-to-year cost of the program would be calculated as follows:

$$PV_C = C_1 + C_2 + C_3$$

Begin by calculating the values of C_1, C_2, and C_3 as follows:

$$C_1 = \frac{\$40,000}{(1+r)} = \frac{\$40,000}{(1+.10)} =$$
$$\frac{\$40,000}{1.10} = \$36,363.64$$

$$C_2 = \frac{\$40,000}{(1+r)} = \frac{\$40.000}{(1+.10)^2} =$$
$$\frac{\$40,000}{1.21} = \$33,057.85$$

$$C_3 = \frac{\$40,000}{(1+r)} = \frac{\$40,000}{(1+.10)^3} =$$
$$\frac{\$40,000}{1.33} = \$30,052.59$$

Add the values of C_1, C_2, and C_3 to compute the total present value of costs of the program over a three-year period:

$$PV_c = \$36,363.64 + 33,057.85$$
$$+ 30,052.59 = \$99,474.08$$

The three-year cost of this program, expressed in the value of today's dollars, is $99,474.

In addition to helping determine direct and indirect benefits, a present-value adjustment can be used to calculate the present and future value of net benefit-cost ratios (see the following sidebar). The present value of benefits (PV_b) is calculated the same way as the present value of costs is, except that monetized program benefits (B_y) are substituted for program costs (C_y) in the formula. Just as in the case of costs, the computation of the present discounted value of an intervention (the value today of payments in the future) requires the use of a discount rate to reflect that future dollars have less value than today's dollars.

For example, suppose your medical self-care program was evaluated and showed a benefit-cost ratio of $1,000 to $750, or a return of $1.33 for every $1 spent. Nonetheless, you wonder if this 33% return on investment (ROI) will be maintained in the future. Chances are, it won't. The main reason is that the actual monetary value of benefit dollars differs over time from that of cost dollars. Thus, it is important to discount each of these values according to how the economy affects them. To do so, these values are subjected to different discount rates when calculating the net benefit-cost ratios of the program.

In the following sidebar, a discount rate of 12% has been tied to benefits based on the premise that any cost savings from the program (1) will take time to accrue and (2) will lose their value proportionately due to higher rates of medical inflation. Essentially,

A SAMPLE FRAMEWORK OF PRESENT VALUE ADJUSTMENT (PVA)

1. Benefits

$$PV_b = \sum \frac{B_y}{(1+r)^y} = \frac{B_1}{(1+r)^1} + \frac{B_2}{(1+r)^2} + \frac{B_3}{(1+r)^3}$$

$$\frac{B_1}{(1+r)^1} = \frac{\$50,000}{(1+.12)^1} = \frac{\$50,000}{1.12^1} = \frac{\$50,000}{1.12} = \$44,642 \text{ (year 1)}$$

$$\frac{B_2}{(1+r)^2} = \frac{\$50,000}{(1+.12)^2} = \frac{\$50,000}{1.12^2} = \frac{\$50,000}{1.25} = \$40,000 \text{ (year 2)}$$

$$\frac{B_3}{(1+r)^3} = \frac{\$50,000}{(1+.12)^3} = \frac{\$50,000}{1.12^3} = \frac{\$50,000}{1.40} = \$35,714 \text{ (year 3)}$$

$$PV_b = \sum \frac{B_y}{(1+r)^y} = \$44,642 + \$40,000 + \$35,714 = \$120,356$$

2. Costs

$$PV_c = \sum \frac{C_y}{(1+r)^y} = \frac{C_1}{(1+r)^1} + \frac{C_2}{(1+r)^2} + \frac{C_3}{(1+r)^3}$$

$$\frac{C_1}{(1+r)^1} = \frac{\$40,000}{(1+.10)^1} = \frac{\$40,000}{1.10^1} = \frac{\$40,000}{1.10} = \$36,363 \text{ (year 1)}$$

$$\frac{C_2}{(1+r)^2} = \frac{\$40,000}{(1+.10)^2} = \frac{\$40,000}{1.10^2} = \frac{\$40,000}{1.21} = \$33,057 \text{ (year 2)}$$

$$\frac{C_3}{(1+r)^3} = \frac{\$40,000}{(1+.10)^3} = \frac{\$40,000}{1.10^3} = \frac{\$40,000}{1.33} = \$30,075 \text{ (year 3)}$$

$$PV_c = \sum \frac{C_y}{(1+r)^y} = \$36,363 + \$33,057 + \$30,075 = \$99,495$$

3. Calculate net benefit-cost ratios

		Year 1	Year 2	Year 3
$\dfrac{\text{Benefit}}{\text{Cost}}$	=	$\dfrac{\$44,642}{\$36,363}$	$\dfrac{\$40,000}{\$33,057}$	$\dfrac{\$35,714}{\$30,075}$
Return on investment (ROI ratio)		$\dfrac{\$1.22}{\$1.00}$	$\dfrac{\$1.21}{\$1.00}$	$\dfrac{\$1.18}{\$1.00}$

a discount rate of 12% represents the high end of the medical inflation range because the evaluator believes that health care inflation in the future may worsen beyond its traditional trend.

On the cost side, dollars spent to fund a health promotion program are weighed less heavily than future benefits for at least two reasons:

• First, due to inflation, a dollar can usually purchase more health promotion resources this year than it can next year.

• Second, economists depreciate the value of cost dollars at a lower discount rate than benefit dollars because cost (worksite health programming) dollars could (if decision makers chose to divert this money) actually be deposited in an interest-bearing account today. There, they would accrue a higher dividend than benefit dollars, which cannot be deposited until they are achieved. Since these cost dollars could be invested for a longer time frame and could generate a larger return, they are discounted more favorably than benefit dollars.

In addition, discount rates assigned to typical cost items are generally 25% to 50% lower than discount rates assigned to benefits. Hence, a discount rate of 10% has been applied to the cost values in table 8.15. Notice that the ROI ratio in table 8.15 gradually drops over time (from $1.22:1 to $1.18:1 in three years) because benefit dollars (discounted at 12%) depreciate faster than cost dollars (discounted at 10%). Thus, the positive ROI will eventually disappear if the medical self-care program merely sustains the initial impact and fails to improve. The prospect of such shrinking ROIs causes many decision makers to ask whether they

could have invested the cost dollars in a different project and earned a high ROI. An organization could answer this question by using a cost-effectiveness analysis (CEA) to compare two different self-care programs against each other or to compare the self-care program against another program. In either case, the CEA could reveal which of the two interventions generated the most benefit for the least cost.

To summarize, BCA is an excellent tool for comparing the value of a program's cost and benefits, provided that all cost and benefit items can be reasonably measured and assigned monetary values. It is also important to incorporate present-value adjustment (PVA) formulas when possible, keeping in mind that the value of today's benefits and costs are affected differently by the economy. The information provided by a well-done BCA and supplemental PVA can be extremely valuable to decision makers as they plan for the future.

What Would You Do?

Upon reviewing HRAs and health-care claims data, you notice an increase in diabetes-related cases and costs from last year. While preparing a program proposal for diabetes education and management, you anticipate that your boss will ask you how the program will be evaluated and when the program will begin to pay off. What type of evaluation framework is most appropriate—a cost-effectiveness, a benefit-cost, or break-even analysis? Which approach would you choose, and why?

CHAPTER 8 WRAP-UP

Key Points

- Up-front planning is essential for avoiding various pitfalls that can compromise the integrity and objectivity of a WHP evaluation.
- Writing clearly delineated goals and objectives requires a good understanding of resources, realistic expectations, and appropriate evaluation protocols.
- Although process- and impact-level evaluations are common in many WHP settings, emphasis on evaluations based on financial outcomes is growing.
- Evaluation designs vary greatly in scope, specificity, and strength. Thus, it's vital to use a design that is commensurate with an evaluator's ability to control certain factors that may influence the WHP program's impact on the desired outcome.

- Protocols for cost-effectiveness analysis and benefit-cost analysis offer WHP practitioners a relatively simple method for assessing the financial value of their WHP efforts.
- The financial value of today's benefits and costs should be adjusted accordingly to determine how they will be influenced by economic forces in the future.

Glossary

benefit-cost analysis (BCA)—A technique designed to determine the feasibility or worth of a product, service, policy or program by quantifying and comparing its costs and benefits.

break-even analysis (BEA)—A technique used to determine how soon a benefit (e.g., sales volume, cost-savings) is needed to offset the cost of a product, service, policy, or program.

comparison group—A group of subjects that is exposed to all the conditions of a study except for the experimental treatment (program) being tested. This group is not matched with (nonequivalent to) the group that does receive the experiment.

control group—A group of subjects that is matched as closely as possible (via random selection) with the experimental group.

experimental design—A study design generally used to test possible cause-and-effect relationship between specific variables. This design includes an experimental group of subjects and a control group of subjects who are randomly assigned to groups and to treatment options.

experimental group—A group of subjects who intentionally receive the experimental treatment (program).

nonexperimental design—A design in which an experimental treatment (program) is given only to an existing group of subjects who are not randomly selected.

present value adjustment (PVA)—The current value of a quantified benefit, discounted at an appropriate interest rate to show its diminishing value in the future.

quasi-experimental design—A design in which preexisting, intact groups are not randomly assigned to either the experimental or the control group. The evaluator may also be unable to control which group will get the experimental treatment.

Bibliography

Brady, W., et al. 1997. "Defining total corporate health and safety costs: Significance and impact." *Journal of Occupational and Environmental Medicine* 39(3): 224-231.

Chenoweth, D. 2001. "Decision points around evaluation." *AWHP's Worksite Health* (Summer): 8-14.

Chenoweth, D. 2002. *Evaluating worksite health promotion*. Champaign, IL: Human Kinetics.

Chenoweth, D., and J. Garrett. 2006. "Cost-effectiveness analysis of a worksite clinic: Is it worth the cost?" *Journal of the American Association of Occupational Health Nursing* 54 (2): 84-89.

Disease Management Association of America (DMAA). *Outcomes Guidelines Project 2009, Volume IV Recommendations.* Georgetown University, Department of Psychology (Glossary). Accessed April 13, 2010. www.psychology.georgetown.edu/resources/researchmethods/glossary/8550.html.

Harvard University. 2010. "Harvard family research project: Selected evaluation terms." Accessed April 12. www.hfrp.org/publications-resources/browse-our-publications/selected-evaluation-terms.

Suchman, E. 1967. *Evaluative research.* New York: Russell Sage Foundation.

Looking Ahead

Now that we've covered several important aspects of preparing and applying program evaluations, it's time to consider how a company's size influences our programming approach. Chapter 9 describes key variables to consider when working with small, multisite, and large employee populations.

Part IV

Managing Essential WHP Considerations

This part of the book offers information for both new and experienced WHP personnel to consider in honing their professional capabilities. Chapter 9 describes the characteristics and challenges of many small and multisite WHP settings. It also outlines how to address these issues as opportunities, rather than threats. Chapter 10 offers resources and tips for aspiring WHP professionals to consider when building their professional knowledge and skills. This section also addresses job seeking and interviewing skills. Collectively, these two chapters serve as an impetus for WHP practitioners at all levels to continuously learn how to stay competitive in today's ever-changing world.

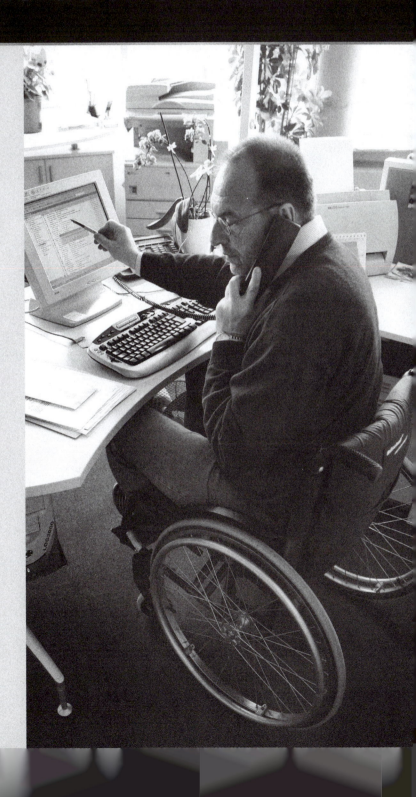

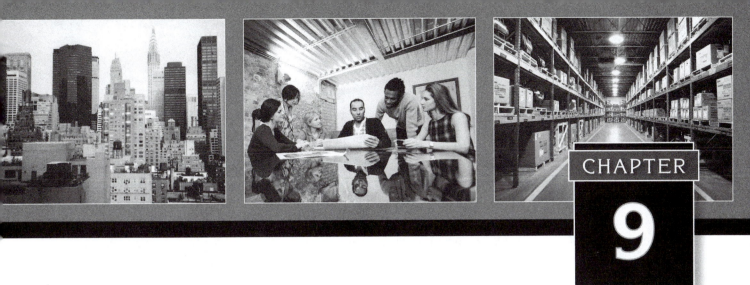

Overcoming Challenges of Company Size

LEARNING OBJECTIVES

After reading this chapter, you will be able to do the following:

- ✔ Identify several barriers that small businesses must overcome to establish successful WHP programs.
- ✔ Describe how some small businesses pool their resources to provide employee health insurance.
- ✔ Explain how a small business may use a release-time staffing arrangement for WHP programming.
- ✔ Compare the process for program planning used in multisite settings with that used in a single worksite.
- ✔ Distinguish differences in scope of evaluating WHP programs between small, single-site settings and multisite settings.

Recent nationwide surveys found that company size was a prominent indicator of the quantity and type of health promotion activities offered at the worksite (Linnan et al. 2008; PriceWaterhouseCoopers 2009). Worksites with more than 750 employees consistently offered far more health promotion activities than smaller worksites. The smallest worksites in these studies consistently offered fewer programs than the larger companies. Thus, most workers, being employed in small businesses, are underserved in regard to health promotion programming.

Small firms (those employing 2 to 500 people) make up more than 95% of all employers in the United States (U.S. Census Bureau 2010). The National Federation of Independent Business estimates that 60% of all businesses have fewer than 4 employees and 80% have fewer than 20 employees. With the advent of downsizing, demographic shifts, and an expanding service sector, more employees find themselves working in smaller worksites. Moreover, many of these worksites are becoming more culturally diverse every day. Thus, they require different strategies from those of traditional WHP programs.

This chapter discusses the challenges involved in planning programs that are accessible and appropriate for employees in multisite organizations, small worksites, and culturally diverse workplaces. Although these challenges are real, skilled WHP practitioners can meet the unique needs of these worksites with an effective plan of action.

SMALL BUSINESSES

Research shows that many **small business** owners are interested in WHP activities, but feel they lack adequate resources to plan and implement them. Many of them cite the following obstacles to overcome in their quest to provide WHP:

• *Productivity demands.* Being preoccupied with productivity and cost issues, many small business owners neglect investments in human capital, such as health promotion.

• *Poor financial support.* Small profit margins may limit funding for some programs.

• *No trained personnel.* Most small worksites lack professionally trained personnel who can develop, administer, and oversee WHP programs and services.

• *Lack of time.* Most small businesses operate with a minimum of workers in labor-intensive jobs with little or no flex time to participate in WHP opportunities.

• *Regulatory overkill.* Some owners of small businesses feel overwhelmed by existing state and federal regulations, so they reject the idea of additional employee-health-oriented programs not mandated by law.

• *Lack of facilities and equipment.* The initial expense of equipping and modifying part of the facility for fitness and health programs often makes small-business owners view WHP as a luxury they cannot afford.

• *Expectations of low participation.* Decision makers may think too few people would participate in WHP to justify the resources needed for a program.

• *Limited space.* Many small-business operations—service stations, convenience stores, fast food outlets—don't have adequate space to offer on-site programs.

• *Geographic dispersion.* Travel obligations of employees working on the road in transportation, consulting, delivery, and

sales positions limit their access to worksite-based opportunities for health promotion.

• *Multisite logistics.* With limited resources, it is difficult to reach small numbers of employees who are working at several satellite locations.

Despite these obstacles, many small businesses have several advantages over large companies in planning and sustaining WHP programs. For example, small businesses have fewer people to accommodate, which mean less expense and less space to manage. Second, small businesses have more of a family-oriented, close-knit community that fosters an environment for more group participation. Third, local health agencies and organizations offering free or low-cost services often prefer to serve smaller companies. Finally, improvements in employee health are more visible to coworkers in small worksites, which increases the chance that others might be more motivated to participate.

Health and Productivity Management

The explicit connection between health and productivity has spawned several relatively new concepts of particular value to WHP program planners and decision makers at all levels. For example, health and productivity management (HPM) operates on the belief that an at-risk workforce is a business risk that poses both direct and hidden costs that affect overall productivity. In fact, strong evidence exists that efforts that improve employees' health status also improve a firm's overall productivity by doing the following:

• Attracting top-notch workers in a competitively global marketplace.
• Reducing absenteeism and lost time
• Boosting retention
• Improving on-the-job decision making and use of time (reduced presenteeism)
• Improving employee morale, which fosters wide-scale loyalty
• Reducing management-labor conflicts by creating a heightened spirit of goodwill between key stakeholder groups

The first step for small businesses to enhance workplace health and productivity is to sponsor an affordable health care plan for employees. Most experts agree that WHP programs, when properly designed and implemented, can help a small business improve its health and productivity profile as well as contain its health care costs. As many small-business owners can testify, strategies to contain their health care costs are particularly challenging, since even one employee's poor health and medical misfortunes might significantly damage the bottom line. Although many small-business owners know the importance of having a good health insurance plan to protect against such risks, fewer than 50% of all small businesses actually provide basic health coverage for their employees. In fact, nearly two-thirds of those without health insurance are in families headed by a full-time worker, most of whom work in very small businesses. In today's inflationary marketplace, the high cost of providing health insurance coverage to employees and dependents is prohibitive for many small-business owners. Consequently, employees at these businesses are forced to personally shop the insurance market for the best deal, often changing insurers every year. Millions of others go without health insurance, forced to risk the devastating consequences of accidents or long-term illness because they simply cannot afford to pay rising health insurance premiums.

Some small companies are helping their employees obtain coverage through **health insurance pooling**. A well-publicized example is a group of small businesses in Cleveland, Ohio, that formed a large pool called the Council of Smaller Enterprises (COSE). COSE is the region's largest support organization for small business. It provides cost-effective group purchasing programs, advocacy on legislative and regulatory issues, and networking and educational resources to help small businesses in northeast Ohio grow. The council consists of more than 17,000 member companies, representing more than 225,000 covered employees throughout northeast Ohio. All COSE members can purchase affordable health insurance coverage because the council has persuaded large insurers to offer their coalition the same advantages given to larger companies. The most important of these advantages is the clout to pressure doctors and hospitals to keep costs down. The COSE arrangement has been a successful cost-control strategy for its members, whose annual premiums typically rise only about one-fourth as much as those in non-COSE businesses. For more information on the council, consult their website (www.cose.org).

Increasingly, the availability and cost of a company's health care plan often depends on employees' health risks. In such a case, a company might only be able to afford insurance that does not pay claims directly tied to a person's choice, such as smoking-induced lung disease or injuries received during motor vehicle accidents in which safety belts were not worn. The company might not be willing to pay the difference if lifestyle choices result in higher risk. In either of these cases, a primary goal of WHP would be to motivate high-risk and unhealthy employees to reduce their risk factors.

Planning

A greater understanding of existing health promotion programs in small businesses is essential if WHP practitioners expect to reach more of this growing sector. According to some experts, securing management support is the key prerequisite for establishing a successful WHP in small business. While some business owners strongly believe in programs to promote employee health, others are less enthusiastic, requiring evidence before they will support WHP efforts. When possible, consult with other WHP personnel in your community to learn why their small-business programs succeed (or why they have failed). For an example of a successful small-business WHP program, see the profile of R.E. Mason Company on page 184.

To plan appropriate activities and programs for health promotion, small businesses should follow the same procedures as larger businesses. The procedural guidelines tied to identification, assessment, planning, implementation, and evaluation (as discussed in chapters 2, 3, 4, 7, and 8) are the same, regardless of the size of a business. Yet, a proposal for WHP should be modified around the unique characteristics of a small business during the general planning process. For instance, WHP planning for small business should provide for the following:

- *A flexible format.* For instance, health-enhancement programs could be offered at the worksite or in a community center for several businesses to use collaboratively.

- *Simple equipment and space needs.* A small business does not need a large-scale exercise room or enough space to accommodate a large aerobics class. Modest arrangements are often enough for employees to achieve their personal health goals.

- *Easy administration.* Again, nothing fancy is required. Programs that are relatively easy to plan and implement are often sufficient at smaller companies. For example, a prework stretching and warm-up routine for the lower back only requires a small area of open space and management support.

WHP programs do not have to be elaborate or expensive to be effective. In fact, most small worksite programs have no fitness facilities and require only a modest amount of money and time to administer. Many small businesses use community health agencies and vendors who can provide personnel, facilities, equipment, and instructional materials at little or no cost. Some of them work with the local chamber of commerce, local health departments, local merchants or trade associations, or shopping malls to hold events and activities. Some affordable small-scale options include the following:

- Sponsor on-site flu shots, blood-pressure checks, diabetes screening, and so on. Check with your local health department, hospital, or nearby university departments of health education, exercise science, and nursing to determine whether any of them can perform such services.

- Provide written materials that provide health-related news bits, such as self-care books, periodic newsletters, and a printed listing of websites.

- Encourage and provide time for employees to exercise either before, during, or after work.

- Provide clean, safe, and accessible stairways to encourage stair climbing rather than use of elevators or escalators.

- Explore suitable outdoor paths for break-time walking.

- Offer financial incentives for employees who walk, ride a bike, take public transit, or carpool to work.

- Offer safe, secure, and free bike storage.

- Provide food choices in vending machines and eating venues that meet healthy nutrition standards (see sidebar on page 183).

For additional strategies for promoting employee health in small business, consult *Healthy Workforce 2010 and Beyond: An Essential Health Promotion Sourcebook for Both Large and Small Employers,* published by Partnership for Prevention (www.prevent.org).

In some areas, small businesses can participate in community health alliances to offer WHP programs and activities to employees. For example, in north Texas, the Small Business Wellness Initiative is a community-collaborative project funded by a grant from the Department of Health and Human Services (SBWI 2010). The mission of the initiative is to enhance the health, productivity, and quality of work life for small-business leaders, their employees, and their communities. Community partners include the Tarrant Council on Alcoholism and Drug Abuse, the North Texas Small Business Development Center, and Organizational Wellness and Learning Systems. For more information on the initiative's model, programs, and services, access its website at www.sbwi.org.

Because most small businesses have a small (or nonexistent) budget for health-promotion programs, employee volunteers or members of management might use an expense management grid (see chapter 5,

HEALTHY VENDING MACHINE POLICY (MINIMUM STANDARDS)

Beverages

50% of beverages offered in each vending machine will include one or a combination of the following:

- Water and flavored water
- Nonfat or 1% low-fat milk (flavored or unflavored)
- 100% fruit or vegetable juice
- Unsweetened regular and herbal tea (hot or cold)
- Coffee
- Other noncaloric beverages, including diet sodas

*Except for water, as product availability allows, beverages shall be no greater than 12 ounces. Juices in 6- to 8-ounce portions are preferable.

*Advertising on vending machines should only include beverages that meet the nutrition standards.

Snack Food

50% of snacks and foods offered in each vending machine shall meet the following criteria:

- <200 calories per snack
- <35% total calories from fat, excluding nuts and seeds
- <7% total calories from saturated fat
- Zero trans fat (<0.5 g per serving)
- <480 mg of sodium
- <35% calories from total sugars with the exception of the following:
- Fruits and vegetables without added sugar
- Unflavored nonfat and low-fat yogurt
- Flavored nonfat and low-fat yogurt with no more than 30 grams of total sugars per 8-ounce (230 g) serving

*Item selection should prioritize whole grains, fruits, vegetables, low-fat dairy, nuts, and seeds.

*Advertising on vending machines should only include foods that meet the nutrition standards.

*Pricing on foods that meet the nutrition standards should be kept as close as possible to the price of foods that do not meet the standards.

---

page 91) as a guide to determine how to best use on-site and community resources. The grid can help a small business explore the feasibility of purchasing, renting, leasing, bartering, or brokering resources. For example, more small businesses are joining together with their peers to form consortiums, cooperatives, or pools to negotiate purchasing products and services at discounted rates. Services might include reduced employee membership fees at local health clubs, YMCAs, and community centers; affordable EAP services for local mental-health clinics; and shared walking trails, school gymnasiums, parks, and athletic fields.

Despite the growing success of small-business pools, many small companies might not have that option in their communities. These businesses must resort to personal arrangements with local providers. If properly structured, these arrangements can benefit both parties. For instance, the partnership between the Wisconsin-based Copps grocery-store chain and the YMCA has become a model for small businesses. Copps contracted with the Y to provide a three-phase WHP program consisting of (1) fitness testing and consultation, (2) health education, and (3) special recreational opportunities. Nearly half of Copps' employees participate in the program. The success of the arrangement has had widespread value, benefiting not only Copps and the Y, but also the entire community. Other area businesses have also established similar programs.

Evaluation

Although they are not as likely as larger companies to have data-management systems for tracking absenteeism, productivity, health care use, and so on, progressive-minded small businesses can monitor certain types of data to evaluate their health promotion efforts. Chapter 8 discusses evaluation procedures that can be modified to suit small-business programs. At a minimum, employee participation should be tracked to evaluate interest in different types of health promotion programs.

The R.E. Mason Company in Charlotte, North Carolina, has a workforce of about 100 employees. In addition to programs initiated by the HR director or the president, programs and activities for health promotion are being developed and implemented by a committee of employees that is made up of a cross section of workers from various departments. Before an activity is launched, the committee seeks final approval from the HR director and the president to assure that budgets are considered and that work time and productivity are not adversely affected.

All managers and employees are reminded of healthy living and of the company's commitment to health and wellness through various avenues: employee newsletter articles, information posted on the intranet site and on bulletin boards, annual health screenings, annual health fairs, weekly exercise classes held in the workout room, and the healthy snack program, among others.

Several incentives presently exist to encourage employee participation in wellness activities. Payroll deductions for health insurance premiums are reduced if employees participate in annual health screenings. The current health insurance carrier allows employees to log into its website and enter weekly points for healthy eating and exercise to earn gift cards and other prizes. Company contests and activities also offer a variety of prizes for participation.

The R.E. Mason Company has earned various statewide awards for its outstanding WHP efforts.

As is common today in the realm of company-sponsored health insurance, the R.E. Mason Company has experienced some rising premiums. It is always looking at ways to control costs. At the same time, the company continually encourages employees and their families to be good consumers of their health care benefits, as a way to reduce both out-of-pocket costs to employees as well as the costs to the plan. For example, they might consider waiting to see a primary care physician instead of going to the emergency room. But, focus on prevention is paramount. The company encourages all employees to pursue preventive health care services, to exercise and eat right, and to generally stay focused on leading a healthy lifestyle.

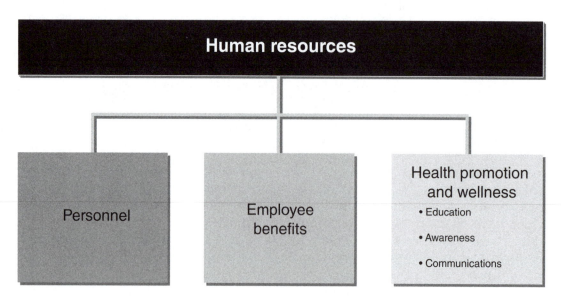

Figure 9.1 The integrated framework for health promotion used at R.E. Mason Company.
Reprinted, by permission, from R.E. Mason Company.

In planning an evaluation, small businesses should not overlook possible assistance from local health associations and the prospects for creating collaborative arrangements. For example, faculty members at a local college may be interested in providing evaluation assistance in exchange for using a small worksite as a research site.

Although small businesses often need to find innovative ways to evaluate their programs, this step should never be neglected. A WHP program that is not evaluated cannot provide evidence that the program should be continued, thereby increasing the odds that management may consider WHP to be expendable.

Even relatively minor attempts to reduce risk can pay off for small businesses. For example, consider two employees with chronic back problems: John works for a large company with 1,000 employees and Michelle works for a small company with 20 employees. From a risk-management and economic point of view, the health care costs associated with John's back problem can be spread among 999 other employees, whereas Michelle's costs are spread among only 19 other employees. Consequently, on a per-capita basis, Michelle's condition increases her company's health insurance risk 50 times more than John's condition, making it increasingly difficult for her company to qualify for—much less afford—today's costly health coverage. Fortunately, today's health-insurance pools (alliances) are closing this gap for many small businesses.

MULTISITE OPERATIONS

As more businesses continue to downsize and relocate their employees at multiple locations, WHP programming has become more challenging for many health promotion practitioners. When working with multisite populations, WHP personnel need to develop programs and policies based on representative data from all sites. The data collected from site to site will often vary, and the program itself may need to change in order to meet each site's unique needs. This tailoring is possible in large part because of the recent development of technology, mail-based initiatives, and online services that have opened up a lot of WHP options for small and multisite operations of all sizes.

Organizational Structure

Generally speaking, multisite businesses fall into two categories of organization: *centralized*, which is the traditional structure, and *decentralized*, a more contemporary organization. Refer to figures 9.2 and 9.3 for models of the two structures.

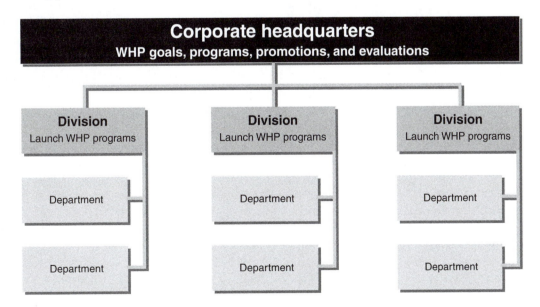

Figure 9.2   A centralized (traditional) organizational structure.

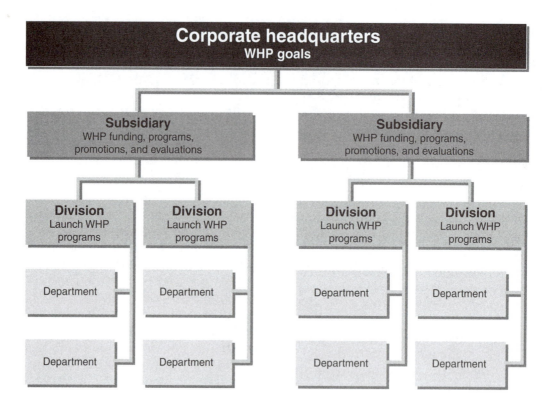

Figure 9.3 A decentralized (contemporary) organizational structure.

Multisite programming varies depending on the organizational structure. If a company is centralized, the headquarters facility generally funds WHP programs, while headquarters staff develop the materials and roll out the program through field coordinators (who may or may not be health professionals). Although a company may be centralized and funded by corporate headquarters, if the local sites are dispersed throughout the country or abroad, cultural and demographic differences can greatly affect health promotion outcomes. In fact, even in a centralized operation, it is not uncommon for headquarters to grant some autonomy for individual sites to tailor their WHP efforts around these unique characteristics.

If a company is decentralized, the local site tends to have more control over WHP programming. The local sites fund programs and generally want more customization. For example, a corporate goal for health management may be to provide a safe and healthy work environment. The operating division

(individual site) may adapt this broad goal by adding specific goals, such as the following:

- Administer a prevention program to reduce back-injury costs by 50%
- Provide healthy food options that make up at least 75% of all items in the cafeteria
- Encourage and help each employee achieve high levels of wellness and productivity
- Establish exercise options at the worksite that will engage at least 50% of all employees in regular activity

Although a decentralized organization often presents more challenges for WHP planners, program considerations are similar for the two structures. In each case, programmers must find a way to modify the WHP planning framework (presented in the preface) to meet the needs of a multisite operation. In the sections that follow, the major components of the framework (identification, assessment, implementation, and evaluation) will be discussed in relation to a company with employees spread among two or more locations.

Identification and Assessment

As is true at a single-site location, planning WHP for a **multisite program** first involves identifying and assessing employee needs and interests. Thus, a thorough strategy for health-risk assessment is essential. It should accurately gauge the prevalence of specific risk factors that warrant a clinical measurement (e.g., obesity, hypertension, smoking, hyperlipidemia, and so on) rather than relying solely on self-report.

When a business has employees at several sites that are hard to reach or are very different, identification and assessment become particularly important. Review chapters 1 and 2 for details about these phases of the process and customize these activities around the unique characteristics and needs of your site. In particular, when conducting multisite programming, the key components within the two phases are to do the following:

- Visit the sites and meet with decision makers, including management.
- Learn current policies and procedures for health and safety.
- Understand the site's operating systems (e.g., manufacturing or services protocol, databases, interdepartmental communication).
- Establish a line of ongoing (future) communication with key personnel.

A first step is to visit the site and talk with key members of management. Depending on the number of locations, you may want to start with a survey to learn about employee demographics, areas of greatest need, shift schedules, cultural diversity, and types of work performed. You can mail this survey before you visit so that you have time to weigh the results prior to meeting with employees and management.

To make your site visit more effective, talk to both management and employees to get an accurate perception of the operation. This is a good time to inquire about what types of community health agencies and resources may be available in the area to assist small and multisite operations with their WHP efforts. Also, discuss safety issues, employee morale, common health problems seen in the workforce, health plan benefits, and whether union representation is involved in employee health issues. If possible, see whether it's possible to observe and possibly work an off-schedule shift. This is a good opportunity to show employees that you are there to help them, not just management.

Along with meeting employees and management, inquire as to whether health-care utilization and cost-data reports are available on site. Such data may reveal specific types of health care services that are commonly used, as well as types and locations of health care providers. This information may be particularly helpful when developing programs for health care consumerism and medical self-care. Finally, try to meet with human resources or WHP personnel at other worksites in the area to learn about their approach and experiences with employee health promotion.

During your site visit, get a copy of an employee handbook or a policy and procedure manual. Review the document, looking at areas that influence the health of the work environment, such as the site's smoking policy, flex-time policy, mandated programs for safety or preventing illness and injury, sick leave and family leave, cafeteria and vending machine options, worksite violence-prevention programs, drug-screening programs, return-to-work programs, preemployment screening process, and other items relevant to employee health.

Understanding a site's operating systems allows more comprehensive WHP planning to occur. The better you develop your programs to align with current organizational systems, the more likely the programs will be accepted and will succeed. During your site visit, talk to human resources or benefits personnel to learn how policies are monitored and modified, when necessary. If an employee union exists, also try to understand the relationship between the union and management and the process they use to reach consensus. Other operating systems to inquire about include safety practices, medical management, communication systems, hiring and training practices, and total quality-management practices. For example, if you don't have good systems in place with sound protocols for delivering on-site or online services, the quality of your programs may be jeopardized.

Implementation

Refer to chapter 7 to review general guidelines for implementing WHP programs. In general, it pays to standardize the way you are implementing the programs in order to create a turn-key operation. Doing so will allow the person in charge of implementing WHP activities to easily adopt and implement WHP activities. Additional steps involved in implementing programs specifically for multisite businesses include recruiting volunteer coordinators, considering the addition of staff to reach all sites, rewriting internal policies and procedures, developing programs to encourage self-responsibility, considering readiness to change, targeting high-risk employees, emphasizing self-care programs, weighing other important considerations, and following up on communication with management, employees, volunteers, and any WHP staff. Each of these steps is discussed in detail in the following section.

Some multisite WHP programs with limited resources are run by employee volunteers who have release time from their official job duties to direct or provide such efforts. By and large, volunteers should have the following qualities:

- Good role models
- Respected by their peers
- Leadership and facilitative skills
- Have a respect for and appreciation of employees' diversity (values, beliefs, lifestyles, and so on)

In the event that a committee of employee volunteers is responsible for directing or staffing WHP activities, it may be useful to develop a charter that can be used to guide and monitor personnel activities. It may include length of membership on the committee, roles and responsibilities, and expectations of communicating between and among various parties. In addition, volunteer committees will need ongoing support and guidance from qualified and respected leaders to ensure responsibility and focus. Possible options may include assistance from the following people:

- Local health department personnel knowledgeable in WHP issues
- Local university faculty experienced in WHP issues
- WHP-savvy representatives from your health plan
- Outside WHP vendor who provides feedback and ideas at regular intervals

During the development and implementation of awareness and basic education programs for employees, someone outside of the health profession can roll out and follow up with many program materials. But as the site matures and more focused education and behavior change programs are developed and implemented, the need for professional assistance arises. Staffing options vary, depending on site funding and demand. Some of these options include the following:

- Providing internships for qualified students from a local university
- Hiring a local vendor skilled in WHP issues
- Hiring and training a local team of professionals to go on site-specific assignments
- Teaming with your current health plan to provide services at a reduced rate

Whatever options are used for staffing, it is important for all staff members to have a clear understanding of corporate-wide WHP goals and how site-specific WHP goals relate to the big picture. For example, provide all on-site staff with customer research data and marketing processes to make sure they understand management's view and level of commitment. This will help them accommodate employees with disabilities and possible liability concerns. The better they fit into the cultural norms, the fewer barriers will exist to compromise participation.

For WHP programs to work in multisite settings, company policies and program interventions must be properly aligned. For instance, smoking policies should support smoking cessation efforts, the cafeteria and vending machines should provide healthy meals consistent with existing nutrition and weight-management programs, employee hours need to be flexible enough to allow participation in health promotion activities, and so on. Worksite health programs that are inconsistent with overall company policies reduce the programs' credibility and practically ensure failure.

Before implementing a program, revisit the initial discussions you had with site management to ensure that the program's goals match up with management expectations.

You might put agreements in writing to reconfirm all parties' commitment to responsibilities, costs, time lines, and follow-up procedures. The more health promotion is integrated with other company functions, the greater the importance of this communication. All parties should be involved on a regular basis. This is particularly true since individual WHP professionals will not have a full-time presence in all sites of a multisite arrangement. Moreover, official job duties of WHP volunteers generally do not include health promotion responsibilities. Thus, it is simply not enough for WHP personnel to have an on-site presence. Make sure you have a good communications plan in place so that employees consistently understand who is responsible for conducting WHP activities at each site.

Many multisite programs do not have the benefit of having an on-site, full-time WHP specialist or health care professional. Although all programs should encourage employee self-responsibility, multisite populations without immediate resources need to be developed and implemented with self-responsibility in mind. Therefore, it's important to plan programs with a facilitative approach, rather than a direct approach. Instead of telling employees what to do to be healthy, motivate them through education about the effects of their lifestyle choices. Give them options they can tailor to meet their goals and to fit their situations and values. As one program director once put it, "We need to adopt the attitude that we may be great coaches, but we cannot ourselves get out there and win the ball game."

In dispersed workforces, organizational change and issues will be different. For example, one site may be in union negotiations, another may be downsizing, and still another may be undergoing a safety audit. Given the changing variables within each organization, program implementation may look different, and timing will vary from year to year on site requests. To ensure that organizational needs are met, develop core content that can be flexible and customized to cultural demands. When assessing an employee's need and readiness to change, factor in physical risk factors, current behavior and habits, psychological factors, and social support. Most health-risk appraisals provide this type of individual assessment. In addition, take the time to research and understand cultural predispositions to certain health risks, as well as correlating lifestyle patterns. At this point, an insightful occupational health nurse or human resources manager can shed some light on how a workforce's demographic, cultural, and lifestyle characteristics may influence employees' willingness to participate in your WHP programs. While tapping these insights, consider what can be done to assess where employees currently exist on the readiness-to-change continuum. This is a good time to reconsider DiClemente and Prochaska's stages of change:

1. *Precontemplation.* Employees are unaware, unwilling, or discouraged when changing problem behavior.
2. *Contemplation.* Employees are considering the prospects of change and are researching information about the pros and cons of the change.

3. *Preparation.* Employees intend to make change in the near future; they have learned valuable lessons from past attempts and failures.

4. *Action.* Employees take action to change behavior.

5. *Maintenance.* Employees attempt to sustain change and avoid relapse.

By assessing and gathering baseline data on employees, you can better develop and implement different intervention options that will appeal to people at their personal level of readiness to change. In particular, try to provide self-responsible options and choices from group programs to individual programs and from corporate-based models to programs based on community organizations or health plans. Understand the culture to know whether tangible incentives extrinsically motivate employees to start behavior change. Consult your volunteer committee and local resources to enhance your programming decisions. Many times you will perceive an employee's readiness to change, but the worksite environment or cultural norms cannot support the process. This is where flexibility and knowledge, as well as utilization of resources, become particularly important. Of course, in today's high-tech worksites, the versatility of Internet and in-house intranet platforms offer additional venues for transmitting new information to employees.

Multisite programs should further implementation efforts of ongoing awareness campaigns, health fairs, and group education programs. While resources remain limited, shifting delivery from untargeted, group-based health promotion to targeting at-risk employees is proving to be a very cost-effective approach. For the greatest effect, consider targeting the at-risk group that is the most ready to change.

Historically, WHP efforts have not adequately addressed relapse, which is the greatest barrier to permanent lifestyle change. Research conducted by StayWell Health Management Systems, Inc. indicates that targeting employees with high risk profiles who are ready to change increases the potential for long-term behavior change (Shumaker et al. 2009). High-risk employees generally require proactive, ongoing support. Note the comparison in table 9.1 of the traditional model with the focused intervention model. Thus, by shifting funds from group-based programming to a high-risk focus, you are more likely to bring about some of your program goals sooner and to sustain long-term results. Yet, in every worksite setting, it is important to provide WHP opportunities to all employees, including those classified as being at low risk. In fact, some research shows that it may be just as important (in terms of cost) to keep low-risk employees at that level as it is to move high-risk employees to moderate- or low-risk status.

Since virtually all employers are justifiably concerned about today's rising health care costs, it's not surprising to find many worksites of all sizes adopting medical self-care programs. When properly designed and administered, these programs can effectively reduce the overall demand for health care by helping employees enhance their decision-making skills, improve their quality of self-care, and communicate effectively with their health care providers.

Motivating employees to be savvy, informed health care consumers is particularly important in multisite operations that have a difficult time reaching all employees at the same time or on a regular basis. Moreover, employers may offer several types of health plans to their employees, especially in multi-state locations, which may vary widely in types of benefits and provider networks. These employees need to learn how to navigate this maze of health care options. With the advent of medical self-care and with growing consumerism, some companies are reporting benefit-cost ratios of 3:1 or better with such initiatives.

Multisite programs differ most in the need for flexibility and creativity in implementation and delivery methods. Factors, such as decentralization, site-driven funding, employee groups that are culturally and occupationally diverse, limited staffing, organizational readiness, and individual readiness, challenge WHP personnel to meet

Table 9.1 A Comparison Between a Traditional and a Targeted Health Promotion Intervention

Traditional	Targeted
Workforce promotion • Posters and flyers • Team meeting announcements • Newsletter articles • Rarely integrated or coordinated with benefits/human resources	***Personalized promotion*** • Individually tailored around an employee's interest, risk, and readiness to act • E-mail and other tech-generated messaging • Integration or coordination with benefits/human resources
Time-based health screening • Annual or scheduled • Based on age and gender, not just risk • Heavy reliance on health-risk assessment questionnaire	***Participation and risk-based screenings*** • Targeting all employees • Screenings focus on risk with follow-up
Generic group programming Same programs and activities for everyone; no consideration of individual needs or interests	***Individually focused programming*** • Individual invitation to specific risk-based programs and activities • Tailored around individual interests • On-site webinar delivery • On-site and off-site activities encouraged
Nonfinancial incentives/rewards • Motivation based on peer/buddy/group support • T-shirts, well bucks, hats, water bottles	***Nonfinancial and financial incentives/rewards*** • Discount on health insurance premium • Accounts for health savings and health reimbursement • Gift cards, well days off, and so on • T-shirts, well bucks, hats, or water bottles
Reactive maintenance Relapse is ignored or addressed only when it occurs	***Proactive support and follow-up*** • Structure programming around each employee's stage of readiness • Regularly assess progress and adapt program accordingly • Personal health and life coaching
"Ex post facto" (after the fact) evaluation • Evaluation planning during or after the program was underway • Heavy tracking of participation; some monitoring of changes in risk factor	***Prospective evaluation*** • Built-in evaluation protocol prior to start of program • Three levels of evaluation (process, impact, and financial outcome) • Integrated system for health-data management • Economic based/ROI

Reprinted, by permission, from StayWell Health Management Systems, Inc.

these multifaceted needs at different times and in customized ways. Niche programming for the local culture is critical. Spending time in their environment, especially with blue-collar employees, cultivates trust and a relevant understanding of their jobs, which is extremely important.

Evaluation

Considerations for multisite program evaluation are often more complex than a single-site evaluation. The following section discusses some issues unique to multisite evaluation.

Throughout the life of the program, management support is essential. The more decentralized the health promotion program is, the more time you find yourself spending to obtain ongoing support and focus for it. It is wise to have a broad base of management support; don't rely on one champion at the site. For example, you may have 40 sites, with 5 to 7 managers at each site. The possibility for turnover and rotation of these

A SUCCESSFUL MULTISITE PROGRAM

The Washoe County School District is one of the largest employers in northern Nevada, providing self-funded health benefits to 6,500 employees and their family members and about 1,000 retirees. In the early 1990s, the district's group insurance committee, which governs the self-funded health plan and includes representatives from the school district's teachers and associations of classified employees, began meeting periodically to discuss how to control health care costs. The district risk manager and benefits coordinator provided the committee with information about the potential of worksite wellness programs to reduce costs. The third-party administrator ran cost reports and provided other financial reports and analyses needed to convince all parties of the need for and potential benefits of this type of program. After 2 or 3 years of discussions and a review of published literature, a focus group agreed to try a wellness program. This subset of the committee developed an outline of the current program.

Approval was sought and obtained from school district leaders and representatives of the employee associations. A fulltime wellness coordinator was hired specifically for this initiative. The program was advertised to employees. The payroll deduction was also arranged, with separate funds earmarked for the wellness coordinator's salary and for program activities and incentives. Other participants include the Washoe County School District's risk manager, benefits coordinator, and members of the group insurance committee, each of whom participates as a part of regular duties in the planning, design, and operations of the program.

A wellness coordinator must have creativity and energy, knowledge and experience in the wellness field, and the ability to communicate effectively using the Internet, mailings, and other tools. The coordinator is responsible for developing and operating the programs, as well as instituting new ones on an ongoing basis. Typically, the Washoe County school district runs 6 or 7 distinct activities per year, repeating some activities every 2 or 3 years. Some programs incorporate a seasonal theme, such as spring gardening contests and weight-loss incentives around the winter holidays. Often, activities incorporate prize drawings, small enrollment gifts (e.g., water bottles, gym towels), payment for success (e.g., $10 per pound lost), and other incentives (e.g., gym scholarships). Some awards are based on team competitions.

Startup costs were negligible because participants in the program's design incorporated the work into their daily activities. The program is cost-neutral, since payroll deductions cover the coordinator's salary and activity costs. It was funded internally by the Washoe County School District by combining interesting programming with financial incentives to encourage the 7,500 employees, spouses, and retirees covered by its self-funded health plan to participate in the wellness program. All employees and retirees covered by the district health plan may reduce their monthly premiums by $40 by getting an annual screening or physical examination and completing a premium discount form by December each year. Employees, retirees, and spouses covered by the district's self-funded health plan are automatically enrolled in the wellness program. They then can review current program activities and participate in those that interest them on a voluntary basis. The premiums of employees and retirees who do not alter their health plan go into the school district's wellness fund, which finances creative programs that promote wellness.

Employees and retirees enrolled in the district's self-funded health plan receive mailings and e-mails that advertise the wellness program and provide reminders about upcoming programs, recipes, and encouraging quotations. Communications encourage people to sign up for activities and to obtain an annual health screening or physical examination from a physician. Employees can receive information and sign up for programs online. They can also track their compliance with activities and self-report their results. For more information on the program, please refer to their website (www.washoe.k12.nv.us/staff/wellness-program).

managers creates an ongoing process of educating management on key issues, focuses, and outcomes.

During the initial period of proposal writing and meeting with management, bring an evaluation plan to base decisions on. Managers who are unaware of the benefits of health promotion and preventive health services may have a difficult time determining and articulating their desired outcome. Lead them by offering options, especially in a multisite environment where decentralized managers are looking for specific goals. An effective and cost-efficient strategy is to facilitate consensus of goals and objectives across all multisite management teams. Work with the organization's business plan and metrics and lay out the evaluation plan within the existing framework. Be realistic in your evaluation plan. Use multisite report-

ing in the data, writing the data parameters you need from each site in order to meet its goals and objectives. For example, you need either to receive health-plan utilization from human resources or you need a copy of the monthly incident report. Reach a consensus with other functional groups on how this data should look when you receive it.

Program tracking is the most critical component of a multisite program and evaluation. The need for a data-management system and clear utilization process to link the integrated program is crucial for evaluation success. Good options for linking systems include using a computer-wide area network, local-area network, integrated health-data management systems (IHDMS), or e-mail to coordinate the multisite data collection (see figure 9.4). For very small multisite locations, a strategy may be to have WHP

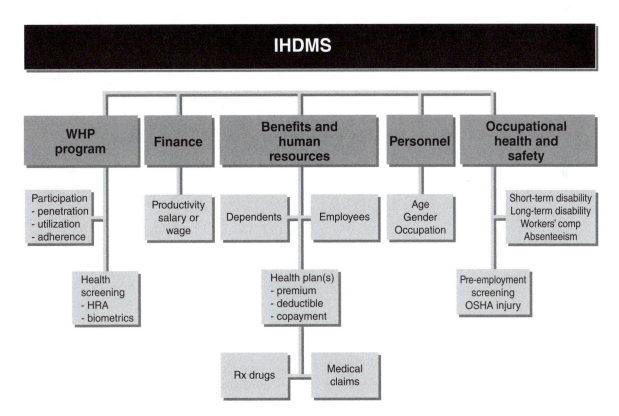

Figure 9.4 A sample framework for an integrated health-data management system.
Reprinted, by permission, from Chenoweth & Associates, Inc.

staff complete a standard evaluation form to send to a centralized data collection site. In any case, the tracking system for evaluation must be clearly thought out, planned, and funded at the outset of the program.

Program effectiveness is usually gauged by the ratio of benefit to cost. With multisite programs, you may be required to report by location. Suppose one of your multiple sites decides to implement a program that includes an initial survey, a health fair with HRAs and screenings, and a high-risk targeted follow-up for 10% of the site employees. How will you measure this one site's return on investment? Does the benefit-cost ratio fit your overall strategy to support the goals and objectives? Or, given the scope of your programs, is it more practical to simply track changes in participation or risk-factor status?

The data-tracking system should enable seamless recording of participation levels. Be prepared to measure specific types of participation based on utilization, penetration, and adherence rates. At a minimum, the number of employees in attendance should be tracked and utilization and penetration should be readily available, if requested. Each independent site should be given feedback as well as aggregate data collected on all multiple sites. It is customary to monitor employee adherence to an activity and track behavior change. It may also be valuable to record how many high-risk employees attended the program and improved.

Planning processes are essential to ensure consistent development and growth of your program. As integration at each multisite heightens, more checks and balances are needed to ensure process efficiency. Process evaluation of each functional group and of the integration links are critical to maximizing outcomes and program influence. Other functional groups collect data alone (e.g., health plan utilization, safety records, and workers' compensation data) or in collaboration with a data-management system. Yet, the overall process of data integration affects outcomes. The opportunity for duplication of services, costs, and low communication grows as the integration spreads without control.

Survey your multisite management customers throughout the life of the program to ensure site-specific satisfaction and to gather feedback. An employee survey measuring the level of commitment and opinions about behavioral change, assessing motivational levels, and providing the opportunity to offer feedback will allow program planners to refocus and insure the program has an influence. An important goal of an evaluation strategy is to provide feedback that you will continually communicate to management and employees.

Multisite program planning requires consistent communication, clarification, and follow-up with management customers. Organizations in continually changing environments have a tendency to work as a single site in a vacuum, which creates barriers for those planning multisite programs and policies. Critical success factors for a multisite program manager include working for high integration, reaching all levels of employees with communications, and consistently building program penetration. You can ensure this by working with them on their shift and in their work environment. Be real and honest with these employees. Ask the customer what is right and wrong with the program and how it can be improved. Customers are your ultimate audience, and their empowering trust to you only comes with real personal presence and experience. See table 9.2 and the following sidebar for details concerning Chevron's multisite health promotion programs.

Table 9.2 Description of WHP Services Offered by Chevron's H&P Advisors to Chevron Worksites Worldwide

WHP services	Description
Planning and assessment	
Annual plan	An H&P advisor discusses your business health needs and describes H&P services available. A plan is made jointly by the H&P business, advisor, and local staff for the delivery of specific services that may involve outside vendors.
Health plan coordination	H&P advisors work with Chevron health plans to evaluate preventive services and maximize their accessibility to their employees and their families; often includes free delivery of health promotion services at the worksite.
Health-risk assessment (HRA)	
Blood pressure/cholesterol screening	A voluntary HRA is provided, which uses medical screening values and a health questionnaire to identify employee health risks. All participating employees receive feedback. Businesses with 50+ HRAs completed receive an aggregate report of group risks. Repeat HRAs and screening annually.
Initial consult	Review H&P business plan and cost/services. Discuss customer needs, business values, and wellness strategy.
Awareness	
Health fair	Coordinate events in which vendors provide materials on various health and wellness topics.
Newsletter articles	Develop and distribute schedules of services and programs or articles within local newsletters focusing on healthy lifestyle topics.
Healthy workplace	
Fitness center	Provide guidance on establishing supervised or unsupervised facilities with aerobic programs and equipment for cardiorespiratory, strength, and endurance exercises.
Vending and nutritional consultation	Provide recommendations to catering vendors regarding healthy choices and alternatives in menu selections. Work with customers to provide healthy vending choices.
Smoking control policy	Written policy against tobacco use on site exists in several locations and is communicated at the site.
Back health	Train supervisors, employees, and ergonomics committees to review correct lifting mechanics, apply National Institute of Occupational Safety and Health (NIOSH) guidelines to work situations, and adapt habits to prevent injury.
Emergency response team/ firefighter physical conditioning	Train ERT and firefighters, including a physical assessment and exercise guidelines applicable to ERT duties, safe lifting, and back-injury prevention.
Office ergonomics	Manage an ergonomic prevention program for employees in discomfort related to their workstations. The program includes workstation evaluations, clinical evaluations, and job-specific conditioning. Provide preventive and clinical interventions for high-risk and discomfort cases (U.S. locations).
Pretask safety stretching	Development of stretching programs for use prior to working or doing physical tasks. Provide on-site stretch and stretching breaks.
Behavior change	
Nutrition and weight control	Provide guidance to work groups on healthy eating (i.e., control-room cooking classes or weight-management programs). Nutrition and weight control are included in enterprise programming to address cardiovascular disease risk.
Physical activity	Provide access to walking programs to increase physical activity. Where possible these activities are integrated with enterprise programming to address cardiovascular disease risk and fitness center activities.
Incentive program	
Consultation/development	Provide guidance on effective, appropriate incentives to motivate all employees to participate in healthy lifestyle activity.
Medical self-care and health care consumerism	An online medical self-care book is made available to all employees and is reinforced through training.
Smoking control	Employees are aware that smoking cessation resources are readily available. Resources are varied and range from self-help materials to one-on-one coaching. Smoking cessation is included in enterprise programming to address cardiovascular disease risk.

Reprinted, by permission, from Chevron Preventive Health Services. © 2011 Chevron U.S.A. Inc.

SATISFACTION SURVEY FROM PREVENTIVE HEALTH SERVICES MANAGEMENT

Thank you in advance for sharing your input on Preventive Health Services (PHS). Your response is very important to our continuous improvement process. Because we are requesting feedback from several different perspectives at many Chevron worksites, we would greatly appreciate it if you would complete this survey yourself and not pass it on to someone else. Please return this survey by October 12th to the address on the other side.

I. Each statement below describes a specific aspect of PHS.

Using the following scale, please indicate how much you agree or disagree with each statement.

Strongly disagree	Disagree	Somewhat disagree	Somewhat agree	Agree	Strongly agree
1	2	3	4	5	6

1. Our PHS advisor has contacted me to describe the range of services PHS provides.

1	2	3	4	5	6

2. PHS is an important resource because it helps my employees be more productive.

1	2	3	4	5	6

3. PHS provides information that helps my employees be more productive.

1	2	3	4	5	6

4. My employees utilize PHS.

1	2	3	4	5	6

5. Our PHS advisor responds to our needs quickly.

1	2	3	4	5	6

6. Our PHS advisor sees goals and priorities to accomplish goals.

1	2	3	4	5	6

7. Our PHS advisor demonstrates the expertise to meet our needs.

1	2	3	4	5	6

8. Our PHS advisor suggests creative solutions to address our needs.

1	2	3	4	5	6

9. Our PHS advisor works effectively with us or our employees to deliver services.

1	2	3	4	5	6

10. Our PHS advisor expresses herself or himself clearly.

1	2	3	4	5	6

11. Our PHS advisor demonstrates effective presentation skills.

1	2	3	4	5	6

12. Our PHS advisor gives us a written annual summary of services delivered.

1	2	3	4	5	6

13. The services offered by PHS have been of benefit to my employees in areas such as employee safety, health, and commitment to the company. Therefore, they are worth the cost.

| 1 | 2 | 3 | 4 | 5 | 6 |

14. I will continue to use PHS.

| 1 | 2 | 3 | 4 | 5 | 6 |

II. We have used the following PHS programs (check all that apply):

❑ Annual wellness program
❑ Back-injury prevention
❑ ERT/firefighter physical conditioning
❑ Fitness facility consultation
❑ Health education
❑ Health fair
❑ Health plan coordination (regarding preventive services)
❑ Health-risk assessment and blood pressure or cholesterol screening
❑ Health Quest University
❑ Nutritional consultation for healthy cafeteria/vending
❑ Initial PHS consultation
❑ Newsletter/health awareness articles
❑ Office ergonomics
❑ Smoking policy development and smoking cessation programs
❑ Other: _____

III. My primary reasons for utilizing PHS are as follows.

Rank the following reasons (with 1 as the most important):

___ Demonstrate commitment to employees and their health
___ Improve safety on and off the job
___ Increase employee morale
___ Increase employee productivity
___ Reduce health-related risks
___ Support incident-free operations
___ Other: _____

IV. Please tell us something about yourself.

Your work type: _____ Human resources _____ Safety _____ Other: _____

V. Comments:

_____
_____
_____

Courtesy of Chevron Preventive Health Services.

What Would You Do?

In your quest to find a summer job, you land a part-time sales position with a small auto parts distributor (50 employees). During your first week, the human resources director distributes a storewide memo announcing that (a) the store's health care costs have increased 25% over the past year, (b) nearly 50% of the increased costs are caused by lower-back injury claims, and (c) all employees will have to contribute $150 more per month to maintain their health insurance benefits. As you size up the situation, the thought of proposing a lower-back stretching program on work time comes to mind. You assume that such a program (a) may demonstrate to the health insurer that the store is committed to reducing its risk of lower-back injury and (b) would buy more time for the store to show that it can lower this risk and associated costs. With your game plan in mind, what obstacles should you consider in selling this proposal to the human resources director?

Read the following descriptions of different worksites, all of which are part of the same corporation, and choose one.

> *Case study 1.* A coal mine in New Mexico employs 85% Navajo American Indians. The total employee population is 375 people (90% men and 10% women). The mine is unionized and works three rotating 8-hour shifts. The mine has three different sites with separate entrances. The union participates in a nationwide health plan negotiated specifically for coal miners, which includes little preventive care. Management will only participate and pay for preventive activities if employees drive the program.

> *Case study 2.* A refinery employs 90% men and 10% women. The total employee population is 1,200 and the average age is 42. The nonunion workforce requires 70% heavy labor done in two rotating 12-hour shifts. A health promotion program has been in place for two years with an on-site fitness facility of 10,000 square feet (3,048 m). The top employee risk factors are poor eating habits, stress, back injuries, high blood cholesterol, and lack of daily aerobic exercise.

> *Case study 3.* In a large city, a cellular phone company has five worksites with a total of 1,500 white-collar employees. The population is 50% male and 50% female, and the average employee age is 34. The majority of employees have a college education, and the company is nonunion. Access to health promotion and risk-reduction programs is limited to the choice of two managed care programs.

> *Case study 4.* Located on the East Coast are 55 offshore oil platforms, which house 15 to 40 employees at each bunkhouse. Each facility has a catered food arrangement, and 17 have functioning fitness facilities. The population is nonunion and is 90% blue-collar males. The employees belong to a traditional indemnity (fee-for-service) plan and emergency care is the most common claim.

After reviewing the strategies for multisite WHP programs described in this chapter, select one of the sites in the case study and create ideas for conducting each of the four activities listed below:

1. Employee research (needs and interests)
2. Marketing
3. Development and implementation
4. Evaluation

CHAPTER 9 WRAP-UP

Key Points

- Small businesses present unique challenges and opportunities for WHP practitioners.

- By joining health insurance pools, small businesses can spread their aggregate risk level, thus enhancing their purchasing power.

- Identifying and assessing employees' needs and interests in multisite operations requires an efficient plan of action.

- As workforce demographics change and more small and multisite operations evolve, WHP programs must be designed to allow for flexible and customized application.

- Evaluating WHP programs and staff performance in smaller and multisite operations can be effectively conducted with proper protocols and resources.

Glossary

health insurance pool—A group of small businesses constituting a single organization in order to spread health risks and negotiate more affordable health insurance.

multisite programs—Programs offered at multiple locations within the same organization that may differ in content, resources, frequency, population, staffing, and other features.

small business—Normally, a privately owned corporation, partnership, or sole proprietorship that has fewer than 100 employees in the United States or fewer than 50 employees in the European Union.

Bibliography

Council Of Smaller Enterprises. 2010. "About COSE." Accessed March 10. www.cose.org/About%20COSE.aspx.

Linnan, L., et al. 2008. "Results of the 2004 national worksite health promotion survey." *Journal of the American Public Health Association* 98: 1503-1509.

Partnership for Prevention. 2010. *"Healthy workforce 2010: An essential health promotion sourcebook for employers, large and small."* Accessed March 5. www.prevent.org.

PricewaterhouseCoopers. 2009. "PwC health and well-being Touchstone survey results." Accessed November 12, 2010. www.pwc.com/us/en/healthcare/publications/pwc-health-and-well-being-touchstone-survey-results.jhtml.

Proschaska, J., J. Norcross, and C. DiClemente, C. 1994. *Changing for good.* New York: William Morrow and Company.

Small Business Wellness Initiative. 2010. "The small business wellness initiative." Accessed November 12, 2010. http://sbwi.org/documents/SBWI_Executive_Summary.pdf.

Shumaker, S., J. Ockene, and K. Riekert. 2009. *The handbook of health behavior change.* New York: Springer.

U.S. Census Bureau. 2010. "Statistics about business size (including small business) from the U.S. Census Bureau: Employment size of firms, 2004." Accessed November 12. www.census.gov/epcd/www/smallbus.html.

Washoe County School District. 2010. "Wellness program." Accessed March 10. www.washoe.k12.nv.us/staff/wellness-program.

Looking Ahead

Now that we've covered several ways to overcome common WHP programming challenges in small and multisite worksettings, it's time to consider how to professionally prepare for a positive influence. Chapter 10 highlights several strategies for building a strong base of knowledge and skills, as well as how to position yourself for a successful career in WHP.

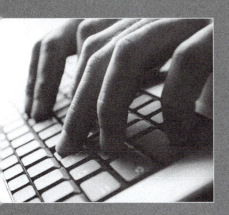
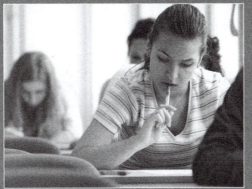
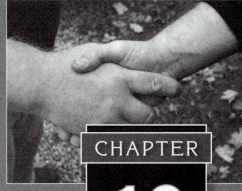

Building a Career in WHP

LEARNING OBJECTIVES

After reading this chapter, you will be able to do the following:

✔ Identify professional skill areas highly preferred by prospective employers.
✔ Describe how certification and professional resources can enhance your career preparation.
✔ List several factors to consider in preparing for a WHP internship.
✔ Construct a quality cover letter and résumé.
✔ Demonstrate good skills in a mock interview.

The number of WHP programs in American worksites grew at an unprecedented rate in the 1980s and 1990s. Corporate health programs continue to grow in the 21st century, although at a slower rate. Much of this continued growth is driven by increasing recognition of their benefits to employee health and productivity. Even as the global marketplace has faced an economic downturn over the past several years, tempting decision makers to pare back on all employee benefits but the core ones, recent surveys show that the overall prevalence of WHP programs has been sustained.

What does the future have in store for WHP programs and aspiring professionals? This question is certainly provocative and timely, considering the turbulent economic times we live in. However, given today's increased emphasis on health and productivity management at many worksites, this field has a promising future, especially for enthusiastic and energetic workers who prepare for it.

According to two independent surveys—one involving nearly 200 WHP program directors from educational, corporate, and hospital settings—certain behaviors, knowledge, and skills are highly desirable. Overall, the surveys reflect an increased emphasis on acquiring a broad background, especially for those hoping to become program managers or directors.

> What are the essential skills for successfully entering today's competitive job market?

ACADEMIC PREPARATION

To meet the growing health-management needs of most employers, many universities offer courses in WHP. Some universities offer undergraduate- or graduate-level concentrations or certificates in WHP as well.

HIGHLY DESIRABLE AREAS OF WHP KNOWLEDGE AND SKILLS

KNOWLEDGE	SKILLS	BEHAVIORS
Accounting/finance	Budgeting	Initiative and work ethic
Behavior modification	Coaching and counseling	Models healthy lifestyle
Benefit-cost analysis/ROI	Communications/presentations	Respects others' views,
Exercise physiology and prescription	First aid and CPR	beliefs, and values
Disease management	Health screening	Safety focused
Federal statutes (e.g., ADA, HIPAA, GINA)	Program evaluation	Strong interpersonal skills
Health plan options and costs	Program planning	Works well individually
Health-risk assessment	Program marketing	and with others
Health and productivity management	Using data to drive programs (e.g.,	
Nutrition	claims data analysis, culture audit)	
Population health management		
Stress management		
Weight management		

Since academic courses typically reflect the philosophies of their faculty, it is important for aspiring WHP professionals to closely compare curricula before enrolling in a particular program. Ask to see copies of syllabuses so that you can evaluate the topics covered in each course. Review this information and talk with a faculty member to determine whether a particular academic program really reflects today's marketplace and your career interests. If possible, select a program with a strong foundation in health promotion that can be complemented with courses in exercise science, business management, and any other ancillary area in which an academic minor or specific **certification** is sought. Overall, a good academic program should provide you with a true perspective of what is happening in WHP locally, regionally, and nationally. It should also offer an internship or practical exposure in a real worksite setting.

To succeed in today's competitive marketplace, you need a strong base of skills in health promotion, exercise science, and business management. A multifaceted background is particularly important; career options evolve, and companies look for one person to serve multiple roles. Having a versatile background can also be the crucial ingredient for moving into advanced positions.

Competitive Academic Programs

In preparing for a career in WHP, work closely with your academic adviser to develop a competitive curriculum that makes full use of your elective hours. For example, avoid filling these credits with easy courses just to boost your GPA. A handful of soft A's won't win you many points in an interview, much less on the job. Today's marketplace is increasingly competitive, so prepare for your future by engaging in a challenging curriculum as well. The following subjects are among the upper-level courses you should consider taking when possible:

A COMPETITIVE ACADEMIC CURRICULUM

BUSINESS
Accounting or finance
Business law
Business statistics
Industrial or personnel psychology
Management
Marketing
Professional speech
Risk management

HEALTH PROMOTION
Accident and injury prevention
Disease management and prevention
First aid and CPR
Health behavior
Health and productivity management
Nutrition
Program evaluation
Program planning
Stress management

EXERCISE SCIENCE

EXERCISE PHYSIOLOGY

EXERCISE TESTING AND PRESCRIPTION

EXERCISE INSTRUCTION

KINESIOLOGY

ALLIED HEALTH
Anatomy and physiology
Medical terminology
Occupational health

To further enhance your job prospects, seriously consider a minor in business administration, occupational safety, allied health, or another area related to WHP. To keep abreast of the ever-changing nature of the current worksite climate, learn as much as you can about as many things as you can. Read widely from publications about health promotion, fitness, and business to keep apprised of today's key issues and trends in WHP.

During your senior year, ask your academic advisor about opportunities for certification, professional conferences, and internships. Also, be sure to sign up with your university's job placement center. Many university career centers sponsor workshops to assist students in writing application letters, creating effective résumés, and successfully interviewing with prospective employers.

Online Programs

With today's accessible and affordable technologies at their fingertips, most universities and colleges are moving swiftly into online delivery of academic courses and programs. In fact, numerous institutions are offering graduate-level programs exclusively in an electronic platform. Although online delivery is expected to grow aggressively in the coming years, some industry observers are understandably concerned about the pros and cons (e.g., quality assurance, student learning, skill development) of moving from the traditional classroom-based delivery to current technology-driven approaches.

In considering the personal benefits and limitations of online options, take time to thoroughly assess the following:

• Personal needs and interests (e.g., your work schedule, learning style, finances, and so on)

• Availability of a reliable academic adviser who can assist you with registration and course scheduling

• Ratio of students to faculty adviser and of students to course instructor

• Credentials and reputation of the institution

• Credentials, experience, and reputation of online instructors

PROFESSIONAL CERTIFICATION

Over the past two decades, the percentage of WHP-related job descriptions that require some type of certification has substantially increased. Thus, your academic program must provide the right type of knowledge and skills to help you qualify for appropriate certifications. For example, if you are pursuing a university program as part of a particular certification, ask a faculty member or your advisor the following questions:

- Which courses will help me to prepare for certifications relevant to my chosen occupation?
- When is the best time to take these courses—independently, in combination, in my senior year, or just prior to an internship?
- Is a study group available to help me prepare for a certification exam?
- Does the university sponsor any on-site certification exams throughout the academic year? If not, what is the closest university offering these exams?
- How desirable are specific certifications in the marketplace?
- What distinguishes one certification from another?
- Once a person earns a particular certification, is an ongoing program (such as continuing education) available to maintain the credentials?

Table 10.1 provides a listing of various certification programs for corporate health and fitness specialists.

Unquestionably, professional certification affords the following key advantages to corporate health and fitness professionals:

- Verifying a participant's minimum level of knowledge, skills, and abilities
- Recognizing the participant's commitment to professional standards
- Aiding employers in identifying reputable candidates
- Assuring that participants receive safe and effective guidance based on national standards
- Facilitating the marketability of the practitioner, both for national mobility and a secure identity as a health fitness professional
- Providing a continuing education system so practitioners remain current in their field

Table 10.1 Selected Certifications for WHP and Fitness Specialists

Organization	Web site address	Certifications
Aerobics and Fitness Association of America	www.afaa.com	Personal trainer, instructor of group exercise, step aerobics, yoga, Pilates, and other specialties
American College of Sports Medicine	www.acsm.org	Health fitness specialist, clinical exercise specialist, registered clinical exercise specialist, certified personal trainer, cancer exercise trainer, inclusive fitness trainer, and specialist of physical activity in public health
American Council on Exercise	www.acefitness.org	Personal trainer, group fitness instructor, lifestyle and weight management consultant, and advanced health and fitness specialist
American Heart Association	www.heart.org/heartorg	Cardiopulmonary resuscitation (CPR), first aid, and use of automatic external defibrillator (AED)
American Lung Association	www.lungusa.org	Freedom from smoking facilitator
American Red Cross	www.redcross.org	Cardiopulmonary resuscitation (CPR), first aid, and use of automatic external defibrillator (AED)
The Cooper Institute	www.cooperinst.org	Personal trainer
International Dance and Exercise Association	www.ideafit.com	Personal trainer, group fitness, and others
National Academy of Sports Medicine	www.nasm.org	Personal trainer
National Commission for Health Education Credentialing	www.nchec.org	Certified health education specialist (CHES)
National Wellness Institute	www.nationalwellness.org	Wellness practitioner

To determine if a particular type or level of certification is appropriate for your career aspirations, you should first consider your particular plans. Specifically, do some research to determine if certification is an absolute necessity or simply advantageous. Simply put, what kind of job do you envision taking when you graduate? For example, if you're self employed, or working as an independent contractor or in a clinical setting, you will likely need professional liability insurance that may intrinsically require you to maintain a professional certification. Thus, it's good to talk with others working in your chosen profession to find out if they are certified, what type of certification they hold, and how their certification has helped them in their careers.

Since there may be multiple organizations to choose from, first consider how the certification will be used (e.g., enable you to work with special populations or in a particular occupational setting, to demonstrate general competency and marketability, or maintain your occupational license). Second, what is expected from the certifying organization? Will you need to engage in networking? Enroll in continuing education? Purchase liability insurance? Finally, are specific types of certification more respected or acceptable by employers in your particular geographic area or type of industry?

Certification Organizations

The *health-fitness instructor* certification is designed for the entry-level practitioner. As such, it is an ideal way for health-fitness professionals to promote themselves as dedicated and knowledgeable in a highly competitive field. Although it is impossible to identify and list all health-fitness certifications in this chapter, you may wish to explore one or more of the following certifying bodies, which happen to be some of the largest and best-known entities:

- American Council on Exercise
- American College of Sports Medicine
- Aerobics and Fitness Association of America
- The Cooper Institute
- Fitness Institute International
- National Academy of Sports Medicine
- National Strength and Conditioning Association
- International Dance and Exercise Association
- Young Men's Christian Association (YMCA)

Of these, three organizations are affiliated with the National Organization for Competency Assurance and are sometimes referred to as the *big three:* the American Council on Exercise (ACE), the American College of Sports Medicine (ACSM), and the National Strength and Conditioning Association (NSCA).

The mission of ACE is to promote active, healthy lifestyles with positive effects on the mind, body, and spirit and "to protect against unsafe and ineffective fitness products and instructions." (American Council on Exercise 2010). ACE offers certifications to become a personal trainer, clinical exercise specialist, group fitness instructor, and lifestyle and weight management consultant through a written, independently proctored exam. Although only the exercise specialist certification requires a bachelor's degree, all certifications have a CPR prerequisite. Additionally, certifications must be renewed no more than two years after completion. Continuing education credits may also be required.

ACSM offers three tracks for the practitioner. For those involved mostly with healthy clients, the health-fitness track includes certifications as a personal trainer or health fitness specialist. The clinical track is offered for professionals involved in rehabilitation of cardiac and pulmonary patients, as well for those who prescribe exercise for patients with chronic diseases like diabetes. The ACSM health-and-fitness certifications include the exercise leader, health fitness instructor, and health fitness director. The clinical track includes certifications as a clinical exercise specialist and a registered clinical exercise physiologist. The specialist track is designed for those working with unique populations or in unique settings.

This track offers certifications as a certified cancer exercise trainer, certified inclusive fitness trainer, and physical activity in public health specialist. As with ACE, all ACSM certifications require a valid CPR card and either recertification after four years or accumulation of continuing education credits. Among the big three certifying organizations, a unique aspect of ACSM certification is their practicum addition to the exam protocol. This is consistent with ACSM's mission of "promoting and integrating. . . practical applications. . . to maintain and enhance physical performance, fitness, health, and quality of life." (American College of Sports Medicine 2010). The practicum section involves one-on-one testing and evaluation.

NSCA, a "worldwide authority on strength and conditioning for improved physical and athletic performance," (National Strength and Conditioning Association 2010) offers two certifications. The personal trainer certification addresses the needs of the fitness instructor. The designation of certified strength and conditioning specialist (CSCS) is for those who develop strength and conditioning programs for athletes. Each require valid CPR cards, but only the CSCS requires a bachelor's degree or current senior status to sit for the written exam.

The ACE certification exams to become a personal trainer, group fitness instructor, lifestyle and weight management consultant, and clinical exercise specialist are now formally being recommended for college credit by the College Credit Recommendation Service, a branch of the American Council on Education. Approximately 1,100 colleges and universities in the United States recognize these credit recommendations. Students, however, must contact the appropriate school official, since each educational institution makes the final decision. Students must successfully complete the exam in order to receive credit. ACE is the first—and currently the only—organization to have academic recognition for fitness-certification examinations.

The myriad of fitness certifications and employer requirements and preferences may initially seem confusing to both current and future health-fitness professionals. However, after examining your professional goals, employment preferences, and geographic considerations, you can more clearly navigate this maze of options and make an informed decision.

Health Coaching

One area that is generating a lot of attention in WHP circles is **health coaching.** Health coaching is a structured, supportive partnership between a participant and a coach. Like traditional coaches, health coaches set goals, identify obstacles, and use personal support systems to motivate behavior change. In particular, health coaches guide patients to talk about what is most troubling to them about their health, what they want to change, what support they have to foster change, and which obstacles they must remove or minimize to achieve better health. Fundamentally, it is not the primary role of the health coach to teach, advise, or counsel clients, but to facilitate positive action.

Given the lack of consistency in how health coaching is defined, practiced, and assessed, it's difficult to determine whether all current versions of the job are evidence based. Today, professionals representing a host of different backgrounds, from nutritionists and fitness trainers to massage therapists and nurses, may refer to themselves as health coaches or wellness coaches. Yet, many have not been exposed to or professionally trained in structured, evidence-based coaching practice.

Since health coaching is currently a relatively new and unregulated discipline, many WHP industry insiders wonder whether popular health coaching training programs are evidence based. An informal review of popular training programs and curricula for health coaches suggests that many are based on models for life coaching. Life coaches use mentoring, values assessment, behavior modification, goal setting, and other approaches to help their clients succeed in life. Moreover, many health coaching programs represent a collection of psychological concepts and techniques, typically with little or no overview of **motiva-**

tional interviewing. Yet, researchers have found that motivational interviewing is the only technique to have been fully described and consistently demonstrated as causally and independently associated with positive behavioral outcomes.

Some of the most publicized training programs for health coaches include the following:

- Whole Health Coaching (www.whole-healtheducation.com/counseling/index.shtml)
- Intrinsic Coaching (www.totallycoached.com/en/home)
- National Society of Health Coaches (www.nshcoa.com)
- Wellcoaches (www.wellcoach.com)
- The Circle of Life Coaching (www.healthandwellnesscoaching.org)

Since there are so many organizations for health coaching training to choose from, it pays to thoroughly research your options to see which one best fits your particular needs.

PROFESSIONAL RESOURCES

A good way to stay apprised of the latest WHP research and trends is to access various professional resources, which range from professional journals and online webinars to seminars and conferences. Many WHP-related journals have abstracts of selected articles that you can access free of charge at their respective Web sites; full articles are available to paying subscribers. Some publishers provide student discounts. A listing of WHP-related publications is shown in table 10.2.

Most of the listed organizations also sponsor conferences that provide excellent opportunities to learn about the latest events, network with others, and explore internship and job possibilities.

Table 10.2 Professional Publications and Web Listings Related to WHP

Publication	Website
ACSM's Health & Fitness Journal	www.acsm.org
American Association of Occupational Health Nurses Journal	www.aaohn.org
American Journal of Health Promotion	www.healthpromotionjournal.com
Benfield Business-Health Leadership	www.thebenfieldgroup.com
Corporate Wellness Magazine	www.corporatewellnessmagazine.com
Employee Benefit Adviser	http://eba.benefitnews.com/
Health & Productivity Management	www.ihpm.org
Health Promotion Practitioner	www.hesonline.com
HERO e-newsletter	www.the-hero.org
HR Magazine	www.shrm.org
IDEA Fitness Journal	www.ideafit.com
IDEA Trainer Success	www.ideafit.com
IDEA Fitness Manager	www.ideafit.com
Journal of Health & Productivity	www.ihpm
Journal of Physical Activity & Health	http://journals.humankinetics.com/jpah
Journal of Occupational & Environmental Medicine	www.acoem.org
Platinum Book: Health & Productivity Management	www.ihpm.org
The Physician & Sports Medicine	www.physsportsmed.com
Wellness Management	www.nationalwellness.org

The University Affiliate Program

A valuable resource for universities preparing WHP practitioners is the **University Affiliate Program (UAP)**, which is created and administered by WELCOA, the Wellness Council of America. UAP is an initiative that provides the latest WHP information for strengthening and enhancing health promotion curricula of participating colleges and universities. Colleges and universities taking part in the UAP are given a complimentary subscription to WELCOA's InfoPoint and related links. These resources are currently utilized by more than 2,500 corporate members as points of reference for worksite health promotion. Published 10 times a year, *Absolute Advantage* includes tips and strategies, unique insights, and real-life studies from some of the best WHP programs in the country. InfoPoint is home to several resources of great value to both students and professionals. Additional areas of interest available at the InfoPoint website include past issues of *Absolute Advantage*, how-to guides, downloadable presentations, case studies, a wellness library, and career center. Colleges and universities interested in becoming UAP members should e-mail their requests to wellworkplace@welcoa.org.

Internships

One of the best ways to enhance your marketability is to get some worksite experience. Many business, industrial, governmental, military, and health care organizations offer internships. These can provide valuable experience in developing and refining your skills in an actual worksite. One student summed up his internship this way:

> This internship has been a wonderful learning experience for me. It showed me that I could interact with a wide array of people and help them meet their special needs. I also benefited from exposure to the employee health screenings that I would not have gotten through the university. This experience helped hone my writing skills. This internship has made me more self-reliant (in part because of my newly developed computing skills) and increased my self-confidence. I have recognized my shortcomings, too—frustration at setbacks and the need to prepare further in advance. Overall, this internship was a period of tremendous growth, both professionally and personally. This is the result of the entire staff carefully preparing our activities for the summer. A contributing factor to my growth was the amount of 'hands-on' experience we (student interns) received.

If you are interested in doing an internship, meet with your academic adviser to discuss opportunities related to your career interest. Since intern responsibilities and employer expectations can vary greatly from site to site, it is important to research each organization's programs, staff members' backgrounds, internship requirements, and other pertinent information well in advance of applying.

INTERNSHIP LISTING ORGANIZATIONS

The number of internship websites is growing rapidly, which can make your search a timely endeavor. Thus, you may wish to begin perusing a sample of websites in your initial quest and then proceed accordingly. Here's a sample listing to get you started:

www.hpcareer.net
www.internshipprograms.com
www.medicalfitness.org
www.wellnessconnection.com
www.internsearch.com
www.hfit.com/internships.asp
www.ltwell.com
www.corporatefitnessworks.com
http://esmassn.org
www.exercisecareers.com
www.healthandwellnessjobs.com

Although each site has its own admission criteria for prospective interns, many worksites typically place the greatest emphasis on the following factors when considering a candidate:

- Ability to perform basic health screenings (e.g., body fat, blood pressure, flexibility)
- Grade point average of B or better in major field of study
- Evidence of a proven work ethic (e.g., volunteering, summer jobs)
- Certification in first aid and CPR
- Good written and verbal communication skills
- Evidence of a healthy lifestyle and image

Some worksites have a specific application form for prospective interns to submit. A sample application may request the following:

- Information about your major and minor fields of study
- Your grade point average
- The type of internship site desired (e.g., manufacturing industry, hospital, small business, managed care organization, community health organization, health club, rehabilitation center)
- Certifications attained
- Dates of your proposed internship
- Number of weekly and total internship hours required by the university
- Major and minor courses completed
- Goals you would like to achieve in an internship
- Your perceived strengths and weaknesses
- Other information that you believe an internship supervisor and staff members should know about you

Some internship sites have a standard application for applicants to complete; others do not. In either case, it's good to prepare a formal **cover letter** that clearly reflects the nature of your interest in a particular organization. (See the following sidebar for a sample letter.)

For many students, an internship is the only real worksite experience they have before entering the job market. Thus, these experiences should be carefully planned within a framework of clearly delineated policies and procedures. For example, when I was directing an undergraduate WHP program at East Carolina University, I developed a student WHP manual with guidelines defining the relationship among student interns, university supervisors, and worksite supervisors. Here is a condensed version of these guidelines:

1. Most worksites require interns to have personal liability insurance coverage. This coverage is typically available through the university's personnel or human resources department at a very low cost.
2. The operating procedures within an internship are subject to both the worksite's discretion and the university's policies.
3. With rare exceptions, interns must pay their own living expenses.
4. Interns should experience the responsibilities of a full-time employee. Thus, a variety of activities are encouraged to foster an appreciation of the commitment required for a full-time job.
5. If travel policies and time allow, a university supervisor will usually visit the employer at least once to observe and discuss the intern's performance. Telephone conversations may replace on-site visits at distant locations.
6. The internship should last at least 10 weeks, with an average workload of 40 hours a week.
7. A successfully completed internship is worth 12 semester hours of academic credit.

SAMPLE FORMAL COVER LETTER

September 1,_____

Robert Smith
Intern Coordinator
Corporate Health Services
612 Modlin Place
Baltimore, MD 00000

Dear Mr. Smith:

I am a senior at (name of college/university) planning to graduate in July _____with a Bachelor of Science degree in Health Promotion and a major concentration in Worksite Health Promotion. Once I complete my coursework this semester, I am required to complete a 400-hour internship in a worksite health promotion setting. Please consider this letter as an expression of my interest in doing a internship with Corporate Health Services in the spring semester of _____.

I learned about Corporate Health Services through an internship database, "Internweb." Since I am from southern Maryland, your company's involvement in corporate health programs caught my eye. I further researched your company to learn that Corporate Health Services has played a leadership role in providing many worksite health promotion initiatives throughout the Delmarva Peninsula over the past 20 years. In reading about CHS' significant role in providing various programs and services in the corporate health field, I am very interested in pursuing an internship with your organization.

I am extremely interested in the field of corporate health and fitness and I have a particular passion for physical fitness, nutrition, health screening, program planning, and delivering presentations. However, I am eager to learn about all aspects of corporate health management. I realize that this is a growing field that requires well-rounded employees. I feel that many of my upper-division courses have prepared me to work well, both on an independent basis and with others in team-oriented situations.
I have also enclosed a résumé with various background information. If any other information is needed, I can be reached at _____-_____, after 11:00 a.m. Monday through Friday. If you prefer to contact me via e-mail, my e-mail address is: _____. I welcome the opportunity to speak with you over the phone or in person about a possible internship with Corporate Health Services.

Thank you for your time and consideration.

Sincerely,
Luke N. Forajob

Sponsoring worksites and universities generally specify responsibilities for student interns. Some common work requirements for interns include the following:

1. Interns should meet with their worksite supervisor early in their internship to complete a basic orientation with a primary focus on these subjects:

   - Organizational (administrative) hierarchy
   - Current health promotion programs and services
   - WHP personnel training, certifications, and experience
   - Problems, needs, and constraints for the existing health promotion program
   - Duties of an intern

2. They may participate in a variety of activities, such as staff conferences, workshops, seminars, and health fairs.

3. They may complete a project planning form before starting a major project to be reviewed with the worksite supervisor on a regular basis.

4. If requested, toward the end of their time, interns may make a formal presentation of their experience to the staff of the sponsoring organization.

To fulfill written requirements for academic credit, the intern is responsible for these duties:

1. Keeping a daily log of major activities and perceptions.

2. Preparing a weekly typed report (based on daily reports) that describes significant events and insights for each week. (One copy should be sent to the worksite supervisor and another should go to the university supervisor. The worksite supervisor and intern meet weekly to discuss each weekly report's contents and strategies for overall improvement.)

3. Preparing a typed final report that includes both descriptive and analytical material. The first part of the final report should include descriptions of the following:

   • The organizational structure of the company

   • The purposes and goals of the company's health promotion program

   • The program components and their functions

   • The major sources of funding for the program

   • The planning process and activities for the major project

The analytical overview of the internship should include insights on your perceptions of the following:

   • What you enjoyed and what aspects of the internship challenged you

   • Major benefits you experienced in doing the internship

   • Suggestions for how the university might improve training experiences before the internship

   • How the worksite might improve the experience for future interns

After completing your internship, submit two typed, bound copies of the final report. Send one to the worksite supervisor and one to the university supervisor.

Common Responsibilities for Worksite Supervisors

1. Provide the recommended orientation for the intern.

2. Assist in planning intern activities and supervising the intern during the internship.

3. Hold a weekly conference with the intern to discuss the intern's performance and specific recommendations for improvement.

4. Discuss the intern's performance with the university supervisor as needed.

5. Complete evaluations in the middle and at the end of the internship. Recommend a final grade to the university supervisor.

Typical Responsibilities for University Supervisors

1. Meet with the prospective intern on several occasions to determine career interests, skills, and weaknesses. Suggest specific preparatory experiences for the internship, explore worksite internship options, and coordinate the application process.

2. Clarify assignments and needs with the intern and worksite supervisor.

3. Make one or more visits to the worksite to review weekly reports and conduct evaluations at the midpoint and end of the internship.

4. Solicit a letter-grade recommendation from the worksite supervisor.

JOB SEEKING

Because competition increases every year, position yourself for the future job market as early as possible. Register with the on-campus career placement office at least six months before you graduate to take advantage of various seminars on preparing application materials, interviewing tips, and job-seeking techniques.

Before graduating, you can enhance your job-searching efforts in various ways. Examples include the following:

- Ask selected faculty members and your employer (if you are working) if they will serve as professional references for you.
- Check the Sunday edition of an area's major newspaper to review the classified section for employment opportunities relevant to your interests.
- Attend a state, regional, or national convention to network with prospective employers and use the on-site job-placement center.
- Attend an on-campus job fair to network with prospective employers and participate in real or mock interviews.
- Check out various job listings on the Internet.

Sample WHP Job-Listing Websites

- http://acsm.healthjobsplus.com
- www.healthpromotionjobs.com
- www.hpcareer.net
- www.phfr.com/jobFinder
- www.wellnessjobs.com
- www.exercisecareers.com
- www.leisurejobs.com

Of course, during your internship, ask your worksite supervisor how you can network with other WHP professionals, which specific skills they're looking for in entry-level candidates, and about steps for enhancing your job-seeking efforts. Network on a regular basis. You never know if current or previous contacts might have the right opportunity for you. The best way to get started is to identify all your personal contacts who may be able to help you (e.g., professors, classmates, family and extended family members, coworkers and employers, and so on). When establishing a connection with contacts, try to meet them in person whenever possible. Be prepared to answer specific questions about your interests and skills, conduct yourself in a personable yet professional manner, and follow up with every contact, thanking them for their time.

Once you identify a job opportunity, prepare a cover letter and related materials to formally apply for a specific position. A cover letter is like a handshake through the mail that serves to introduce you to a prospective employer. In preparing a cover letter, be sure to do the following:

- Address the cover letter to a specific person with the appropriate title. If necessary, contact the organization for this information.
- Customize the letter to address the full scope of each job description. For example, if the job calls for an enthusiastic, organized person, be sure to address these attributes in your cover letter.
- Use a professional format and focus on proper spelling and punctuation.
- Use a font style and size that are large enough to easily read.
- Use the same style and weight of paper for your cover letter and résumé to reflect consistency.
- Close your letter with a legible signature.

Although a cover letter for a job application is similar to the an internship cover letter, it is important to customize each type of letter accordingly. For example, if a job description requests that candidates possess knowledge and skills in a particular area, then it's important to highlight your relevant capabilities in your cover letter and résumé. A cover letter should be accompanied by a résumé with a succinct, informative profile of your background, skills, and professional interests. As a general rule, if the content does not help build your case as a potential employee, it does not belong in the résumé. A well-rounded résumé contains the following information:

- *Personal identification information.* This includes your name, present address, and phone number with area code. You may want to list a permanent address if your current address is temporary.
- *Education.* List your degree (including the date it was granted and the institution from which it was earned), your major (and minor, if appropriate) field of study, your grade point average (overall and in your major), and any internship and student-teaching experience.
- *Course work.* List the upper-level courses you took that pertain to the job description.
- *Employment.* List your paid work history, including summer employment, part-time positions during school, and any full-time positions. In each entry,

list your job title, major responsibilities, and beginning and ending dates for each position.

- *Professional references.* If the job position requests references, list the names and contact information of appropriate references.

Prior to your interview, learn as much as you can about your potential future employer, such as the following:

- Company size (number of employees and number of sites)
- Potential growth of the company
- Products, programs, and services the company provides
- Organizational structure of company headquarters and division offices or plants
- Management style (authoritative, participative, or a mixture)
- Union status and the relationship between the union and management
- Recent news about the company
- Company's philosophy on health promotion
- Established health promotion programs and facilities
- Major health problems of the organization's workforce
- Organizational structure and level of integration of health, fitness, and safety personnel
- Potential growth of health promotion programs

You can find some of this information in the company's annual report, which may be available on the company's website or in a business directory at your local library (e.g., Standard and Poor's Directory). Also, access the organization's website for a possible link to its employee health programs, activities, facilities, and staff members.

In preparing for an interview with prospective employers, review the following tips. In particular, consider possible questions that interviewers may ask and think about how you would answer them. After practicing on your own, have a friend or classmate play the role of an interviewer and ask you typical questions (along with a few surprise questions). Also, prepare several questions that you can ask the employer. Write them down and bring them to the interview. Finally, bring an extra copy of your résumé, a typed list of your references, a bound portfolio of examples of your work, existing letters of recommendation, and questions that you plan to ask the interviewer.

Interview Like a Professional

- Dress professionally and arrive a few minutes early for the interview.
- Greet the interviewer with a handshake and pleasant smile.
- Maintain good posture and a calm disposition throughout the interview.
- In case your interviewer is not as organized as you are, bring along a clean copy of your résumé to have on hand.
- Give the interviewer enough time to ask each question completely. Take a moment or two to think about the question before responding.
- Be honest about past and present employment activities, academic performance, courses taken, and perceived weaknesses or limitations.
- If asked to comment on past employers, make only positive comments.
- Avoid using technical terms. It is better to be perceived as down to earth than pretentious.
- Avoid using hand motions and other gestures to emphasize everything you say. These may be distracting to the interviewer.
- Avoid asking about salary and benefits until you have been offered a job.
- End the interview with a summary statement of the skills you have to offer and your interest in the position.
- Send a mailed letter of appreciation to the interviewer two days after the interview or sooner.

While beginning in an entry-level position, you should strive to expand your knowledge and skills, especially in high-demand competency areas (see tables 10.3, 10.4, and 10.5).

Table 10.3 Major Job Function: Business Skills

Subfunctions	Competencies
A. Technological applications	1. Identify organizational and management-data needs common to a WHP program.
	2. Recommend and assist in the application of appropriate computer hardware and software and other technologies for a WHP program.
B. Facilities, equipment, and materials	3. Coordinate an effective system for inventory control in a WHP program.
	4. Coordinate a schedule of equipment and facility maintenance for a WHP program.
	5. Respond to policies, procedures, and government regulations related to the environmental, structural, and safety issues which assure safe and optimum delivery of health promotion services.
	6. Evaluate needs and recommend appropriate equipment and space.
	7. Evaluate needs and recommend appropriate educational material.
C. Budgeting and purchasing	8. Assist in the budgeting process through review and input.
	9. Assist in the development of a budget presentation.
	10. Assist in the application of proper financial management practices to maintain a health program budget.
	11. Coordinate appropriate purchasing processes with vendors and monitor the quality of products and services received.
D. Program policies and procedures	12. Adhere to administrative and program policies in the worksite environment.
	13. Recommend changes to update policies and procedures based on current standards or changes within the worksite environment.
	14. Effectively communicate these policies and procedures to other staff and to vendors of the program.
	15. Adhere to organizational and professional standards concerning confidentiality of information.
E. Communications	16. Identify communication channels within an organization.
	17. Write appropriate management communications (memo and reports) with accepted business writing form.
	18. Describe and demonstrate the skills necessary to deliver an effective oral presentation.
	19. Describe and demonstrate the ability to utilize different communication styles that can be used with various audiences (management, professional, employee, dependents).
	20. Write appropriate marketing communication pieces for a health promotion program (press releases, brochures, newsletters, flyers, bulletin boards).
	21. Conduct effective meetings through a variety of methods (facilitating skills, small-group dynamics).
	22. Demonstrate effective interpersonal communication and conflict-resolution skills.
F. Quality management and assurance	23. Participate in and support recognized and accepted standards of programming quality.
	24. Assist in the identification of evaluation criteria for the quality management and assurance process.
	25. Assist in the application of evaluation data to ensure continuous program improvement using customer-focused initiatives and strategies.
	26. Identify potential liability areas and assist in legal and risk management.
	27. Identify health and safety issues in the organization.
G. Marketing	28. Collect and analyze appropriate marketing data (e.g., surveys, interviews, focus groups, market databases) for the health promotion program.
	29. Assist with the marketing process to implement appropriate offerings for health promotion programs.
	30. Coordinate appropriate marketing strategies for the target population.

Subfunctions	Competencies
	31. Assist in assessing of the effectiveness of marketing strategies, and make recommendations for improvement.
H. Business planning	32. Assist in the development of the mission, goals, and objectives of a health promotion program that are linked to the program-needs assessment and marketing analysis.
	33. Coordinate employee input for the planning process with an employee advisory committee, employee focus groups, and so on.
	34. Implement the action steps of the program to carry out the goals and objectives.
	35. Assist in the identification and development of outcome measures to assess the program's success in attaining established goals and objectives.
	36. Propose new concepts, directions, and opportunities for the health promotion program.
	37. Obtain and continue to update knowledge of new trends in the delivery of health promotion services.

Table 10.4 Major Job Function: Program Coordination

Subfunctions	Competencies
A. Needs assessment	1. Assist in conducting an audit of the organization's priorities and external and internal resources.
	2. Identify and recommend an appropriate needs-assessment methodology for a WHP program.
	3. Conduct a needs assessment for a program.
	4. Collect, analyze, and synthesize the results of the needs assessment, then link these results with the marketing analysis findings.
	5. Summarize and document the results of the needs assessment.
	6. Define the target populations for the program offerings.
B. Program design	7. Assist in the development of the program design using needs assessment and marketing analysis data.
	8. Identify and interpret the results of important studies and apply those results to program design.
	9. Identify relevant program models and apply findings to program design.
	10. Plan individual program components that complement the organizational culture, structure, and environment.
	11. Develop a plan for individual program components that effectively account for action steps, resource allocation, assignment of personnel, and time frames for accomplishing program strategies.
	12. Develop a marketing strategy for individual program components.
	13. Design incentive and motivational reinforcements for individual program components.
	14. Assist in the selection of an appropriate evaluation design that is consistent with the program's goals, objectives, and resources.
C. Program implementation	15. Follow operational and administrative policies and procedures.
	16. Promote program services and activities.
	17. Deliver program services and activities to assure maximum accessibility and utilization.
	18. Apply process evaluation procedures and modify the program appropriately.
D. Program evaluation	19. Utilize the appropriate methods of data collection and analysis.
	20. Interpret the data, draw conclusions, and make recommendations.
	21. Disseminate the results of an evaluation to the appropriate people within the organization.

Table 10.5 Major Job Function: Human Resources Skills

Subfunctions	Competencies
A. Staffing	1. Recommend staffing needs based on a plan for a health-promotion program.
	2. Assist in writing a job description.
	3. Recommend performance standards.
	4. Assist in reviewing applications and résumés.
	5. Assist in conducting a job interview and evaluating candidates for the job.
	6. Assist in evaluating references during the hiring process.
	7. Understand and apply and organization's policies and procedures for hiring and terminating staff.
	8. Orient new health promotion employees to the job, program, and worksite culture.
B. Staff training and development	9. Provide or support staff training and development through the development of training objectives, curricula, and evaluation criteria.
	10. Promote personal and career development among staff.
	11. Provide a work environment that is conducive to learning.
C. Human resources administration	12. Motivate staff to enhance productivity.
	13. Maintain open communication channels.
	14. Use appropriate leadership styles for specific situations.
	15. Assist in determining the criteria for selection of consultants and vendors.
	16. Assist in evaluating the performance of consultants and vendors.
D. Professional development	17. Establish credibility as a role model, expert, and advocate for worksite health promotion.
	18. Develop a personal career plan to promote self-development.
	19. Develop professional links with mentors in the field of WHP.
	20. Demonstrate service to the profession and community.

What Would You Do?

At the beginning of the final year of your academic program, you meet with your adviser to discuss internship options. You would like to pursue an internship in a worksite that offers a comprehensive health promotion program, preferably in another city. Yet, when sharing your interest with the advisor, you feel that his sense of such well-rounded internship experiences is quite limited because his primary focus is internships based at fitness centers. To expand his knowledge of today's diversified internship marketplace while also taking personal responsibility for seeking a suitable experience, what would you do?

CHAPTER 10 WRAP-UP

Key Points

- In today's ever-expanding market of educational and skill-building opportunities, it's important to thoroughly research all available options.
- An appropriate certification enhances your ability to secure and maintain viable employment.
- Health coaching is becoming more prevalent in many WHP settings. Yet, some training and certification programs appear to lack an appropriate level of evidence-based standards.
- Quality-oriented internships offer aspiring WHP practitioners a valuable platform for starting a successful career.
- Proper research and practice can enhance your confidence for successful interviewing.

Glossary

certification—Procedure by which an accredited or authorized agency assesses and verifies the qualifications of a student in accordance with established requirements or standards.

cover letter—A typed letter designed to reflect an applicant's interest in and qualifications for an internship, job, or similar position of opportunity.

health coaching—A structured, supportive partnership between a coach and client that effectively motivates behavior change.

motivational interviewing—A directive, personal counseling style for eliciting behavior change by helping clients to explore and resolve perceived obstacles.

University Affiliate Program (UAP)—WELCOA's multifaceted website with resources for college students and faculty.

Bibliography

American College of Sports Medicine. 2010. "About ACSM." Accessed December 15. www.acsm.org

American Council on Exercise. 2010. Accessed December 14, 2010. http://acefitness.org/

Black, S. 2008. "So, you want to be a medical fitness facility director?" *ACSM's Health & Fitness Journal* 12(2): 28-30.

Butterworth, S., A. Linden, and W. McClay. 2007. "Health coaching as an intervention in health management programs." *Disease Management and Health Outcomes* 15: 299-307.

Duke University Center for Integrative Medicine. 2006. "Health coaching." Accessed May 3, 2010. http://dukehealth1.org/int_med/healthcoach.asp.

Eickhoff-Shemek, J. 1999. "Examining the benefits of professional certification." *AWHP's Worksite Health* (Fall): 18-19.

In Focus. 2010. "Realizing the promise of health coaching." Accessed May 3. www.healthsciences.org/Infocus/index.html.

Karch, R., and M. Rose. 2004. "Measuring up." *WELCOA's Absolute Advantage* 3(3): 46-49.

Nagle, E., P. Pierce, K. Abt, and L. Bernardo. 2009. "Mentoring the future health and fitness professional." *ACSM's Health-Fitness Journal* 13 (1): 13-19.

National Strength and Conditioning Association. 2010. Accessed December 10, 2010. http://www.nsca-lift.org/

Rager, R., S. Horowitz, and T. Adams. 2001. "A competencies framework: Intermediate level." *AWHP's Worksite Health* 8: 32-36.

Rojas-Guyler, L., R. Cottrell, and D. Wagner. 2006. "The second national survey of U.S. internship standards in health education professional preparation: 15 years later." Poster session, American Alliance for Health, Physical Education, Recreation, and Dance, National Convention, April 26th.

Rollnick, S., and W. Miller. 1995. "What is motivational interviewing?" *Behavioural and Cognitive Psychotherapy* 23: 325-334.

Snelling, A. 2004. "The journey...from good to great." *WELCOA's Absolute Advantage* 3 (3)" 37-41.

"WELCOA's university affiliate program." 2004. *WELCOA's Absolute Advantage* 3 (3): 30-35.

Looking Ahead

After graduating from college, most WHP and fitness personnel assume entry-level positions with limited roles and responsibilities. However, today's worksites need WHP personnel who can assume broadly defined roles and responsibilities. This is particularly true for those who are working as program managers or program directors, since they often monitor large-scale WHP operations on a daily basis.

Although many WHP positions in management and direction have traditionally been held by those with master's degrees or a good decade or more of experience, it's not uncommon to find younger, qualified workers in these positions today. Seek out higher-level posts and take advantage of opportunities to expand the scope and specificity of your personal and professional development.

APPENDIX A
PERSONAL HEALTH QUESTIONNAIRE

Please complete the following questionnaire and return it to _____. We will then contact you to schedule your first consultation. If you have any questions, please call _____.

ALL INFORMATION IS CONFIDENTIAL

Employee ID#:_____

Name:_____

Sex: ❏ M ❏ F Birth date: _____   Dept./title: _____

Phone: Home (_____) _____   Work (_____) _____

Emergency contact (name & phone #): _____

Activity Profile

Level of intensity or exertion (please circle one)   Low   Moderate   High

  1. Level of physical activity at work.   1 2 3 4 5

  2. Level of physical activity at leisure.   1 2 3 4 5

  3. Do you currently exercise regularly? ❏ No ❏ Yes

  4. Number of times per week. 1-2 3-4 5-6 Over 6

  5. How long do you exercise (minutes)? <15 15-30 30-45 >45

  6. Briefly describe your exercise program: _____

_____

If you answered No to question 3, when was the last time you exercised, and what type of activity did you do? _____

_____

Biomedical Profile

  1. Name(s) of your physician(s): _____

  2. Date of last complete medical exam: _____

  3. Do you know your resting blood pressure? ❏ No ❏ Yes What is it? _____

  4. Do you know your resting heart rate? ❏ No ❏ Yes What is it? _____

  5. Do you know your blood cholesterol level? ❏ No ❏ Yes What is it? _____

  6. Do you know your ratio of total cholesterol to HDL cholesterol? ❏ No ❏ Yes What is it? _____

  7. Do you know your body fat percentage? ❏ No ❏ Yes What is it? _____

From D. Chenoweth, 2011, *Worksite health promotion,* 3rd edition (Champaign, IL: Human Kinetics).

8. Do you have, or have you ever had, any of the following? Check all that apply.

Condition	Past	Present	Condition	Past	Present
Angina	❑	❑	Rheumatic fever	❑	❑
Extra heartbeats	❑	❑	Dizziness/fainting	❑	❑
Arthritis	❑	❑	Scarlet fever	❑	❑
Heart attack	❑	❑	Emphysema	❑	❑
Asthma	❑	❑	Stroke	❑	❑
Heart murmur	❑	❑	Epilepsy	❑	❑
Back pain	❑	❑	Varicose veins	❑	❑
High blood pressure	❑	❑	Muscle weakness	❑	❑
Bronchitis	❑	❑	Muscle pain	❑	❑
Leg cramps	❑	❑	Bone injuries	❑	❑
Cancer	❑	❑	Bone pain	❑	❑
Pneumonia	❑	❑	Surgery*	❑	❑
Diabetes	❑	❑	Shortness of breath	❑	❑

*Date of surgery: _____ Type of surgery: _____

9. Explanation/comments on any of the above: _____

_____

10. Other diseases/injuries/medical problems you have (past or present): _____

_____

11. Do you have any medical problem or injury that might make it difficult to exercise? ❑ No ❑ Yes

If yes, explain: _____

_____

Health Inventory and Lifestyle

1. Height: _____ Weight: _____ Weight at age 21: _____

2. What do you consider to be a good weight for you? _____

3. Have you ever been on a diet prescribed by a doctor or registered dietitian? ❑ No ❑ Yes

How many pounds did you lose? _____ In how many weeks? _____

4. Do you currently smoke tobacco products? ❑ No (Skip to #8) ❑ Yes What type?

❑ cigarettes; packs per day _____ ❑ cigars; number per day _____

❑ pipe; pouches per day _____

5. How many years have you smoked? _____

6. What is the primary reason you smoke?_____

7. Have you ever tried quitting? ❑ No ❑ Yes

By what method _____

8. Do you currently use smokeless tobacco?   ❑ No ❑ Yes

9. Do you drink alcoholic beverages?   ❑ No (Skip to #9) ❑ Yes   What type?

   ❑ beer; cans per day _____   ❑ wine; glasses per day _____   ❑ liquor; shots per day _____

10. What types of caffeinated beverages do you drink?

   ❑ caffeinated coffee; cups per day _____   ❑ tea; glasses per day _____

   ❑ colas; cans per day _____

11. Place a check mark beside those foods you eat at least once a day.

   ❑ Whole milk   ❑ Hard cheese   ❑ Eggs   ❑ French fries   ❑ Butter
   ❑ Ice cream   ❑ Chocolate   ❑ Fast food   ❑ Deep-fried foods   ❑ Cake/pie/doughnuts
   ❑ Cold cuts   ❑ Chips   ❑ Sausage/ham/bacon

12. How much stress do you have in an average day?
   ❑ More than the average person   ❑ About the same as the average person
   ❑ Less than the average person

13. How do you manage stress? _____

   _____

Personal Interests

Please list the types of health improvement programs in which you would like to participate:

_____

_____

_____

_____

_____

_____

Thank you.

Your feedback will help us plan programs and activities to help you achieve your personal health goals.

APPENDIX B
LIFEGAIN HEALTH CULTURE AUDIT™

The Lifegain Health Culture Audit™ is an anonymous survey that assesses the level of cultural support for healthy lifestyle choices. It examines five dimensions of culture: (1) shared values, (2) norms, (3) cultural touch points including formal and informal policies and procedures, (4) peer support, and (5) work climate. It is a tool for planning and evaluating culture change. The instrument is tailored to the goals of the wellness initiative and the language of the cultural environments being examined. Further information about the instrument and its use is available from Judd Allen, Ph.D. at JuddA@healthyculture.com. The copyright for the Lifegain Health Culture Audit is held by the author and unauthorized use is strictly prohibited.

The following confidential and anonymous survey measures the level of cultural support for healthy lifestyles at work. It's your chance to share your views about the social environment among the people you work most closely with. This may mean your peer group or work area, but it applies to any combination of people you work with frequently. Your feedback through this survey will help to develop initiatives that support better health and wellness for all employees. Your opinion is helpful even if your feelings are neutral or if you are unsure.

Note: There are no incorrect answers. We are asking for your opinion.

Please indicate your level of agreement with each statement using the following scale:

1 = Strongly disagree, 2 = Disagree, 3 = Neither agree nor disagree, 4 = Agree, 5 = Strongly agree

1 2 3 4 5   Living a healthy lifestyle is highly valued among the people I work most closely with.

1 2 3 4 5   Supporting employee wellness is among the top priorities at work.

1 2 3 4 5   My immediate supervisor models a healthy lifestyle.

1 2 3 4 5   The use of resources such as time, space and money shows a commitment to supporting healthy lifestyles.

1 2 3 4 5   The physical work environment (such as available food choices, accessible stairways, changing rooms and bike racks) supports healthy lifestyles.

1 2 3 4 5   The people I work most closely with are taught skills needed to achieve a healthy lifestyle.

1 2 3 4 5   Among the people I work most closely with, new employees are made aware of the organization's support for healthy lifestyles.

1 2 3 4 5   The people I work most closely with are rewarded for efforts to live a healthy lifestyle.

1 2 3 4 5   Among the people I work most closely with, participation in healthy activities is a primary way to renew friendships and to meet new people.

1 2 3 4 5   Among the people I work most closely with, we have one or more traditions or rituals that symbolize our commitment to healthy lifestyles.

1 2 3 4 5   Among the people I work most closely with, people regularly assess how they are doing in terms of living a healthy lifestyle.

1 2 3 4 5   The people I work most closely with have a sense of community (for example, people really get to know one another, feel as if they belong and care for one another in times of need).

1 2 3 4 5   The people I work most closely with have a shared vision (for example, people feel that the organization's conduct is consistent with their personal values and people are clear about how they fit in with the big picture).

1 2 3 4 5   The people I work most closely with have a positive outlook (for example, people enjoy their work, celebrate accomplishments, adopt a "we can do it" attitude and bring out the best in each other).

1 2 3 4 5   My immediate supervisor supports employees' efforts to adopt healthier lifestyle practices.

From D. Chenoweth, 2011, *Worksite health promotion*, 3rd edition, (Champaign, IL: Human Kinetics). Copyright Judd Allen and Human Resources Institute LLC. Further information is available from the author at JuddA@healthculture.com. 802-862-8855.

1 2 3 4 5   My immediate coworkers support one another's efforts to adopt healthier lifestyle practices.

1 2 3 4 5   My housemates support one another's efforts to adopt healthier lifestyle practices.

1 2 3 4 5   My friends and family (living outside my home) support one another's efforts to adopt healthier lifestyle practices.

Health Norms

Please indicate your level of agreement with each statement using the following scale:

1 = Strongly disagree	3 = Neither agree nor disagree	5 = Strongly agree
2 = Disagree	4 = Agree	DK = Don't know

Among the people I work most closely with, it is a norm (expected) for people to

1 2 3 4 5 DK   Get adequate sleep (seven plus hours) most days.

1 2 3 4 5 DK   Achieve a balance between work, rest and play.

1 2 3 4 5 DK   Practice some form of stress management technique (such as yoga, meditation or prayer).

1 2 3 4 5 DK   Not smoke.

1 2 3 4 5 DK   Be physically active (such as taking a brisk walk for at least 30 minutes most days).

1 2 3 4 5 DK   Maintain a healthy weight.

1 2 3 4 5 DK   Eat foods at work that are low in fat and refined sugar and high in whole grains, fruits and vegetables.

1 2 3 4 5 DK   Drink alcohol moderately if at all (that is, not more than 14 drinks per week or more than 2 drinks on a single day).

1 2 3 4 5 DK   Get help with addictions and mental or emotional problems early on.

1 2 3 4 5 DK   Not come to work sick.

1 2 3 4 5 DK   Stay current on recommended health screenings and vaccinations.

1 2 3 4 5 DK   Not speed.

1 2 3 4 5 DK   Use safety belts.

1 2 3 4 5 DK   Organize work to avoid injury (such as office layout, lighting, lifting and safety gear).

1 2 3 4 5 DK   Form and maintain friendships at work.

1 2 3 4 5 DK   Treat all people with respect and fairness regardless of sex, age, race, disability or sexual orientation.

1 2 3 4 5 DK   Celebrate accomplishments.

APPENDIX C
ENVIRONMENTAL CHECKSHEET

Nature of Work

1. Percentage of workers doing physical labor: _____%

2. Percentage sitting most of time: _____%

3. Percentage of workers

   standing: _____%   sitting: _____%   lifting: _____%

Behaviors

1. Percentage of workers operating video display terminals (VDTs): _____%

   Are VDT stations equipped with

   ❑ filtered screens?   ❑ wrist/hand rests?   ❑ indirect lighting?

   Are they positioned appropriately for employees' height, reach, and posture? _____

   If not, what improvements are necessary? _____

2. Percentage of workers walking, standing, or sitting with poor posture: _____%

3. Percentage of workers doing a lot of lifting: _____%

   Percentage lifting over 10 pounds per lift: _____%

4. Percentage of workers smoking on the job: _____%

   in other areas where smoking may be permitted: _____%

5. Other significant behaviors (list):_____

Environmental Health and Safety Hazards

1. Is the work environment noisy? _____

   If so, where? _____

2. Is the work environment   ❑ hot?   ❑ cold?

   If so, where? _____

3. Is the lighting adequate? _____

   If not, where? _____

4. Are fumes, vapors, or mists in the air? _____

   If so, describe: _____.

5. Are employees exposed to substances that are toxic or caustic (burning)? _____

   If so, describe: _____.

   Are employees properly protected? _____

6. Are employees around flying objects? _____

   If so, where? _____

   Are employees properly protected? _____

7. Are employees likely to injure themselves due to excessive lifting or improper lifting? _____

   If so, where? _____

From D. Chenoweth, 2011, *Worksite health promotion,* 3rd edition (Champaign, IL: Human Kinetics).

8. Are any areas slick (oily, wet)? _____

   If so, where? _____

9. Do areas exist where employees may fall? _____

   If so, where? _____

10. Do any areas exist where employees may be caught in, on, or between machinery? _____

    If so, where? _____

Safety Promotion and Injury Prevention

1. Are warning devices posted at high-risk areas? _____

   If not, where are they needed? _____

2. Are visible posters displayed to motivate safety practices? _____

   If not, where are they needed? _____

3. Are safety records posted? _____

   If not, what is a central location for all employees to see? _____.

4. Do workers in high-risk areas wear proper clothing, safety gloves, hard hats, goggles, and protective shoes? _____

   If not, where are they needed? _____

Summary

1. Nature of work for most employees is ❑ physical or ❑ mental.

2. Most significant behaviors displayed among workers include:

   A. _____

   B. _____

   C. _____

3. Degree of risk associated with health and safety hazards:

   A. High _____* B. Fair _____* C. Low _____

   *Reasons: _____

   _____

   _____

   _____

   _____

   _____

Signature (Investigator): _____Date: _____

From D. Chenoweth, 2011, *Worksite health promotion,* 3rd edition (Champaign, IL: Human Kinetics).

APPENDIX D
MAINTAINING EXERCISE EQUIPMENT

The durability of a fitness facility and equipment is best preserved by maintaining a temperature near 70 °F (~21 °C) and humidity level lower than 50%. Ask exercisers to put a towel over computer control panels to protect them from perspiration. Place electronic equipment in locations with adequate ventilation to reduce heat overload. Monitor equipment use to ensure that it is being used properly. Misuse is probably the biggest contributor to broken or malfunctioning equipment, so provide mandatory orientation sessions for all users.

The furnishings of the facility should not only be practical but also contribute positively to the exercise environment. Fans help a facility's air conditioner circulate air more efficiently; large ceiling fans are more attractive than floor models. Mirrors should be shatterproof, especially in the weight room.

The lighting of the facility should be bright enough for safety, yet as pleasant and energy-efficient as possible. When properly positioned, windows provide natural, inexpensive lighting. Consider energy-efficient bulbs, which are more expensive up front, but more cost-efficient in the long run because they use less energy and last longer. Windows should be ideally positioned to absorb sunlight for solar heat during winter months without causing glare. Select lighting panels that provide dim lighting during off-peak hours to cut energy consumption. Mercury-vapor fluorescent bulbs work well for racquetball and basketball. Avoid surface-mounted fluorescent lights because they cause glare. If you have locker rooms, recessed fluorescent lighting provides a nice ambience.

Efficient ventilation in the shower room is essential for providing comfort, containing heating and cooling costs, and maintaining the overall health of the facility. A heating, ventilation, and air conditioning (HVAC) system that ventilates at least 40 cubic feet per minute is necessary to minimize excessive heat and moisture in showers and locker rooms.

If your company can afford lockers, full-size lockers are desirable to hang dresses and suits, whereas stacked lockers are adequate for leisure clothing. A good locker has vents for air circulation, is easy to clean, is purchased from a reputable manufacturer, includes a service contract, and can be purchased at a discount when bought in bulk.

Many experts recommend surfacing your facility with a wood spring-coil floor or a polyurethane mixed-foam floor with padding or carpeting treated with stain repellant to prevent mildew. Rubber is also popular; although it is slightly more expensive than carpet or wood, it lasts longer. The cost per square foot for synthetic foam generally runs from $4.50 to $10, good carpeting from $3.50 to $5, wood from $8 to $15, and rubber from $9 to $17. If your site will include a basketball court, the best surface is polyurethane-finished wood (maple, beech, or birch), pure polyurethane, or polyurethane with acrylic resin. Prices for these surfaces run from $10 to $15 per square foot. For a racquetball court, choose a wood surface of maple, beech, or birch, costing from $10 to $15 per square foot. For high-traffic surfaces, the best choice is a synthetic-fiber carpeting of nylon or olefin, which runs from $5 to $10 per square foot. To avoid fraying, unraveling, and packing down, select a cut-pile version with a low pile height and tight gauge construction. Choose action backing over jute backing to avoid moisture buildup and mildew. When choosing exercising flooring, consider how well a particular surface compares to established performance standards. One of the most common international protocols that many flooring vendors use is the DIN standard 18032, Part 2. DIN is a nongovernmental organization established to promote the development of standardization and related activities in Europe with the goal of facilitating the international exchange of goods and services.

In the weight room, high-quality wood is a good surface. Rubber mats (with trip-free beveled edging) should be placed under each piece of equipment and in the free-weight areas to absorb sound and cushion dropped weights.

In the locker room area (if your company can afford this amenity), carpeting provides comfort, economy, safety, and easy maintenance. The carpet should have antifungus protection and be regularly wet-vacuumed and treated with stain repellant. The color or pattern should minimize the sight of visible stains. In the shower and drying area of the locker room, the best shower surface is slightly abrasive, nonslip tile. Tiles set in mortar are less likely to fall out than tiles glued to waterproof gypsum board. Soft brown is a popular color and doesn't show stains as much as white. Shower walls should be tiled and sealed with epoxy. Epoxy sealant is relatively inexpensive and can be steam cleaned.

If you're lucky enough to afford a facility with an indoor track, choose synthetic surfaces such as rubber or a vinyl laminated to a sponge-rubber cushion. Latex, full-poured urethane, and vented urethane also work well. Corners should be banked slightly to minimize stress on the lower leg. (Remind users to alternate direction on a daily basis to reduce stress on one side of the body.)

If your company plans an outdoor fitness trail, your best selections for surface materials are decomposed granite, limestone quarry particulates, crushed coral, and wood chips. When constructing a trail, cut a 3.5-inch deep trough with a landscaping tractor. The dirt wells up on the sides of the trough, creating a natural border that holds the surface material in place. Fill the trough with 2 inches of compacted gravel, and top it with a surface material to make the trail level with the ground. Locate the trail away from office buildings so that workers are not distracted by people passing by. For one-way traffic only, a 4-foot path is adequate. You'll need a 7-foot path or bigger for two-way traffic. Provide distance markers and perhaps a bench or par course along the trail. Finally, develop procedures to enhance personal safety for all trail users. For example, require all individual users to sign their name in addition to their departing and expected return times in a highly visible location for staff members to regularly monitor. A video surveillance system may also be appropriate in specific settings.

INDEX

Note: The italicized *f* and *t* following page numbers refer to figures and tables, respectively.

ABOUT THE AUTHOR

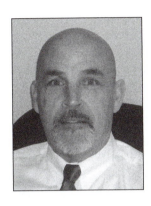

David H. Chenoweth, PhD, has designed, implemented, and evaluated worksite health programs in the public and private sectors for more than 30 years as president of Chenoweth & Associates, Inc. He is a frequent speaker to various business and health care groups and has authored eight books, including *Planning Health Promotion at the Worksite*, *Health Care Cost Management*, and *Evaluating Worksite Health Promotion*. Dr. Chenoweth is a professor emeritus at East Carolina University, where he developed one of the first academic worksite health promotion programs in the United States.

Dr. Chenoweth is a member of the International Association for Worksite Health Promotion and the American College of Sports Medicine. He has also chaired the Business and Industry Committee of the North Carolina Governor's Council on Physical Fitness and Health and is a fellow of the Association for Worksite Health Promotion. In 2004, he was invited by the European Union to consult on worksite health promotion.

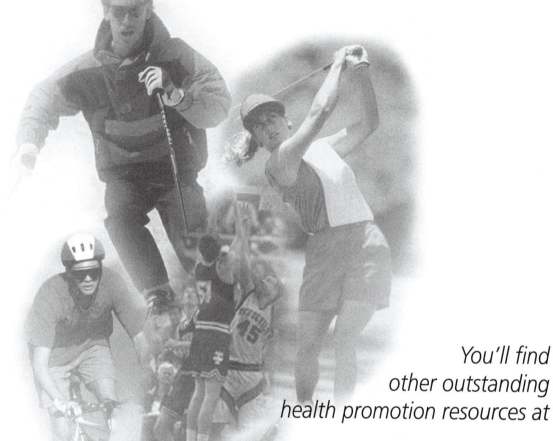